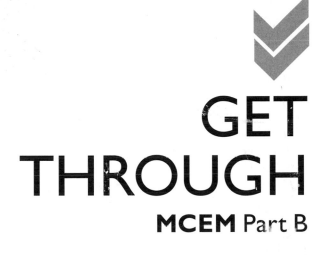

GET THROUGH

MCEM Part B

D0318047

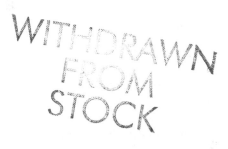

GET THROUGH

MCEM Part B:
Data Interpretation Questions

EDITED BY

Mathew Hall BM BCh PhD MCEM
Specialty Doctor in Emergency Medicine
Princess Royal University Hospital
Kent, UK

Sam Thenabadu MBBS MRCP DRCOG DCH Dip Clin Ed FCEM
Consultant Adult & Paediatric Emergency Medicine
Princess Royal University Hospital
Kent, UK

Chet R Trivedy BDS FDS RCS (Eng) MBBS PhD MCEM
Research Fellow
London Emergency Academic Research Network (LEARN)
London School of Emergency Medicine
London, UK

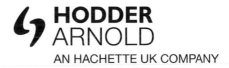
HODDER
ARNOLD
AN HACHETTE UK COMPANY

First published in Great Britain in 2012
Hodder Arnold, an imprint of Hodder Education, a Hachette UK company,
338 Euston Road, London NW1 3BH

http://www.hoddereducation.com

Hachette UK's policy is to use papers that are natural, renewable and recyclable
products and made from wood grown in sustainable forests. The logging
and manufacturing processes are expected to conform to the environmental
regulations of the country of origin.

Whilst the advice and information in this book are believed to be true and accurate
at the date of going to press, neither the author[s] nor the publisher can accept
any legal responsibility or liability for any errors or omissions that may be made. In
particular (but without limiting the generality of the preceding disclaimer) every
effort has been made to check drug dosages; however it is still possible that errors
have been missed. Furthermore, dosage schedules are constantly being revised
and new side-effects recognized. For these reasons the reader is strongly urged to
consult the drug companies' printed instructions before administering any of the
drugs recommended in this book.

British Library Cataloguing in Publication Data
A catalogue record for this book is available from the British Library

Library of Congress Cataloging-in-Publication Data
A catalog record for this book is available from the Library of Congress

ISBN 978-1-853-15872-8

1 2 3 4 5 6 7 8 9 10

Development Editor: Sarah Penny
Production Manager: Joanna Walker
Cover Design: Helen Townson
Project Manager: Aileen Castell, Naughton Project Management

Typeset in 10/12pt Minion by Phoenix Photosetting, Chatham, Kent
Printed and bound by CPI Group (UK) Ltd., Croydon CR0 4YY

What do you think about this book? Or any other Hodder Arnold title?
Please visit our website: www.hodderarnold.com

CONTENTS

Colour Plate appears between pp208 and 209

CONTRIBUTORS

Arif Ahmad MBBS
Associate Specialist in Emergency Medicine
Princess Royal University Hospital
Kent, UK

Harith Adil Tawfiq Al Rawi MBChB DCH FRCS Ed FCEM
Consultant Emergency Medicine
St Thomas' Hospital
London, UK

Mitesh Davda MBBS MRCS FCEM
Consultant in Emergency Medicine
Princess Royal University Hospital
Kent, UK

Shumontha Dev BSc (Hons) MBBS MRCS (Ed) FCEM
Consultant in Emergency Medicine
Guy's and St Thomas' Hospitals NHS Foundation Trust
London, UK

Mathew Hall BM BCh PhD MCEM
Specialty Doctor in Emergency Medicine
Princess Royal University Hospital
Kent, UK

Elaine Harding MBBS MRCS FCEM
Emergency Department Consultant
University Hospital Lewisham
London, UK

Jane Richmond BSc (Hons) MBBS MRCS FCEM
Consultant in Emergency Medicine
Croydon University Hospital
London, UK

Sam Thenabadu MBBS MRCP DRCOG DCH Dip Clin Ed FCEM
Consultant Adult and Paediatric Emergency Medicine
Princess Royal University Hospital
Kent, UK

Emma Townsend MBBS BSi DRCOG MRCP FCEM
Consultant in Emergency Medicine
Tunbridge Wells Hospital
Tunbridge Wells
Kent, UK

Malcolm Tunnicliff MB BS MRCSEd FCEM DipMedTox
Consultant and Clinical Lead in Emergency Medicine
King's College Hospital
London, UK

Chet R Trivedy BDS FDS RCS (Eng) MBBS PhD MCEM
Research Fellow
London Emergency Academic Research Network (LEARN)
London School of Emergency Medicine
London, UK

PREFACE

The College of Emergency Medicine (CEM) sets a structured answer question (SAQ) paper as part of the both its membership (MCEM) and fellowship (FCEM) examinations. These papers examine the whole breadth of the current Emergency Medicine curriculum in the form of short clinical scenarios, followed by a series of questions probing the candidate's clinical knowledge and data interpretation skills. Many candidates find negotiating CEM examination SAQs particularly challenging, in part due to the immense amount of material potentially examined at each diet but also the often unappreciated need for strict examination technique when answering each and every question. The aspiring candidate's problems are further compounded by the marked absence of helpful resources focused on the MCEM and FCEM SAQ examinations, particularly the lack of any practice materials.

We have written this book, *Get Through MCEM Part B: Data Interpretation Questions*, to fill that void. There follows more than 160 practice SAQ questions exploring all the corners of the CEM curriculum but focused on the most commonly examined areas. The authors and contributors have used their extensive experience teaching emergency medicine trainees to construct an informative, up-to-date and effective exam practice text. All areas of the curriculum relevant to the MCEM Part B exam are covered, all possible data interpretation included and a whole chapter is devoted to exam technique with advice on answering individual SAQs to gain maximum marks. Each question is followed by a detailed yet focused answer and discussion of the topic and further reading is recommended where relevant. Each chapter starts with a rundown of the important topics to revise and points to the knowledge necessary to succeed, including referencing many of the important guidelines used in everyday Emergency Department (ED) practice. All in all, we present an essential study guide and practice question book for all those serious about passing the MCEM Part B exam.

All though primarily aimed at those sitting the UK MCEM Part B examination, we believe this book should serve a wider audience and provides a learning resource not only for UK emergency medicine trainees but also all doctors at all levels of training in all countries who deal with acute emergencies in the unselected patient population presenting to their hospital. We hope you find this book useful for both exam revision and, more importantly, improving your knowledge and skill in the practice of Emergency Medicine.

Mathew Hall
Sam Thenabadu
Chet R Trivedy

ACKNOWLEDGEMENTS

It is a pleasure to thank all my colleagues in the Emergency Department at the Princess Royal University Hospital whose everyday debate and discussion of clinical cases has added much in so many ways to the content of this book. In particular, a big thank you to Dr Andrew Hobart for contributing those radiographs and ECGs I just couldn't find anywhere else and to Peter Morris for trawling through our PACS archive for 'just the right' X-ray image to include. I am also very grateful to Dr Donald Adler for his invaluable help with sourcing the dermatology photographs. My thanks also go to all our colleagues from the Bromley Emergency Courses team who have been a constant encouragement throughout the writing of this book and, in particular, to Dr Ian Stell who originally inspired us to write it. My greatest debt, however, goes to my wife, Kim, and two children, Zach and Sophia, who have been constantly supportive throughout this project, despite losing me for many long hours to the word processor!

Mathew Hall

Many thanks to my colleagues who have tolerated my often over-enthusiastic approach to medical education and desire to improve the delivery of high-quality emergency medicine, to my parents for making me believe in pushing myself on to do more, and most importantly, to my wonderful tolerant and ever-understanding wife Molly who has suffered hours on end of me discussing cases with her – couldn't have done it without you.

Sam Thenabadu

For me a career in emergency medicine isn't just a job, it's a much loved hobby which I am privileged to get paid for, and it has given me great pleasure and satisfaction to be involved with this publication. I hope trainees planning to sit the CEM examinations will find it a useful resource. I am grateful for the support of all my colleagues for their time and support. I would like to say a special thank you to Tim Harris, Geoff Hinchley, Ian Stell and Chris Lacy for their extraordinary commitment to trainees, academia and being great role models. I would like to dedicate this book to my late father Mr Ramesh H Trivedy to whom I owe more than I can ever hope to repay.

Chet R Trivedy

LIST OF ABBREVIATIONS

(n.b. these are abbreviations used regularly in this book and is not meant to represent the list of abbreviations approved by the College for use in the MCEM exam)

A-a	alveolar-arterial	DIC	disseminated intravascular coagulation
ABG	arterial blood gas		
AFB	acid fast bacilli	EBV	Epstein barr virus
AIDS	acquired immunodeficiency syndrome	ED	Emergency Department
		ELISA	enzyme-linked immunoabsorbant assay
ALS	Advanced Life Support		
AP	antero-posterior	FBC	full blood count
APLS	Advanced Paediatric Life Support	g	gram
		GCS	Glasgow coma score
ATLS	Advanced Trauma Life Support	GFR	glomerular filtration rate
		GI	gastrointestinal
AV	atrio-ventricular	ICP	intracranial pressure
bd	twice a day	IM	intramuscular
BE	base excess	ITU	intensive therapy unit
BiPAP	bi-level positive airways pressure ventilation	IV	intravenous
		IVI	intravenous infusion
BMI	body mass index	IVU	intravenous urethrogram
BNF	British National Formulary	kPa	kilopascals
BSA	body surface area	LBBB	left bundle branch block
BTS	British Thoracic Society	LFT	liver function tests
CEC	Clinical Effectiveness Committee	LMP	last menstrual period
		LP	lumbar puncture
CEM	College of Emergency Medicine	MC&S	microscopy, culture and sensitivities
CK	creatinine kinase	MCPJs	metacarpophalangeal joints
COPD	chronic obstructive pulmonary disease	MCV	mean corpuscular volume
		mg	milligram
CPAP	continuous positive airway pressure	mcg	micrograms
		MRC	medical research council
CRT	capillary refill time	MRI	magnetic resonance imaging
CSF	cerebrospinal fluid	MRSA	methicillin resistant *staphylococcus aureaus*
CT	computed tomography		

MSE	mental state examination	qds	four times a day
MSU	mid stream urine	RCOG	Royal College of Obstetrics and Gynaecology
NAI	non-accidental injury		
NBM	nil by mouth	RCP	Royal College of Physicians
NICE	National Institute for Clinical Excellence	RCPCH	Royal College of Pediatricians and Child Health
NIV	noninvasive ventilation		
NPIS	National Poisons Information Service	RSV	Respiratory Synctial Virus
		RTA	road traffic accident
NSAIDs	nonsteroidal anti-inflammatory drugs	sc	subcutaneous
		SI	sacro-ileac
OCP	oral contraceptive pill	SIGN	Scottish Intercollegiate Guidelines Network
OPG	orthopantamogram		
od	once daily	SIRS	systemic inflammatory response syndrome
PA	postero-anterior		
PCI	percutaneous coronary intervention	SLE	systemic lupus erythematosis
		TB	tuberculosis
PEA	pulseless electrical activity	TCA	tricyclic antidepressant
PEFR	peak expiratory flow rate	tds	three times a day
PICU	paediatric intensive care unit	TFT	thyroid function tests
PIPJ	proximal interphalangeal joints	U&E	urea and electrolytes
		URTI	upper respiratory tract infection
po	per os (by mouth)		
pr	per rectum	UTI	urinary tract infection
PSA	prostate specific antigen	VZV	varicella-zoster virus
pv	per vaginum	WCC	white cell count

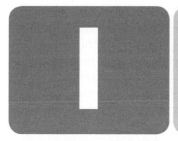

INTRODUCTION

Mathew Hall, Sam Thenabadu and Chet R Trivedy

The College of Emergency Medicine Part B membership examination (MCEM Part B) tests the data interpretation skills of aspiring emergency physicians in the form of short answer questions (SAQs). The typical SAQ will have a short clinical scenario called the 'stem' and then a series of questions either relating directly to the scenario in the stem or possibly of a more general nature (Box 1.1). Clinical data is frequently included in the stem but may also be put into any of the questions which follow. Questions aim to test candidates' clinical knowledge and patient management skills.

Box 1.1 Structure of a typical MCEM SAQ	
A 63-year-old man with known emphysema arrives by ambulance complaining of shortness of breath and worsening exercise tolerance over the past two days. His initial observations are pulse 98 bpm and regular, blood pressure 156/88 mmHg and respiratory rate 26/min.	{The stem}
On chest auscultation, he has poor air entry and audible wheeze.	

His arterial gas on air is shown below
    pH   7.48
    pCO_2 4.9 kPa
    pO_2 7.7 kPa
    BE   −2.9.
	{Including data}

a. Interpret the arterial blood gas given above. [1]	{Questions a–d}
b. Give 2 causes of acute exacerbation of COPD. [2]	
c. Give four treatments you would give this man initially. [4]	
d. Give three indications for empirical antibiotics in an exacerbation of COPD. [3]	

At the time of writing, the MCEM Part B exam contains 16 SAQ questions to be answered in two hours. In recent diets of the Part B exam, SAQs set by the College of Emergency Medicine (CEM) have become standardized with each having a stem and four related questions. Each question is designed to be answered by a short-list of the most appropriate responses, each response a single word or few words in length, or by a brief descriptive sentence at most. All marking is positive, meaning that marks are never removed for wrong answers – no matter how wrong!

It is fair to say that the more clinical experience a candidate has, the better prepared they will be for the MCEM Part B exam. Simply put, the more ECG's they have seen, more trauma X-rays reviewed and, in the final analysis, more patients they have managed, then the more likely a candidate is to recognize the clinical scenarios and data presented in SAQ questions. So, as with any postgraduate medical exam, the best preparation is through abundant clinical contact, asking for help when new territory is encountered and then, in academic time, further reading to consolidate learning.

In addition, however, revision books like this one have an important part to play in exam preparation. Practice questions help fill gaps in candidates' knowledge – things they may not have seen in clinical practice – as well as drawing attention to areas of particular importance and which are, therefore, more likely to be examined. Importantly, answering mock questions also allows candidates to develop and hone the specific skills required for success in exams and which are not necessarily learnt elsewhere. In the case of the Part B SAQs we suggest these are:

- extracting the important or key information from the clinical scenario/ question stem
- interpreting clinical data appropriately
- writing clear, concise and precise answers to all questions
- time management.

This book presents 160 practice questions for the MCEM Part B exam and, in so doing, provides a valuable revision aid for the most important areas of the CEM syllabus. Furthermore, when used with the advice given in the next two sections of this chapter – 'answering SAQ questions' and 'How to use this book' – these questions inculcate the exam skills and techniques listed above and that can make all the difference between pass and fail in the exam itself.

Answering SAQ Questions

Unlike MCQ style questions, where answers are given as a single mark in a box indicating true or false, SAQs challenge the candidate with an empty line or answer box in which anything can be written. Indeed, over and above possessing the knowledge to answer the question correctly, a certain amount of exam technique is also required to encapsulate that knowledge into a short answer containing exactly what the examiner hopes to see to award maximum marks. This section starts with some simple exam tips and then tackles the more difficult topic of exactly how to answer the question!

As you will have been told many times before, always read the questions carefully. The clinical scenarios presented as stems are usually fairly straightforward and are certainly not designed to catch you out. Pay attention to the key points in the clinical description:

- is the patient well or unwell and requiring resuscitation?
- what are the salient features of the history and/or examination?
- if observations are given what do they indicate about the patient?
- is there anything about this patient which might influence your approach,

both to diagnosis and/or management, e.g., pregnancy, diabetes, renal failure or particular medications or allergies?

- look at any data included with the stem to see what light it may throw on the clinical scenario, in particular – does it indicate a certain diagnosis is likely?

Importantly, however, do not panic at this stage if you are either unclear about what the clinical scenario is getting at, or how to interpret the data given. Wait to see what the questions actually ask for. Often, further information is given as part of the questions while, in many other cases, the question can be answered without relying on the stem to provide the crucial insight.

Read each question carefully and think what exactly is being asked for. This is more important than it sounds – consider the following:

- does it ask for symptoms, signs or features of a particular condition? Each has different medical meanings. Symptoms are the problems which the patient notices or experiences. Clinical signs are observed or elicited by the examining doctor and are therefore objective. Features can be either.
- treatments versus management. Treatments are specific interventions designed to improve outcome. Management is a broader concept encompassing all actions necessary to effectively deal with a patient within a given healthcare setting. Thus, management includes, for example, disposal of the patient from the care of the Emergency Department, as well as resuscitation status decisions, both clearly aspects of care of which would not normally be considered treatments
- risk factors vs causes. Risk factors increase the probability of an event occurring. Causes have a direct causal relationship to a specific event. For example, hyperlipidaemia is a risk factor for myocardial infarction through its promotion of atheromatous coronary artery disease but rupture of the atheromatous plaque is a cause.

Then, look for how the question asks for the answer. Again, this is often overlooked – consider the following:

- give, list or describe. Make sure you do as requested.
- often a question asks for a specific number of responses. For example, 'list three causes of chest pain' or 'give four complications of myocardial infarction'. Most importantly, make sure you answer with **exactly** the number of responses requested. Giving too few guarantees lost marks but giving too many also has pitfalls. If the question asks for a list of three causes of chest pain, and the candidate writes a list of five in response, only the first three will be marked and the last two ignored, whether right or wrong. Thus, the best approach is to give exactly the number of responses requested and make sure they are the ones you consider most likely to be correct.
- guidance is sometimes given on exactly how the question is to be answered. For example, 'what specific treatment would you give to this patient (include the **dose** and **route** of administration of any drugs in your answer)?' Alternatively, 'write a **four-point** management plan for this patient.' Make sure you do exactly as the question asks to gain all allotted marks.

- there are different ways of asking about given data. For example, asking for the abnormalities in a dataset differs from requesting an interpretation of the data. Consider the example of an arterial blood gas: pH 7.13, pCO_2 2.3 kPa, pO_2 12.9 kPa, BE −19, lactate 7.8 mmol/L. The abnormalities on this blood gas are acidosis (pH below 7.35 and base excess below − 2.0 units), hypocapnia (pCO_2 below 4.0 kPa) and raised lactate (lactate above 2.0 units). However, the interpretation of the blood gas is 'metabolic (lactate) acidosis with respiratory compensation'.
- similarly an ECG of 'fast AF' has the abnormalities of tachycardia, irregular rhythm and absent P waves but should be interpreted as showing atrial fibrillation with fast ventricular response.

Now let us look at the difficult issue of how to actually formulate an answer. The most effective approach can be summarized as being **concise** and **precise**. Concise in so far as writing the minimum required to supply the answer and precise so as to avoid ambiguity, misunderstanding or doubt about what you mean.

Table 1.1

Concise	Precise
All answers or responses should be single words or names and at the most a brief sentence or two.	Use medical terminology, e.g., 'myocardial infarction' not 'heart attack'
Sentences should be used only where necessary to convey meaning or give a description where a word or medical term alone does not suffice.	Avoid all but the most common and widely accepted abbreviations and acronyms, e.g., 'blood glucose' not 'BM', 'percutaneous coronary intervention' not 'PCI', 'middle cerebral artery' not 'MCA'. In recent diets of the exam, a list of acceptable abbreviations has been given to candidates as part of the instructions.
If you find yourself writing a short essay in answer, **stop** and think again.	
Use lists, bullet points and enumeration wherever possible.	
In recent diets, the MCEM Part B exam answer sheet gives boxes for your answers. The size of the box is probably a good indication of how much they expect you to write in answer and further, writing outside of the box may be disregarded by the examiner. Thus, ignore the answer boxes at your peril!	Do not answer 'I would assess the ABCs' to every question. If any of the airway, breathing or circulation is under threat, the question will likely make this clear and you will be required to state **how** you will perform the relevant assessments.
	Try to avoid generic terms such as 'IV fluids' or 'analgesics'. Say exactly what fluid you would give (e.g. '0.9% saline' or '5% dextrose') or give an example, 'analgesia, e.g., codeine phosphate 30 mg PO'. Similarly answer 'proton pump inhibitor, e.g., omaprazole PO' instead of 'antacids' or 'PPI'.
	Prescribe oxygen correctly (see the introduction to Chapter 3)

Now let's look by way of example at the SAQ given in Box 1 earlier in this chapter, to which we have added a possible model answer.

Question 1

A 63-year old man with known emphysema arrives by ambulance complaining of shortness of breath and worsening exercise tolerance over the past two days. His initial observations are pulse 98 bpm and regular, blood pressure 156/88 mmHg and respiratory rate 26/min. On chest auscultation, he had poor air entry and audible wheeze.

His arterial gas on air is:

pH   7.48
pCO_2 4.9 kPa
pO_2 7.7 kPa
BE   −2.9.

a Interpret the arterial blood gas given above. [1]
b Give two causes of acute exacerbation of COPD. [2]
c Give four initial treatments you would give this patient. [4]
d What are the indications for empirical antibiotics in an acute
  exacerbation of COPD. [3]
                                                                [10]

Answer to Question 1

a Hypoxia (pO_2 below 8.0 kPa) with normal pH and pCO_2. Type I respiratory failure.
b Lower respiratory tract infection.
  Pneumothorax.
c Oxygen via fixed delivery device aiming for saturations 88–92%.
  Salbutamol nebulisers 5 mg repeated as required
  Ipratropium nebulisers 500 mcg
  Oral prednisolone 30–40 mg.
d Increased sputum production
  Consolidation on the chest X-ray
  Clinical signs of pneumonia.

Here is another example requiring short sentences as answers:

Question 2

A 33-year-old man has suffered a laceration across the middle of the palmar aspect of his wrist in an accident with a broken window at work. He is haemodynamically stable with good capillary refill to the distal digits but you are concerned there may be nerve or tendon damage.

a Describe two tests you could perform looking for damage to the median
  nerve at the wrist. [2]

b Name two tendons which might be injured by a laceration at this location. [2]

c Your examination indicates no nerve or tendon damage has occurred. What further investigation is required before closure of the wound. [1]

d After closure of the wound with interrupted sutures, what advice regarding wound care will you give before discharge? [5]

[10]

Answer to Question 2

a Test thumb abduction (abductor pollicis brevis) by placing hand flat, palm upwards then ask the patient to lift the thumb to point towards the ceiling against resistance, test for sensory loss over the radial 3½ digits on the palmar surface of the hand.

b Flexor carpi radialis. Flexor digitorum superficialis.

c Soft tissue X-ray looking for glass in the wound.

d Keep the wound clean and dry until the stitches are removed.

Do not cover the wound with waterproof dressings or coverings.

Remove stitches at your GP practice in seven days.

Seek medical advice, if the wound shows signs of infection (hot, red, swelling, pain or discharge).

After the sutures have been removed apply moisturising cream to encourage healing.

How to use this book

The practice questions in the following chapters are arranged by subject, allowing you to focus on one area of the curriculum at a time. Chapters include a list of key topics to revise, as well as the kinds of data particularly relevant to that subject. We also suggest some further reading, for example, pointing out key guidelines and other material to help with developing data interpretation skills.

The SAQs themselves contain stem, data and a series of between four and six following questions. We have sometimes used more questions per stem than the College (which now use mostly four questions per stem), to allow each SAQ and the corresponding answers, to include as much relevant information as possible and, therefore, for the book to cover as much relevant material as possible. We provide an example marking scheme with each question.

It is difficult to write 'model' answers for SAQ style questions which are also useful for general learning and revision. In addition, for this style of question there may be any number of model answers, all of which, may be equally valid. Limiting our discussion to a model answer only, would considerably restrict the learning and revision goals of this book, particularly if we are adhering to our rule of being concise but precise, and giving only the number of responses requested. Thus, the editors have chosen not to give model answers to each SAQ and, instead, to provide as thorough a discussion of the answer as space allows. Of course we give clear direction as to what the right answers should be, but we also try to cover as many other possibilities as we can, and give as much background knowledge and understanding as is relevant.

With the above thoughts in mind, we suggest the following approach to using and getting the most out of this book:

1 Pick a chapter and read through the introduction to familiarize yourself with the important areas for revision and also the common types of data which may be seen.

2 Attempt some questions. Write down the answers as if you were in the exam and try to be concise and precise as we have outlined above.

3 Turn to the answer(s) and read them through marking your work as you go.

4 Return to any wrong or incomplete answers you have given and right down a correct or full one. Again, pay attention to exam technique and ask yourself 'even although I sort of knew the right answer, could I have made what I had written even clearer for the examiner'? Remember the examiner will only see and mark what you have written on the answer paper and not what you wanted to say but remained in your mind!

5 As you become more practised at answering the questions, start to impose a time constraint. In the current Part B exam you will have around seven minutes to answer each question. Discipline yourself to complete each practice SAQ with a written answer in a similar amount of time. Many candidates run out of time in this exam and it is a sure way to fail.

6 Use the references and suggestions for further reading to fill any gaps in your knowledge and broaden your revision.

From all of the Editors, Good luck!

2

RESUSCITATION

Harith Al Rawi

Introduction

Core topics
- management of cardiac arrest
- cardiac arrest in special circumstances (e.g., pregnancy, hypothermia)
- post-arrest management
- peri-arrest situations
- broad complex tachycardia
- narrow complex tachycardia
- bradycardia
- Advanced Paediatric Life Support (APLS)
- the comatose patient
- the shocked patient
- anaphylactic shock.

Thorough knowledge of Advanced Life Support (ALS)[1] and Advanced Paediatric Life Support (APLS)[2] as well as Advanced Trauma Life Support (ATLS)[3] principles and skills is important to succeed in this section, and the respective manuals are a useful revision resource. Pay particular attention to treatment algorithms, formulae and practical procedures, as well as to resuscitation in special circumstances, such as in pregnancy or the newborn.

Case 1

You receive advance warning that a paramedic crew are bringing a 65-year-old man in cardiac arrest. The patient has been intubated on scene but the crew were unable to gain intravenous access, so he has received no drugs. They will be arriving in four minutes.

a On arrival, the man has no pulse and the monitor shows electrical activity at a rate of 50 bpm. His airway is secure and intravenous access is obtained quickly. Outline your management in the first two minutes after arrival (give three important steps). [3]
b List eight reversible causes of cardiac arrest. [4]
c After one cycle of CPR, he recovers a weak radial pulse at a rate of 70 bpm. Name four investigations you would like do as part of his post resuscitation care. [2]
d The patient remains ventilation-dependent and arrangements are made for transfer to the ITU. What further treatment might be initiated in the Emergency Department (ED) to improve outcome after cardiac arrest. [1]
[10]

Case 2

You are the ED Registrar when a priority call comes through regarding a pregnant woman who is in the advanced stages of labour in the ambulance. Estimated time of arrival is two minutes.

a What further information do you want to know from the ambulance crew regarding this woman's pregnancy? [3]
b The woman has just delivered the baby in the back of the ambulance and the baby is rushed into the resuscitation room limp, with poor respiratory effort and a heart rate of 50 bpm. Outline your immediate actions to resuscitate this baby. [5]
c Despite your initial resuscitation, the heart rate falls to 40 bpm. Describe the correct technique for performing CPR on a newborn baby. [3]
d What is the preferred route for drug administration in the newborn? [1]
[12]

Case 3

An 18-year-old woman is brought to your ED by blue light ambulance. Her parents returned from an evening out to find her unconscious on her bedroom floor. Her parents say that she has been dating a boy known to be a heroin addict. On arrival, she is maintaining her own airway but is largely unresponsive to verbal stimulae. She localizes to pain but does not open her eyes and cannot verbalize any sounds.

Initial observations are; heart rate 105 bpm, blood pressure 85/40 mmHg and oxygen saturations 99% on oxygen via reservoir mask.

a What is her Glasgow coma score (GCS)? [1]
b Apart from heroin overdose, give four possible causes for coma in a
   young woman. [4]
c Name three bedside investigations you would perform straight away in
   this patient. [3]
d Other than coma, give two clinical signs of serious heroin overdose. [2]
e How would you manage a suspected heroin overdose in this patient
   (give doses and routes of any medication given)? [2]
   [12]

Case 4

A 55-year-old woman is brought into the resuscitation room following a collapse preceded by palpitations. She is conscious and has the following observations, heart rate 166 bpm, blood pressure 100/60 mmHg, respiratory rate 20/min and oxygen saturations 100% via reservoir. Below is her ECG (Figure 2.1).

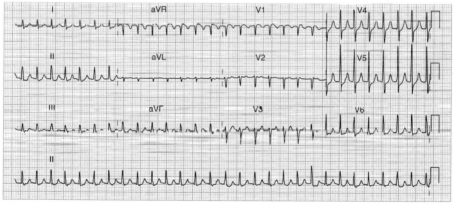

Figure 2.1

a What is your interpretation of the ECG above (Figure 2.1)? [2]
b Give four signs or symptoms of cardiovascular instability you would look
   for in this patient. [4]
c List three drugs you could use to treat this arrhythmia in a stable patient
   (with doses and routes). [3]
d If this patient were to become cardiovascularly unstable, what treatment
   would be indicated? [1]
   [10]

Case 5

A 75-year-old man, known to suffer from recurrent falls, has collapsed in the supermarket and is brought in by the ambulance service. He is drowsy but able to answer questions and you are informed of his initial observations by the resuscitation nurse: heart rate 34 bpm, blood pressure 80/60 mmHg, respiratory rate 20/min and oxygen saturations 95% on oxygen via face mask.

a What is the initial management of bradycardia in an adult patient
   (give drugs with dose and routes)?   [2]
b In a patient with bradycardia, what features of the presentation and/or
   ECG indicate a higher risk of asystole (give four)?   [4]
c He fails to respond to your initial management. Name two further
   pharmacological options for treating this patient.   [2]
d He remains bradycardic and hypotensive. Briefly describe how you would
   perform external cardiac pacing.   [4]
                                                                              [12]

Case 6

A six-year-old girl is brought into the ED following two days of fever and vomiting. Her mother says that, despite treatment with anti-emetics by the GP, she has been unable to drink and has now become lethargic and is passing no urine. On examination, she is very drowsy and has a markedly prolonged capillary refill time (CRT).

a What volume of fluid would you give as a bolus to this child?   [1]
b Two attempts at cannulation fail. Describe the landmarks for placing an
   intraosseous needle.   [3]
c As soon as venous access is obtained, give two bedside investigations you
   would perform.   [2]
d She improves with your initial fluid bolus. Assuming she is now 5%
   dehydrated calculate the volume of maintenance fluids to be given over
   24 hours.   [4]
                                                                              [10]

Case 7

A 40-year-old man is seen in the ED after a sudden collapse accompanied by sudden shortness of breath at his GP practice. He has recently been discharged from hospital following one week's inpatient treatment for cellulitis of his right leg. His initial observations are heart rate 110 bpm, respiration rate 40/min, blood pressure 70/40 mmHg and oxygen saturations 70% on 15 L oxygen via reservoir mask:

a What diagnosis would you consider most likely as a cause of his collapse?   [2]
b What bedside investigation can be performed to confirm this diagnosis
    and what will it show?   [2]
c Name two emergency treatments you would you give to this man in the ED.   [2]
d Shortly after providing emergency treatment, your patient becomes
    unresponsive and you cannot feel a pulse. List four **immediate** actions. [4]

                                                                             [10]

Case 8

A 33-year-old woman with a known peanut allergy is rushed in to the ED by her
husband. She became suddenly unwell with shortness of breath while eating in a
Chinese restaurant. She has a widespread urticarial rash and looks frightened.

a List five clinical features which might indicate a compromised airway in
    this patient.   [5]
b During your assessment, you note her blood pressure is 75/45 mmHg and
    she is becoming increasingly tachycardic. What treatments will you give
    (include routes and doses of any drugs given)?   [4]
c Despite your treatments, she develops marked airway compromise.
    Outline three further steps you would take.   [2]
d You discover from her husband, she takes propranolol for anxiety.
    What additional treatment might you try now?   [1]

                                                                             [12]

Case 9

An 18-year-old boy is brought in to the ED having been involved in a fight,
and struck on the side of the head by a blunt object, where there is now a large
haematoma. You are asked to see him immediately because, although he is
conscious, he is clearly 'not right'. You find him agitated and confused, repeating
the same statements over and over in response to your questions. All his triage
observations and blood glucose are within normal range.

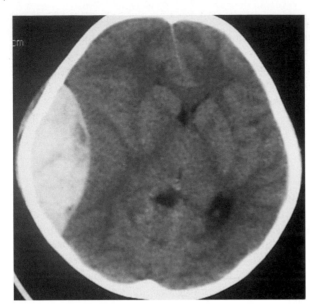

Figure 2.2

a Give five indications for immediate CT imaging of the brain as they appear
   in the NICE guidelines on head injury.   [5]
b Describe the abnormality in the CT image for this patient (Figure 2.2).   [2]
c What anatomical structure has been damaged to cause this appearance?   [1]
d He deteriorates on return from the CT scanner, and his Glasgow coma
   score is now 8/15. Give the two major steps in providing definitive
   treatment to this patient.   [2]
                                                                            [10]

Case 10

A 23-year-old man and 20-year-old woman have been rescued from a burning
house by the fire service. The man had attempted to tackle the blaze and, in doing
so, suffered severe burns to his arms and torso. He has no burns to his face. The
woman appears to be unhurt but has been exposed to thick smoke.

a Give three clinical features of a full thickness burn.   [3]
b The man has burns to the whole of his anterior chest and abdomen, as
   well as to the entire front of both arms. Using a common methodology,
   estimate the percentage burn in this man.   [2]
c Calculate the fluid required to be given to this man in the first eight hours of
   resuscitation after the burn. Assume he weighs 80 kg.   [3]
d Although the woman rescued from the fire appears unhurt, what
   investigations would you carry out to ensure she does not require any
   further treatment as a result of smoke inhalation.   [4]
                                                                            [12]

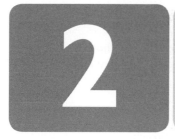

RESUSCITATION – ANSWERS

Case 1

a Be sure to know the ALS algorithm for cardiac arrest.[1] This man is in cardiac arrest with a non-shockable rhythm, so initiate chest compressions immediately, and continue for two minutes before re-assessing rhythm. Give 1 mg adrenaline (10 mL of 1 in 10 000 adrenaline) every three to five minutes. Also give IV fluids, e.g. two bags of 500 mL gelofusin via rapid infuser. Remember routine use of atropine is no longer recommended for pulseless electrical activity and asystole.

b ALS asks us to consider eight reversible causes of cardiac arrest – the four 'H's and four 'T's:

hypoxia	tension pneumothorax
hypovolaemia	tamponade
hyper/hypokalaemia	thromboembolism
hypothermia	toxic and metabolic (drugs, glucose and acidosis)

c **Immediate** post-resuscitation care should include the following investigations:

- blood pressure
- ECG
- arterial blood gas
- chest X-ray.

d Therapeutic hypothermia improves outcome post-cardiac arrest. The International Liaison Committee on Resuscitation (ILCOR) states in their 2002 consensus statement[4] 'Unconscious adult patients with spontaneous circulation after out-of-hospital cardiac arrest should be cooled to 32–34° C for 12–24 hours when the initial rhythm was ventricular fibrillation (VF)'. This has recently been updated to include all cardiac arrest patients with return of spontaneous circulation, regardless of initial rhythm. Local protocols should be followed to achieve this with input from the ITU team who will take over care of this patient.

Case 2

a Although infrequently required in practice, knowledge of newborn resuscitation is essential to the ED doctor. If the situation allows, it is useful to know the following before delivery of the baby:

- gestational age
- any complications of pregnancy
- the position of the baby in the uterus (vertex or breech)
- colour of the amniotic fluid (dark green fluid suggests the presence of meconium).

b Newborn babies should immediately be assessed for breathing (rate and quality), heart rate (fast, slow, or absent), colour (pink or cyanotic/pale) and muscle tone (kicking and crying or floppy and silent). Babies with poor colour and/or inadequate breathing, tone or heart rate are in need of resuscitation with the following measures in order of escalation:[2]

- first, call for experienced help
- dry and stimulate the baby and place in a warmed squad/resuscitaire
- open the airway by positioning the head in the neutral position. Jaw thrust if poor tone
- remove visible secretions from the mouth with gentle suctioning. More vigorous suctioning is required only where thick meconium is obstructing the airway
- if breathing remains inadequate or heart rate below 100 bpm, give five breaths via bag-valve mask to aerate the lungs
- re-assess breathing and heart rate. Continue ventilation at 30–40 breaths/min with supplemental oxygen, until regular adequate breathing is established
- if heart rate falls below 60 bpm initiate chest compressions.

c Neonatal chest compressions are given using the hand encircling technique.[2] Place both hands around the baby's chest with fingers posteriorly and opposing thumbs pressing on the sternum, just below the line of the nipples. Compress the chest to one third of its depth at a rate of 100 bpm and at a ratio of 3:1 with ventilation breaths.

d Central venous access via umbilical vein cannulation is the route of choice for drug delivery during newborn resuscitation. Again, the Advanced Paediatric Life Support (APLS) manual describes the procedure.[2]

Case 3

a No verbal response and no eye opening both score 1 on the Glasgow coma score (GCS), whilst localizing pain scores five. Thus her GCS is 7/15. Below eight is considered coma.

b A useful working differential for coma in a young person might include:

Table 2.1

Neurological	Toxicological
CNS infection (meningitis/encephalitis)	Alcohol excess
Sub-arachnoid haemorrhage	Illicit drug overdose (benzodiazepines, opiates, MDMA and others)
Traumatic brain injury	Therapeutic drug overdose (benzodiazepines, tricyclic antidepressants, lithium and many others)
Seizure and post-ictal states	Carbon monoxide poisoning
Raised intracranial pressure (space occupying lesion, hydrocephalus, blocked shunt)	
Endocrine	**Other**
Hypoglycaemia	Shock (all forms)
Diabetic ketoacidosis	Arrhythmia
Addisonian crisis	Encephalopathy
Hypothyroid coma	Severe depression

c Bedside investigations in an unconscious young woman would include:

- blood glucose measurement
- ECG for arrhythmia, or signs of tricyclic poisoning
- arterial blood gas, mostly for acidosis and lactate level, but looking at the other parameters too, for example, pO_2, pCO_2, BE, HB and CO level
- urinary toxicology testing
- urine for dipstick and pregnancy testing.

d Apart from reduced GCS, opiate overdose is evidenced by respiratory depression and small (pinpoint) pupils. The signs of intravenous drug use such as track marks over peripheral veins may also be a valid clue!

e Treat heroin overdose with naloxone. Give in 0.4–2 mg boluses intravenously and assess response after two to three minutes. Repeat doses (up to maximum 10 mg) can be given. Patients in whom naloxone gives only brief relief from harmful opiate toxicity will require a naloxone infusion.

Case 4

a The ECG (Figure 2.1) has the following features: regular rhythm, narrow complexes and absent P waves. The interpretation is supraventricular tachycardia (SVT).

b The ALS guidelines[1] list the following as signs of cardiovascular instability in patients with a tachyarrhythmia:

- reduced conscious level
- systolic blood pressure <90 mmHg
- chest pain
- heart failure.

c Initial treatment of SVT in a stable patient should involve vagal manoeuvres. Perform carotid sinus massage (after confirming the absence of carotid bruit) or valsalva manoeuvre (in children blowing through a 20 mL syringe against the plunger). Then move on to drugs:

- 6 mg of adenosine by rapid bolus injection. If unsuccessful, repeat with 12 mg adenosine
- further pharmacological options include a rate limiting calcium channel blocker (verapamil 5 mg IV)
- or a beta-blocker (e.g., metoprolol 5 mg IV)
- or amiodarone 300 mg IVI over 20–60 minutes (then an infusion of 900 mg amiodarone over 24 hours, if required).

d Unstable patients with tachyarrhythmia should be treated with synchronized DC cardioversion. In the emergency situation, this will require sedation with adequate airway protection.

Case 5

a Symptomatic bradycardia is initially treated with atropine 500 mcg IV, repeated if necessary or where there is no response up to maximum 3 mg.

b Clinical features indicating a higher risk of asystole are:

- recent asystole
- mobitz II AV block
- complete heart block with broad QRS
- ventricular pause >3 seconds.

c The ALS algorithm[1] recommends intravenous infusion of adrenaline 2–10 mcg/min for atropine resistant bradycardia. Others to consider include:

- isoprenaline
- aminophylline
- dopamine
- glucagon (if β-blocker or calcium channel blocker overdose)
- glycopyrrolate can be used instead of atropine.

d Bradycardia unresponsive to drug treatment requires electrical pacing. Ideally, a temporary pacing wire should be inserted as soon as possible but, to buy time in an unstable patient, transcutaneous pacing in the ED may well be necessary. To provide this:

- conscious patients will need IV analgesia (morphine sulphate) and/or light sedation
- place the electrode pads in AP or right anterior- left lateral configuration
- select demand mode on the defibrillator/pacer
- select a pacing rate ideally between 60–90 bpm
- set the pacing current at the lowest setting and gradually increase the current until electrical capture occurs on the monitor and a palpable pulse is felt.

Case 6

a Initial fluid therapy for a shocked child is 20 ml/kg of 0.9% saline. Calculate the child's weight using the formula (age+4)*2, thus (6+4)*2 = 20 kg. Thus, a bolus of 20 ml × 20 kg = 400 ml 0.9% saline should be given by IV (or intraosseous) injection.

b An intraosseous needle is inserted into the flat medial surface of proximal tibia, one to two cm below the tibial tuberosity.

c The following urgent bedside investigations should be done in a shocked child:

- capillary blood glucose measurement for hypo or hyperglycaemia
- urine dipstick for ketones or glucose
- venous or capillary blood gas for pH and lactate levels.

d Using 20 kg as the estimated weight of the child (you should have calculated this in answer to part **a.** above), the volume of maintenance fluid to be given over 24 hours calculated as follows (Box 2.1):

Box 2.1. Calculating paediatric maintenance fluids

- 100 mL/kg for the first 10 kg +
- 50 mL/kg for the second 10 kg +
- 20 mL/kg/ for each subsequent kg above 20

Thus, maintenance fluid = (10 × 100) + (10 × 50) = 1500 mL over 24 hours
In addition, the fluid deficit must also be made up over 24 hours which in this case is calculated by the formula:

Fluid deficit in mL = %dehydration × 10 × weight in kg
$$= 5\% \times 10 \times 20 \text{ kg}$$
$$= 1000 \text{ mL over 24 hours}$$

Thus, total fluid required over 24 hours for this 20 kg child = maintenance fluid + deficit
$$= 1500 \text{ mL} + 1000 \text{ mL}$$
$$= 2500 \text{ mL/24 hours}$$

Rather than normal saline, 0.45% NaCl + 5% dextrose is a more common paediatric maintenance fluid.

Case 7

a Collapse with sudden shortness of breath in a patient with recent risk factors for venous thromboembolism strongly suggests pulmonary embolism (PE) as the most likely diagnosis. In addition, this patient is haemodynamically unstable and to obtain both marks the diagnosis is massive PE.

b Bedside echocardiography is useful in the diagnosis of massive PE where right heart dilatation is the clear sign.

c Treat massive PE with thrombolysis; protocols vary but where cardiac arrest is imminent, the British Thoracic Society (BTS) recommends 50 mg alteplase bolus. The circulation should also be supported with IV fluids – give 1 L 0.9% saline stat.

d The patient is now in cardiac arrest.

- put out a cardiac arrest call
- start CPR at a rate of 30:2 with ventilation via a bag valve mask
- as help arrives, attach a monitor and assess the rhythm
- secure the airway as soon as possible and change to continuous CPR
- give adrenaline 1 mg IV (if PEA/asystole).

Case 8

a Assessment of a patient with acute anaphylaxis begins with the airway. Features to look for include:

- difficulty speaking or change in voice (hoarseness)
- inspiratory stridor
- swelling of the face, tongue or oropharynx
- drooling of saliva
- respiratory distress
- cyanosis.

b The emergency treatment of anaphylactic shock is:

- 500 micrograms (or 0.5 ml of 1 in 1000) adrenaline intramuscular (IM)
- 10 mg of chlorphenamine IV
- 100–200 mg of hydrocortisone IV
- 1 L 0.9% normal saline stat.

c The airway is now in danger and must be secured urgently. Fast bleep an anaesthetist and get the difficult airway trolley and surgical airway equipment ready. Repeat doses of IM adrenaline should be given after five minutes, if there is no response to the first dose. Give nebulised adrenaline 5 mg of 1 in 1000 as a temporising measure to reduce airway swelling.

d Glucagon 1–2 mg IM or IV can be effective where the response to adrenaline is limited due to β-blockade. Remember glucagon is also the treatment for β-blocker overdose.

Case 9

a NICE guidance on head injury 2007[5] recommend immediate CT imaging of the brain in patients presenting to the ED with the following features:

- GCS <13 at the time of initial assessment
- GCS <15 when assessed two hours post-injury
- suspected open or depressed skull fracture
- clinical signs of basal skull fracture

- post-traumatic seizure
- focal neurological deficit
- more than a single episode of vomiting
- amnesia or loss of consciousness since the injury **and ANY** of the following:
  age > 65 yrs
  coagulopathy (e.g., on warfarin)
  dangerous mechanism of injury (e.g., fall from >1 m or more than five stairs).

b The CT brain image of this patient (Figure 2.2) demonstrates an area of high density in the right parietal region consistent with the appearance of an acute extradural haematoma. In addition, there is mass effect with evidence of midline shift.

c Acute extradural haemorrhage results from traumatic rupture of the middle meningeal artery which runs underneath the temporal bone between it and the dura mater.

d This young man has an expanding extradural haematoma with deteriorating consciousness. It is necessary to secure the airway (rapid sequence induction and intubation with ventilation) and immediate referral to a neurosurgeon for evacuation of the haematoma (which may require transfer to a tertiary centre).

Case 10

a From the ED perspective, burns are most usefully classified into partial or full thickness. Partial thickness burns involve the epidermis and/or dermis of the skin, whereas full thickness burns extend deeper than the basement membrane of the dermis and into subcutaneous tissue. Features of a full thickness burn are:

- white, leathery, blackened and charred, translucent appearance
- non-perfused (thrombosed vessels)
- anaesthetic (no pain felt with pressure from sterile needle)
- dry with absence of blistering.

b Ideally a burns chart (e.g., Lund and Browder chart, appropriate for age) should be used to determine the body surface area burnt, but with the information given in the question, we can also use the commonly employed 'rule of nines' to estimate the extent of the burn as follows:

Table 2.2

Area burnt	% body surface area in an adult
Head	9%
Whole arm	9%
Torso front	18%
Torso back	18%
Whole leg	18%

Thus, this man has burns extending across his whole anterior torso (18%) and the front of both arms (4.5% each arm). Therefore, a rough estimate of the burn area is 27% body surface area. The 'rule of nines' tends to overestimate the burn surface area, compared to the more accurate Lund and Browder chart.

c   Above 15% body surface area (BSA) burns in adults (above 10% in children) is considered major burns and requires IV fluid resuscitation. The guide to volume of fluid required in the first eight hours from the time of burn injury may by calculated using the Parklands formula as set out in the ATLS manual[3] (Box 2.2):

Box 2.2. Parklands formula

24 hour fluid requirement $= 4 \times \%$ BSA burn $\times$ weight (kg)

$ = 4 \times 27 \times 80 = 8640$ ml for this man

Give half over the first 8 hours and the remainder over the next 16 hours.

Thus, he should be given 4320 ml over the first eight hours from the time of the burn.

---

d   Smoke inhalation from a fire, in a contained space, may cause direct thermal injury and swelling to the upper airway, irritation and bronchospasm of the lower airway, pulmonary oedema, carbon monoxide poisoning and cyanide poisoning (from combustible plastics). You must look around the patient's nose and mouth for soot, oedema, and singed nasal hairs as well as in the mouth for soot, oedema and carbonaceous sputum, and assess their voice. Even apparently well individuals such as the woman in this question involved in a house fire, should have the following tests for any occult injury:

- peak flow measurement
- arterial blood gas (occult hypoxia warns of further respiratory compromise)
- carbon monoxide measurement (often as part of blood gas analysis)
- chest X-ray for signs of interstitial oedema.

Also, be alert to the possibility of cyanide poisoning from burning household plastics. There is no rapid test for cyanide poisoning but clinical signs include headache, lethargy, confusion and coma. Where strongly suspected, hydroxycobalbumin (cyanokit) is the antidote.

Further Reading

1.   The Advanced Life Support Group (2010) *Advanced Life Support*, 6th edn. Resuscitation Council (UK).
2.   Advanced Life Support Group. (January 2006) *Advanced Paediatric Life Support: The Practical Approach*, 4th edn. BMJ books and Blackwell Publishing.
3.   American College of Surgeons Committee on Trauma. (2008). *Advanced Trauma Life Support for Doctors*, 8th edn. American College of Surgeons.
4.   Nolan JP, Morley PT, Vanden Hoek TL, *et al.* (2003) *Therapeutic hypothermia after cardiac arrest*. An advisory statement by the Advanced Life Support Task Force of the International Liaison Committee on Resuscitation. *Resuscitation;* **57** 231–35. Also found at www.ilcor.org/data/ILCOR-hypothermia.pdf.
5.   NICE Guideline CG56. (2007) Head Injury: Triage, assessment, investigation and early management of head injury in infants, children and adults. www.nice.org.uk/Guidance/CG56.

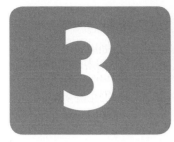

3

CARDIAC EMERGENCIES

Sam Thenabadu

Introduction

Core topics

- chest pain
- acute coronary syndromes
- cardiac chest pain in special circumstances, e.g., cocaine, pregnancy
- tachyarrythmias (atrial fibrillation, ventricular tachycardia, supraventricular tachycardia, Wolff-Parkinson-White syndrome)
- bradycardias/atrio-ventricular blocks
- heart failure
- acute pulmonary oedema
- aortic dissection
- aortic stenosis
- endocarditis and prophylaxis against endocarditis
- pericarditis and pericardial effusion
- malignant hypertension
- syncope
- postural hypotension
- side-effects of cardiac drugs and polypharmacy
- cardiomyopathy
- congenital heart disease.

The ECG is clearly the key piece of data to be able to interpret for this chapter, and if you are not confident reading ECGs now is the time to revise this. We suggest, as a minimum, you should be able to systematically interpret the normal resting ECG[1] and, also, have a working knowledge of the ECG abnormalities of the common cardiac diagnoses.[2]

In addition, the chest X-ray is an important cardiac investigation and knowing the radiological anatomy of the heart and mediastinum as well as the abnormal X-ray appearances of cardiac disease is essential.[3]

Below are a series of MCEM style SAQs on some of the core cardiology topics. In addition, questions on the emergency management of the basic tachyarrythmias (VT, SVT) and bradycardias are to be found in the resuscitation chapter (*see* Chapter 2).

Case 1

A 58-year-old female presents to the ED with abrupt onset of palpitations five hours previously. She only has hypertension in her past medical history and takes bendroflumethiazide. Her observations on arrival are heart rate 170 bpm, blood pressure 135/75 mmHg, respiratory rate 18/min and oxygen saturations 97% on air. Apart from the fast heart rate, she seems otherwise well. You are shown an ECG taken at triage (Figure 3.1).

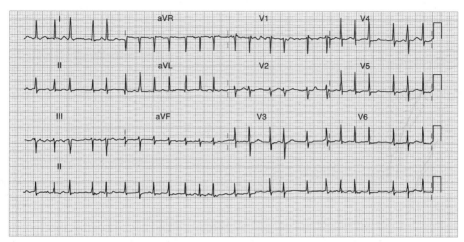

Figure 3.1

a What three abnormalities are present on the ECG (Figure 3.1) and what
  is the ECG diagnosis? [3]
b Give four common causes for this diagnosis. [2]
c Give three pharmacological treatments, with routes and doses, which could
  be used to control **rate** in this patient. [3]
d Give four blood tests you would request in the ED to look for a possible cause
  of this ECG abnormality. [2]
e Briefly outline your approach to **rhythm** control in this patient. [2]
  [12]

Case 2

A 67-year-old Asian male with a history of diet-controlled diabetes and tablet-controlled hypertension presents with a 15 minute episode of left-sided chest pain radiating to his left arm after exertion earlier that evening. He was mildly nauseated and sweaty with the pain, which subsided after sitting and resting at home. In the department, he has a further episode of chest pain, this time, at rest. The nurse looking after him places him on oxygen and performs an ECG (Figure 3.2).

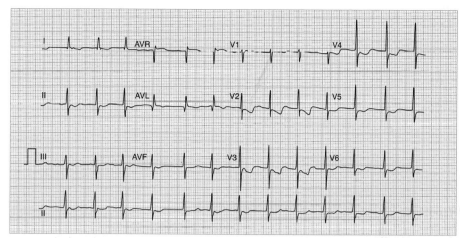

Figure 3.2

a Give three abnormalities present on this patient's ECG (Figure 3.2) which suggest acute ischaemia. [3]

b You prescribe treatment with aspirin and clopidogrel. Which specific anti-platelet pathways do each these drugs utilize? [2]

c Name four other drug treatments that can be used in the initial treatment of acute coronary syndrome (ACS) in this man. [4]

d You are referring him to the medical consultant who asks for his TIMI risk factors. Give four risk factors that are specified within the TIMI score. [2]

e Despite these treatments, he experiences further cardiac pain with accompanying 'dynamic' changes on repeat ECG. What further treatment options exist for him now? [2]

[13]

Case 3

A 62-year-old male presents to the ED with sudden onset central chest pain. He describes the pain as severe and 'ripping' in nature and it radiates between his shoulder blades. He is a known hypertensive but is non-compliant with medication and he smokes heavily. His observations at triage are: heart rate 115 bpm, blood pressure: 205/110 mmHg, respiratory rate 26/min and oxygen saturation on air 95%. An ECG is performed which demonstrates left ventricular hypertrophy (LVH) but no acute ischaemic changes.

a What is the likely diagnosis in this patient and briefly describe its pathophysiology? [3]

b Give two findings on clinical examination that would support your diagnosis. [2]

c For the likely diagnosis you give in answer to part a. above, give four immediate management steps you would initiate in this patient. [4]

d Give three imaging techniques that can be used to **confirm** your diagnosis. [3]

e How would you sub-classify this condition and what is the major implication for treatment arising from your sub-classification system? [2]

[14]

Case 4

A 72-year-old man with a history of rheumatic fever as a child presents to the ED with an episode of collapse and brief loss of consciousness, while walking up a short hill that morning. His observations are heart rate 72 bpm regular, blood pressure 100/85 mmHg, respiratory rate 22/min and oxygen saturations 96% on air. On examining his cardiovascular system, you hear an ejection systolic murmur (ESM) at the left sternal edge.

a Give a differential diagnosis of three conditions which may have caused this man's collapse. From the information given, what would be the most likely diagnosis in this patient?   [4]
b What is the classic triad of symptoms in the diagnosis you give above as most likely?   [3]
c Apart from those found at auscultation, what clinical signs might support your diagnosis (give two)?   [2]
d Name two abnormalities of the ECG associated with this diagnosis.   [2]
e The patient begins to complain of chest tightness in the ED. Name one drug that you would use, and one drug you would avoid, in treating this patient's chest tightness.   [2]

                                                                                           [13]

Case 5

A 38-year-old Nigerian lady, who is 32 weeks pregnant, presents to the ED with central chest pain radiating to her left arm. She has essential hypertension and a strong family history of ischaemic heart disease at an early age. An ECG is performed and shown below (Figure 3.3):

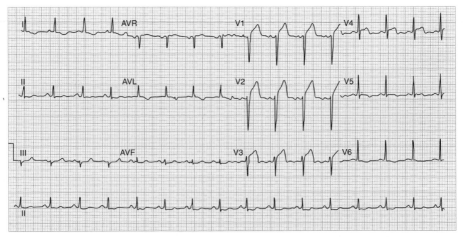

Figure 3.3

a   Give four causes of chest pain which are more likely in a pregnant patient
    than in non-pregnant patients of the same age.   [4]
b   What were the two leading cardiac causes of maternal death in the last
    'Confidential enquiry of maternal deaths in the UK'?   [2]
c   Give two abnormalities of the ECG given above (Figure 3.3) and, on the
    basis of this ECG, what is your final diagnosis in this particular patient?   [3]
d   What is the most appropriate definitive treatment for this patient with the
    final diagnosis you give?   [1]
e   Give four further management steps in the ED management of this patient.   [4]
                                                                                     [14]

Case 6

A 24-year-old male presents to the ED with a two-hour history of crushing central
chest pain and increasing shortness of breath. His partner confides in you that he
has been 'snorting cocaine' at a club tonight, but is not a regular user. He is agitated
but not combative and agrees to have his ECG done (Figure 3.4).

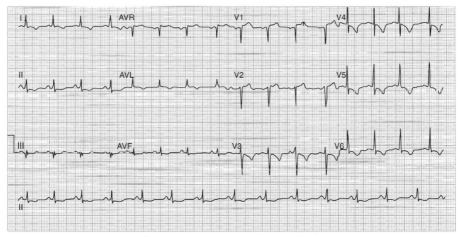

Figure 3.4

a   Interpret the ECG above (Figure 3.4) commenting on the rhythm and any
    abnormalities present.   [4]
b   Briefly outline the pathophysiology of the cocaine-induced chest pain in
    this man.   [2]
c   What is the initial drug of choice to use in this patient?   [1]
d   Name three further drugs that could be used in this situation.   [3]
e   Which common cardiovascular drug should be avoided and why?   [2]
                                                                                     [12]

Case 7

A 27-year-old male attends the ED with a one-week history of fevers, rigors and intermittent pleuritic chest pain. He smells strongly of alcohol and has multiple needle marks in his right forearm and ante-cubital fossa. On examination, he looks unwell and is pyrexic with a temperature of 38.8 °C. You are concerned that he may have infective endocarditis (IE).

a Name three groups of patient most at risk of developing IE?   [3]
b What is the most common organism seen in IE associated with intravenous
   drug use?   [1]
c Which heart valve is most likely to be affected in this patient, and give two
   further clinical features of IE specifically of this valve?   [3]
d List the investigations you would perform in a patient with suspected IE.   [5]
e After appropriate specimens have been taken, what initial antibiotic therapy
   would you prescribe for a patient with first presentation of IE?   [2]
                                                                                                   [14]

Case 8

A 42-year-old Jamaican man is brought by his wife to the ED with a 6-hour history of blurred vision. His wife is concerned that he was complaining of a headache yesterday and now appears to be slightly confused. He has no medical history of note but smokes 30 cigarettes a day and drinks approximately 30 units of alcohol per week. His observations at triage are heart rate 110 bpm, blood pressure 230/130 mmHg and oxygen saturations on air 96% and temperature 37.4 °C.

a Define severe hypertension in terms of blood pressure readings.   [1]
b Give four clinical features of hypertensive encephalopathy.   [2]
c Apart from hypertensive encephalopathy, give three other hypertensive
   emergencies. Briefly describe one test that can be performed in the ED to
   look for each emergency you give.   [6]
d Outline the major steps in the management of this patient with hypertensive
   encephalopathy in the ED.   [3]
e Name four general lifestyle advice points recommended by the NICE
   guidelines that you would give any patient with hypertension.   [2]
                                                                                                   [14]

Case 9

A 26-year-old man comes to the ED with a three-day history of central sharp chest pain radiating to his neck. He describes it as worst when waking in the morning and worse on breathing in. At triage, he does not look unwell and his observations are: heart rate 110 bpm, blood pressure 110/65 mmHg, oxygen saturations on air 96% and temperature 38.2 °C. His ECG is taken at triage and shown below (Figure 3.5).

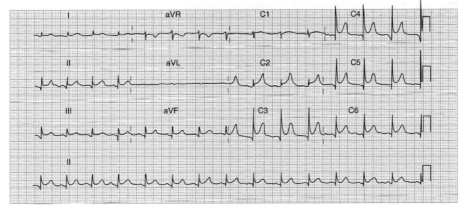

Figure 3.5

a Describe the abnormalities on the ECG (Figure 3.5) and give a likely
   diagnosis in this patient. [3]
b What classic clinical sign would you look for on examination? [1]
c Give three blood investigations, with your rationale for requesting each, in
   this patient? [3]
d What treatment would you initiate in this patient? [1]
e If this patient also complained of dyspnoea, what complication may be
   present? Give three clinical signs and three investigations used to evaluate
   the presence of this complication. [4]

[12]

Case 10

A 70-year-old male with known heart failure presents to the ED with a two-day
history of worsening shortness of breath. His carer tells you he is non-compliant
with his heart medications, as he feels it causes him to urinate too frequently. At
first assessment, he is acutely dyspnoeic and distressed. His initial observations
are heart rate 130 bpm irregular, blood pressure 170/95 mmHg, respiratory rate
28/min and oxygen saturation 86% on room air. His chest X-ray, obtained in the
resuscitation room, is shown in Figure 3.6.

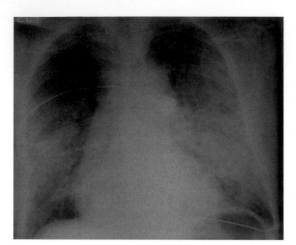

Figure 3.6

a Describe the abnormal appearances in the chest X-ray (Figure 3.6).   [2]
b Give four clinical signs of heart failure you might expect to find on
   examination.   [2]
c Name four cardiac precipitants of decompensation in known heart failure
   patients.   [2]
d How would you treat this man emergently? Include, as part of your answer,
   three pharmacological treatments (with routes of administration) you
   would initiate.   [5]
e The patient's ECG shows atrial fibrillation with rate varying from 130–150.
   How would you control this patient's heart rate?   [1]
f You obtain an arterial blood gas sample after one hour of medical treatment:

pH	7.28
pO_2	7.4 kPa
pCO_2	6.0 kPa
HCO_3	13.5 mEq/L
BE	−9.2

What further treatment could you initiate for this patient in the ED?   [2]
                                                                              [14]

Case 11

A 30-year-old male presents to the ED with acute onset palpitations and shortness of breath. His sister who is accompanying him states that he is known to have 'Wolff-Parkinson-White Syndrome' (WPW). He is alert although uncomfortable, with a pulse of 180 bpm and a blood pressure of 135/75 mmHg.

a What characteristic abnormalities would you see on the resting ECG of a patient with WPW? [2]

b Briefly describe the cardiac abnormality underlying WPW. [2]

c When an ECG is performed, this patient is seen to be in atrial fibrillation (AF) with a ventricular rate 180–200 bpm. Name two anti-arrhythmic drugs that must be **avoided** in this situation and give your reason why. [4]

d How would you treat this patient including the names of two antiarrhythmic drugs that **could** be safely used (doses not required)? [4]

e Despite initiating medical therapy, the tachycardia increases to rate 240 bpm and the patient's blood pressure falls to 85/50 mmHg. What will you do now? [2]

[14]

Case 12

A 35-year-old lady presents to the ED with a two-hour history of intermittent palpitations. She has a 20-year history of depression and takes antidepressants but is otherwise normally well. Her observations on arrival are, heart rate 200 bpm, blood pressure 95/60 mmHg, oxygen saturations on 96% on room air. A rhythm strip is recorded and a section of which is shown below (Figure 3.7):

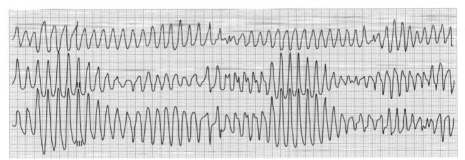

Figure 3.7

a What is the ECG diagnosis (Figure 3.7)? [2]

b What is the first-line emergency treatment of this condition? [2]

c Give three possible pharmacological precipitants and three non-pharmacological causes for this condition. [6]

d How do you calculate the QT interval on the normal resting ECG? [2]

e If your initial management is ineffective, what are the next two treatments? [2]

[14]

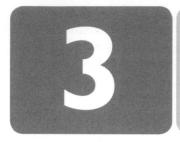

CARDIAC EMERGENCIES – ANSWERS

Case 1

a The ECG (Figure 3.1) demonstrates a tachycardia of rate 120–160. The rate is irregular and no P waves are seen. The ECG diagnosis is atrial fibrillation (AF) with fast ventricular response.

b Causes of AF are legion but some of the most common which should be considered in patients presenting to the ED include:

Table 3.1

Cardiac Precipitants AF	Non-Cardiac Precipitants AF
Ischaemic heart disease	Hyperthyroidism
Heart failure	Pulmonary embolus
Hypertension	Sepsis
Valvular heart disease (commonly mitral)	Alcohol excess or withdrawal
Sick sinus syndrome	Hypokalaemia
Pericarditis	Hypothermia
Cardiomyopathy	Drug use (cocaine)

c ALS guidelines[4] suggest the following pharmacological interventions for rate control in AF (NICE recommendations are similar[5]):

- β-blockers are usually first-line (e.g., metoprolol 5 mg IV or bisoprolol 5 mg PO)
- calcium channel antagonist (e.g., verapamil 5 mg IV) if β-blockers are contraindicated or poorly tolerated (e.g., asthmatics)
- digoxin 500–750 mcg IV or amiodarone 300 mg IV over 30–60 minutes followed by an infusion of 900 mg over 24 hours are used where there is evidence of heart failure.

d Specific blood investigations in a patient with new onset AF include:

- U&Es to identify potential electrolyte disturbances
- thyroid function tests for hyperthyroidism
- Ca^{2+} and Mg^{2+} levels (low levels of both lead to acute rhythm disturbance)
- FBC/CRP to identify occult infection.

e Treatments for atrial fibrillation aimed at rhythm control (i.e., returning the patient to sinus rhythm) are possible where less than 48 hours has elapsed from the onset of AF to presentation. In the woman in this question, the tachyarrhythmia symptoms arose five hours previously and so rhythm control, as soon as possible, is an appropriate treatment goal. Much new onset AF will spontaneously cardiovert to sinus rhythm and this can be encouraged with simple measures such as IV fluid rehydration and correction of any electrolyte imbalance.

Where specific measures are required to achieve cardioversion, advice should be sought from a cardiologist or the on-call medical consultant. Elective DC cardioversion under sedation is often chosen, as it is highly effective in acute onset AF. Chemical cardioversion with flecainide can be attempted in patients **without** previous heart disease or structural abnormality or, where flecainide is contraindicated, amiodarone can be tried.[4, 5]

Case 2

a The patient's ECG (Figure 3.2) indicates widespread ischaemia with downsloping ST depression with T wave inversion in leads V2–V4, horizontal 1 mm ST depression leads V5–V6 as well as ST depression in lead II. The diagnosis is acute coronary syndrome.

   The term acute coronary syndrome (ACS) is a descriptor of the signs and symptoms consistent with ischaemic chest pain, occurring at rest. Based on ECG findings and biochemical markers of cardiac muscle necrosis, ACS can be divided into the following more specific diagnosis:

Table 3.2

Diagnosis	ECG changes of ST segment elevation, new onset LBBB	Biochemical evidence of cardiac necrosis, i.e. positive troponin
ST segment elevation myocardial infarction (STEMI)	Yes	Yes
Non ST segment elevation myocardial infarction (NSTEMI)	No	Yes
Unstable angina	No (although may have other ECG changes of cardiac ischaemia)	No

b Common to the immediate treatment of all three diagnoses within acute coronary syndrome is to give aspirin 300 mg PO stat and clopidogrel 300–600 mg PO stat. Both of these drugs are anti-platelet agents. Aspirin irreversibly inactivates the platelet cyclo-oxygenase (COX) enzyme which synthesizes thromboxane A2, a chemical mediator involved in platelet aggregation. Clopidogrel antagonizes the ADP receptor on the platelet cell surface and so inhibits the ADP triggered intracellular pathway for platelet aggregation.

c This patient's ECG does not have ST elevation and, therefore, he has either unstable angina or NSTEMI. Further emergency treatments for both these diagnoses are initially similar and include the following:

   ● opiate analgesia (i.e., morphine 2.5–10 mg IV titrated to pain)

- GTN sublingually followed, as required, by an intravenous infusion
- low-molecular weight heparin (e.g., enoxaparin 1 mg/kg s/c)
- β-blocker (e.g., metoprolol 50 mg PO).

Giving oxygen might also be an answer here, but you are told that the patient is on oxygen in the question, and so it is unlikely that you would be rewarded with a mark!

d The Thrombolysis in Myocardial Infarction (TIMI) investigators[6] developed a validated risk scoring system for estimating the risk of myocardial infarction (MI) or death within 14 days in patients with ACS (Box 3.1).

Box 3.1. TIMI score

The following factors score one point:

- age >65 years
- three or more coronary artery disease risk factors (smoking, hypertension, hyperlipideamia, family history of ischaemic heart disease, diabetes)
- known coronary artery disease
- already taking aspirin
- crescendo angina
- ST deviation on ECG >1 mm
- elevated cardiac troponin

Score zero to two gives a 3% risk of MI or death after 14 days, score four is a 7% risk, while a score six to seven gives a 19% risk.

The TIMI score can be used to identify ACS patients at high-risk who require more aggressive therapy; either treatment with a glycoprotein IIb/IIIa inhibitor and/or urgent percutaneous coronary intervention (PCI) or, conversely, those at low-risk who might be safely discharged after a negative cardiac biomarker result (e.g., normal 12 hour troponin).

e Ongoing chest pain and/or dynamic changes on the ECG (deepening ST depression or new T-wave inversion) despite medical therapy for ACS also indicates critical ischaemia, and that the patient is at high-risk of myocardial infarction. Further treatment measures are required.

- GTN IV infusion, if one is not already being given
- glycoprotein IIb/IIIa inhibitor (e.g., abciximab, tirofiban)
- percutaneous coronary intervention (rescue PCI).

Case 3

a Ripping or tearing chest pain radiating to the back, particularly between the shoulder blades, should raise suspicion of acute thoracic aortic dissection. Acute thoracic dissection follows a tear in the intima of the aortic lining, allowing blood to enter the vessel wall and 'dissect' through the smooth muscle media, creating a false lumen.

b Clinical signs to look for in the patient suspected of acute thoracic dissection include:

- new murmur of aortic regurgitation (involvement aortic root)
- unequal upper limb pulses or blood pressures (brachial artery involvement)
- paraplegia (spinal artery occlusion)
- oligo/anuria (renal artery occlusion)
- rarely, hoarseness of voice (recurrent laryngeal nerve impingement).

c Immediate management of acute dissection should occur in the resuscitation room with specific interventions including:

- oxygen 15 L via reservoir mask (they are critically ill)
- treat pain generously with IV opiate analgesia, and nausea with anti-emetic as required (making the patient comfortable will also help lower the blood pressure)
- where complete rupture of the aorta occurs, death is swift by massive haemorrhage in the unprepared: obtain large bore intravenous access along with cross-match for six to ten units blood as soon as the diagnosis is suspected
- lowering the blood pressure removes the major driver for progression of the dissection; in the emergency room a GTN IV infusion (high rates may be required up to 10–20 mg/hour) is likely to be the quickest and easiest method to achieve this. Where time and invasive monitoring are available, IV labetalol is the optimal choice of anti-hypertensive in hypertensive emergencies such as this.

d Most EDs in the UK will investigate suspected thoracic aortic dissection with contrast CT angiography of the thoracic and abdominal aorta (sensitivity and specificity around 96%). Trans oesophageal echocardiography (TOE) in skilled hands may also be used with similar accuracy of diagnosis. The gold standard technique for diagnosis has become MRI imaging, which is said to have a sensitivity and specificity of 98% respectively. Disadvantages of MRI are both access out-of-hours, and it takes time – time during which a potentially unstable patient is outside a critical care area.

e Trans-oesophageal echo or CT/angiography will, in most cases, provide a definitive diagnosis and categorization of an acute thoracic aortic dissection is either by using the Stanford or DeBakey classification systems; the Stanford method is simplest:

Stanford Type A	Involves the ascending aorta
Stanford Type B	Does not involve the ascending aorta

The importance of this classification is that type A dissections are generally addressed surgically, and type B treated medically, although this distinction has become less absolute with the advent of endovascular aortic stenting procedures now offered by major vascular centres. As soon as the diagnosis is confirmed on imaging, discuss all cases with the cardiothoracic and/or vascular surgeons as local policy dictates.

Case 4

a Syncope on exertion has a wide differential but conditions to think of include:

- acute coronary syndrome
- aortic stenosis
- hypertrophic obstructive cardiomyopathy (in the younger patient)
- vasovagal syncope.

However, this patient has a prior history of rheumatic fever placing him at risk of valvular disease and, coupled with the ESM noted on auscultation and narrow pulse pressure, indicates the likely diagnosis to be aortic stenosis (AS).

b The classic triad of symptoms in AS are angina, dyspnoea and syncope. These symptoms are most pronounced on exertion, and prognosis is very poor once they develop. Without surgical intervention, death commonly occurs within a three-year period. Other serious manifestations of AS include congestive cardiac failure, arrhythmia and sudden death.

c Peripheral signs of AS are found as the stenosis becomes more severe (i.e., the pressure gradient across the valve at echocardiography is greater than 50 mmHg) and include:

- narrow pulse pressure
- slow rising pulse
- poor volume brachial/femoral pulse
- left ventricular heave
- palpable aortic thrill.

d An ECG is likely to have signs of left ventricular hypertrophy and a strain pattern due to pressure overload (ST depression and T wave inversion I+AVL, V5–6). Sinus rhythm is predominantly seen, but the presence of AF suggests associated mitral valve pathology.

e β-blockers are the mainstay of treatment in the acute treatment of angina in a patient with aortic stenosis. Reducing the work of the heart reduces the pressure gradient across the aortic valve and lessens symptoms.

Nitrates and ACE inhibitors should be avoided by non-specialists, as both drugs cause systemic vasodilation, reduce preload and thus increase the pressure gradient over the valve, thereby worsening symptoms.

Case 5

a As in all patients, acute chest pain in the pregnant woman can originate from cardiac, respiratory, gastrointestinal or musculoskeletal systems. However, pregnancy increases the risk of a number of specific cardiovascular conditions which should perhaps be given more consideration, when assessing the heavily pregnant patient with chest pain. These conditions include:

- gastro-oesophageal reflux disease (relaxation smooth muscle lower oesophageal sphincter)

- pulmonary embolus (pregnancy is an established major risk factor)
- angina and acute coronary syndrome (increased cardiac workload in pregnancy)
- thoracic aortic dissection (caused by hypertensive disease in pregnancy)
- puerperal cardiomyopathy (a dilated cardiomyopathy occurring in the last month of pregnancy)
- angina caused by anaemia (low-oxygen carrying capacity in profound anaemia of pregnancy).

b   The report of the Confidential Enquiry into Maternal Deaths in the United Kingdom 2000–2002[7,8] reported a total of 44 deaths due to heart disease in pregnancy. Puerperal cardiomyopathy and myocardial infarction were the two leading causes of cardiac death followed by thoracic aortic aneurysms and pulmonary hypertension. The reduction in childhood rheumatic heart disease has caused a decline in valvular disease that classically worsens during pregnancy and which used to cause significant cardiac co-morbidity in pregnant women.

   The 'Confidential Enquiry into Maternal Deaths'[7,8] also suggests the four leading risk factors for cardiac disease in pregnancy to be: hypertension, obesity, a positive family history of inherited cardiac disease, and, unsurprisingly, increased maternal age.

c   The ECG (Figure 3.3) demonstrates a normal sinus rhythm, normal axis but with ST segment elevation in leads V1–V4 and reciprocal ST segment depression in leads I and AVl. The ECG diagnosis is an acute anterior ST elevation myocardial infarction (STEMI).

d   Percutaneous coronary intervention (PCI) is the definitive treatment for pregnant women with acute MI and can be performed with lead shielding, to minimize foetal radiation exposure. The thrombolytic agent, tissue plasminogen activator (tPA) does not cross the placental barrier into the foetal circulation, and can be used as an alternative for coronary recannulization where PCI is not available. tPA does, however, substantially increase the risk of maternal haemmorhage and should be used only after weighing the risks and benefits in the individual patient.

e   Other steps in the management of this patient with myocardial infarction in the third trimester of pregnancy:

- oxygen to maintain saturations 94–98%
- anti-platelet therapy (aspirin 300 mg PO and clopidogrel 300–600 mg PO)
- involvement of senior obstetric help to instigate foetal monitoring and offer obstetric advice
- if necessary, improve cardiac output by wedging of the woman in the left lateral position to relieve pressure on the inferior vena cava and maximize preload.

Most drugs used in managing cardiac ischaemia are safe in pregnancy, including aspirin, clopidogrel, GTN, low-molecular weight heparin and β-blockers. Glycoprotein IIb/IIIa inhibitors have also been given to a small number of pregnant women. Cardiovascular drugs to be avoided in pregnant patients are ACE inhibitors, angiotensin receptor antagonists and statins.

Case 6

a The ECG (Figure 3.4) demonstrates sinus rhythm (rate 90 bpm); 1–2 mm ST segment elevation in leads V1–V2 with ST segment depression in the inferior leads (II and aVf). Deep T-wave inversion is also seen in leads V4–V6 and I and aVL. Thus, there is evidence of myocardial ischaemia likely secondary to cocaine-induced vasospasm, but also of an evolving ST elevation myocardial infarction.

b Cocaine-induced cardiac ischaemia is increasingly common with chest pain, hypertension, tachycardia and agitation all present in the acute presentation.

Cocaine is a sympathomimetic and induces vasoconstriction by preventing catecholamine reuptake in the central and peripheral nervous system, and stimulating the release of norepinephrine from adrenergic nerve terminals. These effects result in coronary artery vasospasm while, at the same time, increasing myocardial oxygen demand through stimulating heart rate and stroke volume. The result is ischaemic pain and associated ECG changes which need aggressive treatment to reverse the vasospasm.

Caution is required in older users, however, as habitual cocaine use causes accelerated coronary artery disease and cardiac ischaemia due to coronary thrombosis may also be present. When in doubt, patients should be considered to have both pathologies and be managed accordingly.

c Benzodiazepines are recommended as first-line agents in cocaine-induced chest pain. Diazepam, oral or IV and titrated to response, eases agitation, reduces cardiac work and relaxes vasospasm. They also help avert cocaine induced seizures.

d Otherwise, manage in the ED with:

- oxygen to maintain saturations 94–98%
- aspirin 300 mg PO
- nitrates sublingually then followed by IV infusion as required to vasodilate the coronary arteries
- where coronary thrombotic disease is also possible and/or there is a poor response to initial treatment with vasodilators, refer to the cardiologist for angiography and PCI.

e β-blockers are to be avoided because of concerns with unopposed alpha action, exacerbating the hypertension and tachycardia of the stimulant drug.

Case 7

a Three major groups of patients at risk of infective endocarditis (IE) are:

- patients with prosthetic heart valves
- intravenous drug users (IVDU)
- patients with structural abnormalities of their native heart valves or of other areas of the endocardium such as ventricular or atrial septal defects.

IE, occurring on normal valves tends to be more aggressive causing rapid valvular destruction and presenting with acute heart failure, while infection of prosthetic valves and structurally abnormal native valves often follow a more insidious sub-acute clinical course. IE associated with IVDU can follow either pattern.

b   *Staph. aureus* is the most commonly associated organism with IE in IV drug users; after which comes streptococci, fungi and gram –ve organisms such as serratia. On native valves in non-IVDU patients, streptococci (*Strep. viridians, Strep. bovis*) and *enterocci* account for over 50% cases.

c   IVDU predisposes to right heart endocarditis and most often tricuspid valve infection. The patient in this question has a pansystolic murmur at the parasternal edge, louder with inspiration – the characteristics of tricuspid regurgitation. Thus, the patient has tricuspid valve endocarditis. Incompetence of the tricuspid valve leads to signs of right heart failure:

- raised JVP
- peripheral oedema
- right ventricular heave
- hepatomegaly, ascites and jaundice.

Septic emboli from the right heart valves lodge in the small vessels of the lung causing:

- lung abscess
- pulmonary infarction and pleuritic chest pain.

d   Investigate suspected infective endocarditis with:

- three sets of blood cultures taken from three separate sites, at no less than 60 minute intervals, and preferably at the height of fevers. Aseptic technique should be used to minimize contamination and blood for culture should not be drawn from IV cannulae
- blood tests for inflammatory markers (WCC, ESR, CRP)
- chest X-ray for cardiomegaly and lung infarction or abscess
- urgent transthoracic echocardiography (trans-oesophageal echocardiography, if available) to diagnose cardiac vegetation and delineate the extent of valve lesion
- urine microscopy may show red cell casts.

Although beyond the scope of this book to discuss, a set of criteria known as Duke's criteria give detailed guidance on the positive diagnosis of IE and are worth knowing.[9]

e   The Royal College of Physicians (RCP) recommends initial therapy of suspected IE with intravenous benzylpenicillin 1.2–2.4 g IV/24 hour in four to six divided doses and gentamicin 3–5 mg/kg IV daily in two to three divided doses.[10] This may need tailoring to the results of microbiological sensitivities once known (usually after 48 hours).

Case 8

a Severe hypertension is considered to be present when the blood pressure is above 200 mmHg systolic and/or 120 mmHg diastolic. Younger Afro-Caribbean patients are most at risk of uncontrolled severe hypertension and most likely to present with a hypertensive emergency.

b Clinical features of hypertensive encephalopathy include headache, visual disturbances, nausea, vomiting, fits, focal neurological signs, confusion and reduced GCS. Papilloedema may or may not be present.

c The term hypertensive emergency describes the condition where high blood pressure (usually severe hypertension as defined above) is causing end-organ damage. Organs, other than the central nervous system, potentially at risk from high blood pressure are:

Table 3.3

Organ	Features	Investigation
Heart	Angina Myocardial infarction Pulmonary oedema	ECG : LVH with strain pattern Acute ischaemic changes Chest X-ray: large heart, pulmonary oedema
Kidneys	Renal failure Oligouria Proteinuria	Urea and electrolytes Creatinine Urine dipstick test for protein
Retina	Flame haemmorhages Exudates Papilloedema	Fundoscopy Visual acuity
Aorta	Acute aortic dissection	CT aortogram or echocardiogaphy

d The two key steps in managing this patient would be: first, exclude an acute intracerebral event such as intracranial bleed or infarct with CT imaging of the brain; and second, lower the blood pressure to prevent further organ damage.

You will note that the presentation of hypertensive encephalopathy is similar in many respects to that of an acute stroke or intracranial bleed, both of which can cause a dramatic rise in blood pressure even in an otherwise normotensive patient. We can look for signs of other end-organ damage (see above) to support our diagnosis of hypertensive emergency but, before treating, we must exclude acute intracerebral events with CT imaging of the brain. This is particularly important as rapidly lowering the blood pressure after stroke or intracerebral bleed, reduces cerebral perfusion pressure and may cause considerable harm!

Most patients can be managed with admission, rest and oral anti-hypertensives such as a β-blocker (labetalol) or a long-acting calcium channel blocker (amlodopine). Where appropriate, a diuretic such as furosemide can be added. The aim is to reduce the blood pressure by 25% or so over 24–48 hours – more rapid reduction is discouraged as it could precipitate stroke or MI. Hypertensive emergencies which threaten life such as hypertensive encephalopathy require blood pressure control within hours. Labetolol IV or sodium nitroprusside IV can be used and require invasive blood pressure monitoring via an arterial line and HDU/ITU level care.

e NICE recommend asking hypertensive patients about and offering advice on:[11]

- diet and exercise patterns
- reducing alcohol intake
- reducing caffeine intake
- reducing salt intake
- smoking and offering cessation advice.

Case 9

a The diagnosis here is acute pericarditis and the ECG (Figure 3.5) demonstrates the marked concave ST segment elevation in all territories which may be seen in this diagnosis.

The description given of the pain is classic of pericarditis: sharp substernal pain made better on sitting forward, sometimes radiating to the base of the neck and sharing the characteristics of pleurisy, in being worsened by movement and respiration. The patient is also typical: a well young man with coryzal illness.

The ECG in acute pericarditis may show concave (saddle shaped) ST segment elevation in the anterior, lateral and inferior leads. These changes may be associated with PR segment depression. Leads AVR, V1 and occasionally V2, show ST depression. The changes should all normalize after resolution of the illness.

The commonest causes of pericarditis are viral infections in the young and uraemia or acute MI/post MI Dressler's syndrome in the older patient.

Table 3.4

Causes of Pericarditis	
Viral	Coxsackie, epstein barr virus, HIV, influenza, mumps
Bacterial	Staphylococcus, pneumococcus, TB, haemophilus
Drugs	Hydralazine, procainamide, anticoagulants, phenytoin
Malignancy	Sarcoma, mesothelioma
Rheumatological	Rheumatoid arthritis, SLE, sarcoidosis, , scleroderma, dermatomyositis, ankylosing spondylitis
Others	Uraemia, Dressler's syndrome, aortic dissection, myxoedema, radiotherapy

b The classic sign in acute pericarditis is of a pericardial friction rub, said to be audible in 60–85% of cases.

c Blood investigations in the ED include:

- FBC, CRP, ESR – while the FBC is often normal, the ESR and CRP will confirm an inflammatory process
- U&Es to exclude uraemia
- CK and troponin to identify an associated myocarditis.

If signs and symptoms continue despite treatment, further tests such as blood cultures, ASO titres, TB testing via sputum for AAFB, viral titres for coxsackie and an auto-antibody screen are appropriate.

d The first-line treatment would be non-steroidal anti-inflammatory drugs. In most straightforward cases, the review by the patient's GP is sufficient follow up.

e The major complication of pericarditis is pericardial effusion which, if large (>200 mL), can compromise cardiac function and produce dyspnoea. Life-threatening cardiac tamponade can occur but is rare in simple inflammatory pericarditis and most common in malignant disease or from penetrating trauma. Thus, a patient with a diagnosis of pericarditis, who also complains of dyspnea, requires further evaluation:

- look for clinical signs of tamponade: muffled heart sounds, raised JVP and hypotension (Becks' triad)
- investigate with an ECG (may have small low voltage QRS complexes where large effusions are present), a chest X-ray (large effusions give a characteristic 'flask' shape to the heart – with progressive accumulation of more pericardial fluid a massive, globular heart may be seen) and definitively with transthoracic echocardiography (detects all but the smallest pericardial effusions and will also diagnose globally blunted cardiac activity in tamponade).

Pericardial effusions, not causing cardiac compromise, are best observed with treatment of the underlying cause. On the other hand, cardiac tamponade must be relieved with needle pericardiocentes performed, if necessary, as an emergency in the ED.

Case 10

a The chest X-ray in heart failure can show cardiomegaly, upper lobe blood diversion, Kerley B septal lines, fluid in the interlobar fissures, bat's wing hilar shadowing and pleural effusions. The chest X-ray given in this question (Figure 3.6) demonstrates both cardiomegaly and bat's wing alveolar oedema, supporting the clinical suspicion of acute pulmonary oedema in this patient.

b We should always be aware of the difference between the clinical signs of left ventricular failure and those of right-sided heart failure, although in practice, a patient such as this with decompensated chronic congestive cardiac failure, will have a generous helping of the features of both.

Table 3.5

Signs of left-sided heart failure	Signs of right-sided heart failure
Audible 3rd heart sound (S3 gallop rhythm)	Elevated JVP
Basal crepitations in the chest	Right ventricular heave
Cardiac wheeze	Peripheral oedema (sacrum, lower leg)
Displaced apex beat	Hepatomegaly and ascites

c There are numerous causes for an acute decompensation in heart failure patients. The most commonly seen are listed below, divided into cardiac and non-cardiac precipitants.

Table 3.6

Cardiac Precipitants	Non Cardiac Precipitants
Acute coronary syndrome	Fluid overload
Arrhythmias – aAF most commonly	Non-compliance with heart failure medication
Worsening valve disease (e.g., mitral regurgitation, aortic stenosis)	Polypharmacy or overdose with negatively ionotropic drugs
Failure prosthetic valve	Anaemia
Hypertension	Thyrotoxicosis
Tamponade	Sepsis

d Treat acute cardiogenic pulmonary oedema as follows:

- sit the patient upright
- oxygen 15 L via reservoir mask (until stable)
- nitrates can initially be used sublingually (two puffs of GTN spray) then converted to an IV infusion for venodilation and reduction of preload (GTN IV infusion 2–20 mg/hour titrated upwards to maximal effect, keeping systolic blood pressure above 90 mmHg)
- IV opiates (morphine 2.5–10 mg IV) act as an anxiolytic, as well as causing venodilation, and reducing myocardial demand
- IV loop diuretics (furosemide 40–80 mg IV) may also be given to transiently produce arteriodilation followed by the diuresis beneficial in fluid overload.

e Heart failure complicated/precipitated by AF with fast ventricular rate should be treated by digoxin, which acts as a mildly positive inotrope. It may also have a role in heart failure with sinus rhythm through the same mechanism.

f This patient is responding poorly to medical therapy and remains acidotic and hypoxic. Further management in the ED is with non-invasive ventilation in continuous positive airway pressure mode (CPAP). CPAP increases the airway pressure splinting open collapsing alveoli and tipping the balance of Starling forces back in favour of fluid reabsorption into the alveolar capillaries. It also reduces the work of breathing and has a positive effect on cardiac output. CPAP should be considered in those patients with cardiogenic pulmonary oedema and acidosis, either from the outset or within one hour, if response to medical therapy is poor.

Case 11

a The classic ECG abnormalities seen in WPW are a shortened PR interval (<120 msec) associated with a slurring and slow rise of the initial upstroke of the QRS complex referred to as a 'delta wave'.

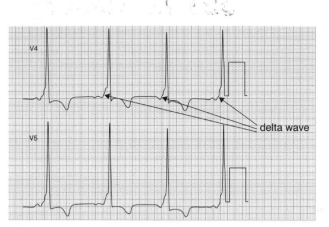

delta wave

Figure 3.8

WPW is divided into type A and type B. These are distinguishable on the ECG by an upright QRS in V1 with type A and, in contrast, a negative QRS in V1 seen in type B WPW.

b A fast accessory conduction pathway, called the Bundle of Kent, exists between the atria and ventricle which can cause pre-excitation of the ventricles and predispose to recurrent tachyarrythmia. All types of tachyarrhythmias may occur in WPW although the most common are the re-entrant SVT and pre-excited AF. It is a congenital condition and a leading cause of tacharrryhmia in young adults.

c AF with fast ventricular response is the most feared of the tachyarrythmias in WPW, as it can occur with rates up to 250 bpm and rapidly deteriorate into VF. It is also difficult to treat! The rule of thumb is that AV nodal blocking drugs must be avoided in WPW with AF or a broad complex tachycardia; thus, calcium channel antagonists, β-blockers, digoxin and, certainly, adenosine are contraindicated.

The reason being, blocking the AV node removes any brake on the abnormal circus current through the pre-excitation pathway. Abnormal conduction is free to accelerate leading to worsening tachycardia, cardiac compromise and ultimately deterioration into chaotic electrical activity. It should be borne in mind that a leading cause of death in WPW occurs through inappropriate treatment of arrhythmia.

d WPW patients with AF and fast ventricular response should be managed as follows:

- apply cardiac monitoring and have full resuscitation facilities close to hand
- give oxygen to maintain saturations 94–98%
- where time permits, discuss with the cardiologist-on-call regarding appropriate drug management
- the aim of drug treatment is to slow the atrial rate (amiodarone) or slow antegrade-conduction through the accessory pathway (flecainide, procainamide)
- a poor response to medical therapy should certainly be discussed with the cardiologist and may require synchronized DC cardioversion to avert the risk of further rhythm deterioration.

e Unstable patients with WPW and tachyarrhythmia are treated along established guidelines with emergency synchronized DC cardioversion.

Case 12

a The ECG (Figure 3.7) shows Torsades de Pointe also known as polymorphic ventricular tachycardia (pVT). Torsades de Point is characterized by rapid rate with oscillation of the QRS electrical activity around the isoelectric baseline on the ECG. Torsade presents with recurrent palpitations, syncope due to hypotension and can progress to VF and cardiac death. It is associated with a long QT on the resting ECG, which can be either congenital or acquired.

b The propensity of Torsades to degenerate into VF requires emergency treatment. First line is magnesium 2 g IV over ten minutes, even if magnesium levels are normal. A magnesium infusion can be used to follow. DC cardioversion is used only after rhythm degeneration into pulseless VT or VF, as it is less effective than magnesium and the Torsade will frequently recur.

c The underlying pathology of Torsades – the long QT, has a large number of causes. There are a variety of rare inherited long QT syndromes which may cause VT or pVT in children, while most cases in adults are due to an acquired long QT interval. Acquired causes of long QT can be divided into drug causes (most common) and non-drug causes as follows:

Table 3.7

Drug Precipitants	Non-Drug Precipitants
Class Ia: quinidine, procainamide	Electrolytes: $\downarrow K^+$, $\downarrow Mg^{2+}$, $\downarrow Ca^{2+}$
Class III: sotalol, amiodarone	Cardiac: MI, myocarditis
Antibiotics: erythromycin, clindamycin	Hypothyroidism
Antihistamines: terfenadine	Hyperparathyroidism
Antifungals: ketoconazole, itraconazole	Anorexia nervosa
Tricyclic antidepressants	Subarachnoid haemorrhage
Antipsychotics: haloperidol, phenothiazines	Toxins: heavy metals, insecticides

d The QT interval is the time from the start of the QRS complex to the end of the T-wave. It varies with rate and so, to allow comparison over different heart rates, a corrected QT interval (QTc) is calculated from the resting ECG using Bazzet's formula: QTc = QT/square root of the R–R interval. Normal QT interval less than 440–460 msec.

e If magnesium fails, isoprenaline is used next to accelerate AV conduction and decrease the QT interval. Overdrive pacing of the tacharrythmia is also used to control Torsades resistant to drug treatment.

Further Reading

1. Hampton JR. (1992) *The ECG made easy.* Churchill Livingstone.
2. Hampton JR. (2003) *150 ECG problems.* Churchill Livingstone.
3. Corne J. (2002) *Chest X-ray made easy.* 2nd edn. Churchill Livingstone.
4. The Advanced Life Support Group. (2010): *Advanced Life Support*, 6th edn. Resuscitation Council (UK).
5. NICE Guideline CG36. (2006) The Management of Atrial Fibrillation. www.nice.org.uk/Guidance/CG36
6. See www.timi.org
7. The Confidential Enquiries into Maternal Deaths in the United Kingdom. Why mothers die: 2000–2002 report. London: RCOG Press. www.cemach.org.uk/getdoc/28695c42-0a1e-4fd6-8601-abd01ad6c162/Saving-Mothers-Lives-Report-2000-2002.aspx
8. CEMACH. Saving Mothers Lives 2003–2005. Reviewing maternal deaths to make motherhood safer. London. (2004) www.cemach.org.uk/Publications-Press-Releases/Report-Publications/Maternal-Mortality.aspx
9. Durack D, Lukes A, Bright D. (1994) New criteria for diagnosis of infective endocarditis: utilization of specific echocardiographic findings. Duke Endocarditis Service. *Am J Med*; **96**(3): 200–9.
10. Advisory Group of the British Cardiac Society Clinical Practice Committee and the RCP Clinical Effectiveness and Evaluation Unit: Prophylaxis and treatment of infective endocarditis in adults: concise guidelines. Found at www.rcplondon.ac.uk/pubs/books/endocarditis/endocarditis.pdf
11. NICE Guideline CG34. (2004) Hypertension. www.nice.org.uk/Guidance/CG34

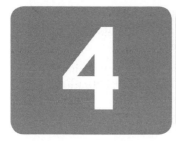

4

RESPIRATORY EMERGENCIES

Mathew Hall and Sam Thenabadu

Introduction

Core topics

- the breathless patient
- airway obstruction
- acute asthma
- pneumonia
- acute exacerbation of COPD
- management of type II respiratory failure
- pneumothorax
- pulmonary embolism
- pleural effusion
- atypical pneumonia
- tuberculosis
- haemoptysis
- acute adult respiratory distress syndrome
- presentation of lung cancer
- pulse oximetry
- acid base and ventilatory disorders.

Respiratory medicine utilizes a large number of investigations any of which may form part of an SAQ. Now is the time to familiarize yourself with the interpretation of the chest X-ray[1], arterial blood gases (ABG)[2], the ECG in pulmonary disease, relevant blood tests (inflammatory markers and D-dimer), lung function tests (particularly peak expiratory flow readings) as well as calculating the alveolar-arterial (A-a) gradient.

Clinical guidelines abound within respiratory medicine courtesy of the British Thoracic Society (BTS) and, to a lesser extent, the Scottish Intercollegiate Guidelines Network (SIGN) and National Institute for Clinical Excellence (NICE). It is not possible in this book to reproduce these guidelines; indeed they are constantly being updated, such that any attempt to reproduce them here would quickly be out-of-date – instead consult the relevant websites for latest versions.

Singled out for specific attention, however, are the BTS guidelines on emergency oxygen use in adult patients[3] which make clear oxygen is a drug and should be prescribed. In summary, they state oxygen should be given, where required, to maintain a target percentage oxygen saturation (% saturation) prescribed for each patient. Acutely ill patients (i.e., most patients requiring hospital treatment) should have prescribed target saturations of 94–98%, **EXCEPT:**

- patients at risk of hypercapnic respiratory failure where oxygen administered using fixed delivery devices (e.g., venturi masks) and target saturations of between 88–92% are more appropriate
- critically-ill patients should have oxygen initially delivered via reservoir mask at 15 L/min
- carbon monoxide poisoning where maximal oxygen delivery is therapy (and pulse oximetry unreliable!).

So, be sure to answer SAQ questions with the correct oxygen prescription – for example, in the critically-ill patient, answer '15 L/min oxygen via reservoir mask' and not just 'high flow oxygen'. There is much more to the guideline and it is well worth reading for clinical use as well as exams!

Case I

A normally fit and well 26-year-old car mechanic presents to the Emergency Department (ED) with sudden onset left-sided chest pain. He has no past respiratory illnesses. He does not report being breathless and has normal vital signs at triage. By the time you see him the following chest X-ray has been taken (Figure 4.1).

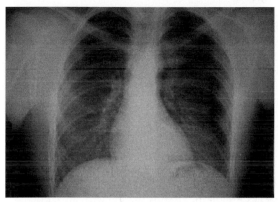

Figure 4.1

a Describe the abnormality in the X-ray (Figure 4.1) and give the radiological diagnosis. [2]
b What clinical signs might be found on examination of the chest to support this diagnosis? [2]
c Outline your management of this young man in the emergency department. [4]
d After your treatment, you decide it is appropriate to discharge this patient from the emergency department. What advice would you give to him? [4]

[12]

Case 2

A 59-year-old man arrives in the ED with heavily productive cough and breathlessness for three days. He can normally walk half-a-mile or so, but now cannot even dress without great effort. He has no formal diagnosis of chest disease but his GP recently sent him for tests where he had to blow into 'lots of tubes'. He shows you his letter from the lung function clinic with the spirometry values shown below:

FVC   2.7 L (normal 5.0 L)
FEV1 1.5 L (normal 4.0 L)

He is alert, although obviously dyspnoeic. Observations include respiratory rate 30/min and oxygen saturations 82% on air. You obtain an arterial blood gas (ABG) sample and the result is shown below:

pH   7.29
pCO_2 8.6 kPa
pO_2 6.8 kPa
HCO_2^- 30.9 mEq/L
BE   +4.1

a Based on the spirometry results and clinical history, what is the likely diagnosis in this man? Give the reasoning behind your answer.   [2]
b Interpret the abnormalities in the arterial blood gas.   [3]
c Outline four initial treatments you would give in the ED.   [4]
d A repeat arterial gas after 30 minutes shows worsening acidosis. What additional therapy is indicated?   [1]
          [10]

Case 3

A 24-year-old woman, who is 16 weeks pregnant, attends the ED with an acute history of worsening chest tightness and wheezing. She is known to have asthma for which she sees her GP infrequently. She tells you she had stopped her regular inhalers after discovering she was pregnant four weeks previously, as she was afraid they might harm the baby. Her observations at triage are heart rate 95 bpm, blood pressure 110/70 mmHg, respiratory rate 26/min, oxygen saturations 94% on room air and initial peak flow of 200 L/min.

a List three features which, if present, would classify a patient as having a severe exacerbation of asthma.   [3]
b How would you initially treat this patient (give dosages and routes of any drugs prescribed)?   [3]
c Give four indications for requesting a chest X-ray in a patient with acute asthma?   [2]
d What patient characteristics are used to calculate their **predicted** peak expiratory flow rate (PEFR)?   [2]
e What would you do next if this patient failed to respond to your initial treatment?   [2]
          [12]

Case 4

A 55-year-old female is referred up to hospital by her GP for shortness of breath. Her X-ray shows a large left-sided pleural effusion and she appears very breathless. She has a temperature of 37.8 °C, heart rate 110 bpm, blood pressure 110/80 mmHg, oxygen saturations 88% on room air and a respiratory rate of 26 breaths/min.

a Give three initial treatments to make this patient more comfortable. [3]
b What clinical signs could you look for when examining the chest to distinguish pleural fluid from consolidation? [2]
c Having satisfied yourself that the patient does have a pleural effusion give four types of fluid that may be present in the pleural cavity. [2]
d You decide to aspirate the chest and obtain a straw-coloured fluid which is sent to the lab for analysis. The lab returns the following results: [7]

Protein   29 g/L (serum protein 54 g/L)
Glucose   3.2 mmol/L
pH   7.3
LDH   167 u/L (serum LDH 205 u/L)
Amylase   97 u/dL

Based on these results, is this a transudate or exudate and briefly give your reason? [3]
e Give a differential diagnosis for this patient based upon your answer to
d. above. [4]
[7]

Case 5

A 68-year-old lifelong heavy smoker comes with his wife to the emergency department. He has coughed up blood on three occasions in the past week and on questioning, says that although he is normally quite breathless on exertion, his breathlessness has worsened considerably over the past few days. His chest X-ray is shown below (Figure 4.2).

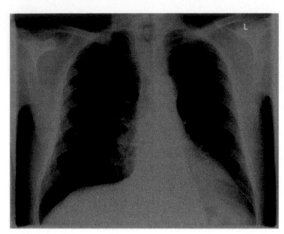

Figure 4.2

a Describe two abnormalities in the chest X-ray (Figure 4.2) and what is the radiological diagnosis? [3]
b Give three systemic and three local signs which you would look for on examination to support the diagnosis of a primary lung malignancy as the cause of this appearance. [6]
c Other than malignancy, give two further common causes of haemoptysis in adults. [1]
d If this patient's X-ray had been normal and he was not breathless, outline your management of a stable patient presenting with minor haemoptysis to the emergency department. [4]

[14]

Case 6

A 29-year-old man presents himself to the ED with a malaise, productive cough and fever with night sweats for over three weeks. He is thin and very unkempt, and lives in a hostel for the homeless. His observations at triage indicate he is cardiovascularly stable although he has reduced oxygen saturations of 94% on air. The triage nurse suspects tuberculosis may be a possibility and, after discussion with you, the patient is given a mask to wear and isolated in a side-room.

a Give three features of the chest X-ray which would support a diagnosis of pulmonary tuberculosis (TB) in this patient. [3]
b What further tests are recommended once TB is suspected in a patient? [1]
c Describe four extra-pulmonary manifestations of *mycobacterium* infection. [4]
d Give four risk factors for developing tuberculosis in the UK that you would ask about. [2]
e Give four drugs which comprise 'quadruple therapy' for TB and give a side-effect for each drug which may cause a patient to seek further medical advice. [4]

[14]

Case 7

A 47-year-old woman attends the ED with acute onset of breathlessness and left-sided chest pain. Her vital signs are heart rate 112 bpm, blood pressure 115/75 mmHg, respiratory rate 22/min and oxygen saturations 94% on air. She is a non-smoker and takes only thyroxine for an underactive thyroid. She has been well recently with no prior respiratory symptoms but does report being treated with warfarin for a previous episode of deep vein thrombosis. Below is her arterial blood gas taken on room air:

pH	7.38
pCO_2	2.6 kPa
pO_2	10.4 kPa
HCO_3^-	23.4 mEq/L
BE	−1.7

a Calculate the Alveolar-arterial (A-a) gradient using the blood gas result. Show your calculations and indicate the significance of your result for this patient, relative to the normal value for the A-a gradient.   [4]
b Give three possible abnormalities of the chest X-ray associated with pulmonary embolism (PE).   [3]
c Apart from previous thromboembolic disease, give four **major** risk factors for PE.   [2]
d What other question must be asked in deciding the clinical probability of PE? [1]
e How would you manage this patient?   [2]

                                    [12]

Case 8

A 39-year-old female comes to the ED complaining of four days of cough productive of green sputum and left-sided pleuritic chest pains. The oral contraceptive pill is her only prescribed medication. She is penicillin allergic. She is fully alert and the triage nurse records the following observations: heart rate 104 bpm, blood pressure 105/55 mmHg, respiratory rate 24/min and temperature 37.7 °C. She is sent from triage for a chest X-ray (Figure 4.3).

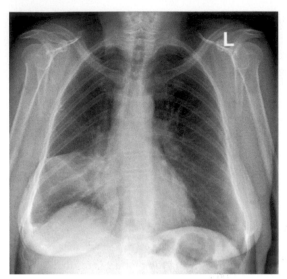

Figure 4.3

a Describe the abnormality on the X-ray (Figure 4.3). [2]
b Give the three most likely pathogens in community acquired pneumonia. [3]
c The patient is alert and oriented. Her blood tests reveal the following:

WCC	15.2×10^9/L
Neutrophils	14.6×10^9/L
N+	129 mmol/L
K+	4.7 mmol/L
Urea	6.4 mmol/L
Creatinine	78 μmol/L
CRP	267 mg/L

What is this patient's CURB65 score and what is her 30-day risk of mortality based on the score you give? [4]
d You decide she is well enough for discharge on oral erythromycin. What common side effects of erythromycin would you warn patients about and what specific advice would this patient need regarding the taking of erythromycin? [3]
e What would you recommend in your discharge summary to the patient's GP? [2]

[14]

4 RESPIRATORY EMERGENCIES – ANSWERS

Case 1

a The left lung margin is visible and there are absent chest markings, indicating a rim of air, between the left lung and chest wall (Figure 4.1). The British Thoracic Society (BTS) pleural diseases guideline 2010[4] divides the size of a pneumothorax into large or small, depending on the presence of a visible rim of air greater or less than 2 cm between the lung margin and chest wall. A 2 cm rim of air equates to roughly 50% loss in lung volume. This X-ray, therefore, demonstrates a large pneumothorax.

b Decreased breath sounds on the affected side will be present with a large pneumothorax, while hyperresonance to percussion, absent vocal resonance and reduced chest expansion may also be noted.

c This patient has no preceding lung disease and, therefore, has a primary spontaneous pneumothorax (PSP). Most large PSP require needle (14–16G) aspiration as first-line treatment, followed by repeat chest X-ray in one hour to assess re-expansion. If aspiration fails, then a small bore (<14 Fr) chest drain should be inserted and the patient admitted to the hospital. If the lung re-expands satisfactorily, then the patient may be safely discharged with advice and an appointment for respiratory out-patient clinic in two to four weeks.[4]

d A patient being discharged following treatment for a pneumothorax should be advised to:

- seek medical help if symptoms (breathlessness or pleuritic pain) recur
- avoid air travel until proven full resolution of the pneumothorax
- avoid underwater diving for life
- stop smoking (smoking is a risk factor for recurrent pneumothorax).

Case 2

a Both the forced vital capacity (FEV) and the forced expiratory volume in 1 minute (FEV1) are reduced but the relative reduction in FEV1 is much greater, giving a FEV1/FVC ratio around 0.55. The normal FEV1/FVC ratio is above 0.7 (typically 0.7–0.8). Values below this indicate airflow limitation and are consistent with chronic obstructive pulmonary disease (COPD). In contrast, restrictive lung disease causes a proportionate reduction in FEV1 and FVC such that the ratio remains within normal limits. Furthermore, the percentage reduction in FEV1 compared to that expected for the patient's sex, age and height allows estimation of the severity of COPD

Table 4.1

Severity of COPD	FEV$_1$ (% of predicted)
Mild	80–90
Moderate	50–79
Severe	30–49
Very severe	<30

Thus, the man in this question has an underlying diagnosis of severe COPD. In addition, from the clinical history, we see that his breathing has suffered an acute deterioration. His full diagnosis is, therefore, an acute exacerbation of severe COPD.

b The arterial blood gas shows (*see* reference 2 for guidance on interpretation):

- respiratory acidosis (pH <7.35 with pCO$_2$ >5.5 kPa and BE >0.0)
- type II respiratory failure (pO$_2$ <8.0 kPa and pCO$_2$ >5.5 kPa)
- renal compensation (HCO$_3$ >30.0 mEq/L).

c Initially, treat an exacerbation of COPD with:[5]

- oxygen via fixed delivery device to maintain oxygen saturations 88–92%
- bronchodilators – nebulized salbutamol 5 mg and nebulized ipratropium bromide 500 micrograms
- steroids – prednisolone 30–40 mg PO
- antibiotics – should be given where an exacerbation of COPD is associated with increased sputum production, consolidation on chest X-ray or signs of pneumonia. Empirical treatment is with an aminopenicillin (e.g., amoxycillin) or a macrolide (e.g., clarithromycin) or both.[6]

d Patients with acute exacerbation of COPD and respiratory acidosis who do not respond quickly (within 30–60 mins) to full medical therapy should receive non-invasive ventilation (NIV). The answer to question 6 in chapter 17 addresses the use of NIV in severe COPD.

Case 3

a Asthma is best managed by classifying an acute attack as one of moderate, severe or life-threatening along the lines of the BTS/SIGN guidelines for the management of asthma:[7]

Table 4.2

Moderate	Severe	Life-threatening
PEFR 50–75% best or predicted Increasing symptoms No features of severe asthma	PEFR 33–50% best or predicted Respiratory rate >20/min Heart rate >110 bpm Inability to complete a sentence	PEFR <33% best or predicted SpO_2 <92% PO_2 <8 Kpa Normal $PaCO_2$ Silent chest Cyanosis Poor respiratory effort Bradycardia, arrhythmia, shock Exhaustion, confusion, coma

b Although pregnant, this patient should be treated exactly the same as any other asthmatic with a severe exacerbation of asthma:

- oxygen to maintain saturations 94–98%
- salbutamol nebulizers (5 mg) repeated three times in one hour
- ipratropium nebulizer (500 micrograms)
- oral prednisolone 40 mg.

c Most acute exacerbations of asthma do not require chest radiography to be managed effectively and to limit unnecessary X-rays in asthma, the BTS recommends the following as indications for chest X-ray:[6]

- suspected pneumothorax
- suspected pneumonia with consolidation
- life-threatening asthma
- failure to respond to appropriate treatment
- requirement for ventilation.

d The predicted PEFR is calculated using the patient's height and age. Different charts are also used for males and females.

e The next step in treating acute asthma not responding to bronchodilators and steroids, is IV magnesium sulphate 1.2–2 g over 20 minutes. Magnesium is also safe in pregnancy (remember it is the treatment for eclampsia!)

Case 4

a Initial symptomatic treatment for a hypoxic, pyrexial patient in pain is:

- oxygen to maintain target saturations 94–98%
- antipyretic (paracetamol 1 g PO)
- analgesia (e.g., codeine phosphate 60 mg PO)

b The table below compares chest signs which might help distinguish between consolidation and effusion (we include collapse for completeness):

Table 4.3

Pathology	Percussion	Breath sounds	Vocal resonance	Added sounds
Consolidation	Dull	Reduced (perhaps bronchial breathing)	Increased	Crepitations
Collapse	Dull	Reduced	Absent	One
Pleural effusion	Stony dull	Absent over effusion	Absent over effusion	Perhaps bronchial breathing or pleural rub above effusion

c Fluid in the pleural cavity may be a transudate, an exudate or may be blood (haemothorax) or pus (empyema).

d The results of the pleural tap indicate an exudate. Traditionally, transudates have a protein concentration less than 30 g/L and exudates greater than 30 g/L but this is not always accurate, particularly where the serum protein concentrations are abnormal, or at pleural fluid protein concentrations close to 30 g/L. Thus, the use of Lights' criteria is recommended,[8] which requires measurement of the pleural fluid, serum protein and lactate dehydrogenase (Box 4.1).

Box 4.1 Light's criteria

An exudate is present when one or more of the following are true:

- pleural fluid protein divided by serum protein is >0.5
- Pleural fluid lactate dehydrongenase (LDH) divided by serum LDH is >0.6
- Pleural fluid LDH >2/3 of upper limit of serum LDH

If none of the above criteria are met, then a transudate is present.
In this question, the pleural fluid protein is 29 g/L but both the pleural fluid protein/serum protein ratio and pleural fluid LDH/serum LDH ratio fulfil Lights' criteria for an exudate.

---

e A pleural exudate has the following common causes:

- malignancy (particularly chest and breast)
- pneumonia
- tuberculosis
- autoimmune diseases (e.g., rheumatoid arthritis, systemic lupus erythematosis)
- pulmonary infarction (secondary to pulmonary embolism)
- trauma (lung contusion).

Case 5

a There is a triangular opacity visible behind the heart shadow (silhouette sign) and the medial border of the left diaphragm is obscured (Figure 4.2). These abnormalities, together with loss of lung volume on the left, indicate the radiological diagnosis of left lower lobe collapse. If a lateral X-ray was also provided, you would see posterior displacement of the oblique fissure. *See* references 1 and 7 for further reading on the interpretation of the chest X-ray.

b Lobar collapse arises from obstruction of a main bronchus and, in adults, the two most common causes are bronchogenic carcinoma and sputum plugging in purulent lung disease. In children, asthma and inhaled foreign bodies are also common precipitants of collapse. Thus, given the patient's age, smoking history and X-ray appearance of collapse, lung malignancy would be strongly suspected. Signs to look for on examination include:

Table 4.4

Systemic features	Local features
Weight loss/cachexia	Horner's syndrome
Finger clubbing	Superior vena cava obstruction
Anaemia	Lymphadenopathy (supraclavicular/axillary)
Wrist pain (hypertrophic pulmonary osteoarthropathy)	Pleural effusion
	Lobar consolidation/collapse
	Hoarseness (recurrent laryngeal nerve palsy)

c The three most common causes of genuine haemoptysis in the UK are lung malignancy, pneumonia and tuberculosis (TB).

d Massive or life-threatening haemoptysis is rare and most patients with a minor haemoptysis, (less than 30 mL blood) but no obvious cause do not need admission. However, it is necessary to perform a chest X-ray (normal in 30% of patients with minor haemoptysis), send blood tests to check for clotting abnormalities and send sputum for acid fast bacilli if TB is a possibility. Most patients – particularly where the haemoptysis lasts more than two weeks, is recurrent, or the patient is a smoker, or over 40 years old – should have urgent chest clinic follow-up for bronchoscopy. Young patients with a single haemoptysis, and evidence of chest infection, might initially be managed with antibiotics and reviewed in two weeks to ensure the haemoptysis has cleared along with the infection.

Case 6

a The classical features of tuberculosis on chest X-ray are apical consolidation, cavitation, hilar lymphadenopathy and calcification. In TB with AIDS or multidrug resistant TB, lobar consolidation is seen. The reticular nodular shadowing of military TB indicates haematogenous spread in tertiary disease.

b NICE guidelines for tuberculosis[9] recommend that once TB is suspected, three sputum samples (including one early morning sputum) are sent for culture and microscopy for acid fast bacilli (AFB). It also recommends taking further aspirate or biopsy samples from non-pulmonary sites where infection may be present (*see* below).

c *Mycobacterium tuberculosis* also causes disease at the following sites, with or without evidence, of pulmonary infection.

Table 4.5

Site	Disease	Localizing signs and symptoms
GI tract	Peritoneal TB	Abdominal pain, ascites, diarrhoea
CNS	TB meningitis	Headache, photophobia, meningism
Lymph nodes	TB lymphadenitis (scrofula is TB of the cervical nodes)	Painless enlarging lymph nodes
Bone (especially spine)	Bone TB (Pott's vertebra)	Back pain, kyphosis (gibbus)
Heart	Acute TB pericarditis Pericardial effusion	Chest pain, haemodynamic compromise, if constrictive pericarditis
Urinary tract	Sterile pyuria Renal TB	Dysuria, haematuria, loin pain

d Risk factors for contracting TB include:

- overcrowding, poor housing or homelessness
- HIV
- other causes of immunosuppression (malnutrition, diabetes mellitus, steroids etc.)
- travel to areas with high prevalence of TB
- close contacts with known TB cases.

e Side-effects are common with anti-tuberculous drugs, due to the nature of the drugs, and the prolonged duration of therapy – two months quadruple therapy, then a further four months with rifampicin and isoniazid, being the recommended regimen for non-HIV, non-multidrug resistant TB. Some of the most commonly seen side-effects are:

Rifampicin	Hepatitis, orange discolouration of urine and other body fluids
Ethambutol	Optic neuritis
Isoniazid	Hepatitis, peripheral neuropathy, agranulocytosis
Pyrazinamide	Hepatitis, arthralgia

Case 7

a The alveolar-arterial oxygen (A-a) gradient is the difference between the partial pressures of oxygen in the alveoli (PAO_2) and in the artery (PaO_2). A quick way to calculate the A-a gradient in a patient breathing room air is shown in Box 4.2.

> **Box 4.2** Quick method for calculating the A-a gradient
>
> A-a gradient = inspired O_2 (kPa) – ($PaCO_2$ × 1.2) – PaO_2
> Where: inspired O_2 in kPa roughly equals FiO_2 (at sea level)
> $PaCO_2$ = partial pressure arterial CO_2 in kPa (from arterial blood gas)
> PaO_2 = partial pressure arterial O_2 in kPa (from arterial blood gas)
> Thus, in this example A-a gradient = 21 – (2.6 × 1.2) – 10.4
> = 7.48 kPa

Normal A-a gradient is 2–4, rising slightly with advanced age. Thus, this woman's A-a gradient is almost twice that of normal, indicating she has a significant abnormality of gas exchange, which could be a result of alveolar membrane disease, interstitial disease or, as seen with PE, a V/Q mismatch.

This quick method of calculating A-a gradients does not take into account variables, such as the atmospheric pressure, or the respiratory quotient and is largely only accurate for FiO_2 below 28%. A more detailed method of calculating A-a gradients with full explanation is given in reference 2, full details of which appear at the end of this chapter.

b The initial chest X-ray is most often normal in patients presenting with early PE. Over 24–72 hours, however, the following abnormalities caused by an obstructed pulmonary vasculature may be seen:

- wedge-shaped infiltrates
- atelectasis
- small pleural effusions
- elevated hemidiaphragm
- oligaemic lung fields (rare and seen in massive PE only).

c The BTS guidelines for suspected acute pulmonary embolism[10] divide risk factors for thromboembolic disease, into major and minor, according to their associated increase in relative risk. The major risk factors have a relative risk increase of 5–20 times and are:

- surgery (major abdominal or pelvic surgery, hip or knee replacement or surgery requiring post-operative intensive care)
- obstetric (third trimester pregnancy, post caesarian section and during puerperium)
- malignancy (abdominal or pelvic malignancy or advanced and metastatic malignancy)
- serious lower limb fractures
- immobility (hospitalization or institutional care)
- previous proven venous thromboembolism.

d Clinical probability of acute PE is assessed by asking two questions: first, is a major risk factor present (see above)? And, second, is there no alternative clinical diagnosis more likely to account for the patient's symptoms?

Table 4.6

	No major risk factors for PE	One or more major risk factors present for PE
Alternative diagnosis more likely than PE	Low probability of PE	Moderate probability of PE
No alternative diagnosis evident	Moderate probability of PE	High probability of PE

e This patient has a major risk factor for PE (previous DVT) and, from the information we are given, no alternative diagnosis. This combination indicates her clinical probability of PE is high and she requires treatment and definitive investigation:

- oxygen to maintain saturations between 94–98%

- treatment dose subcutaneous low molecular weight heparin (e.g., enoxaparin 1.5 mg/kg sc)
- referral to the in-patient medical team for further imaging, either VQ scan or CT-pulmonary angiogram (CT-PA), depending on local policy and chest X-ray appearance (a VQ scan is only useful where the chest X-ray is normal).

A D-dimer cannot be used to reliably exclude PE in high probability patients and should not be requested in this group.

Case 8

a The chest X-ray (Figure 4.3) shows right middle lobe consolidation. Remember obscuration, or a lack of distinction of the right heart border, indicates pathology in the right middle lobe. *See* references 1 and 7 at the end of the chapter for further reading on interpretation of the chest X-ray.

b In UK adults, the three most common pathogens in community acquired pneumonia (CAP) are *Streptococcus pneumoniae* (most common with 30–50% cases and rising in severe pneumonia), *Haemophilus influenzae* and *Mycoplasma pneumoniae*. *Staphylococcus aureus* and Klebsiella species are also common and may give a cavitating lesion on X-ray. Then the atypical organisms, *Legionella pneumophila*, Chlamydia species and *Coxiella burnetii* (Q fever) account for most other cases.

c The British Thoracic Society (BTS) guidelines for community acquired pneumonia (CAP)[11] suggest a simple five point scoring system, the CURB65 score, to risk stratify CAP in relation to mortality. The elements of the CURB65 score are:

Confusion (AMTS >8)	1 point
Urea >7 mmol/L	1 point
Respiratory rate >30/min	1 point
Blood pressure <90 mmHg systolic or <60 mmHg diastolic	1 point
Age >65 years	1 point

This patient's CURB65 score is one (her only positive score is for a diastolic blood pressure less than 60 mmHg). To enable CURB65 to be useful, we must consider the correlation with mortality:[12]

Table 4.7

CURB65 score	0	1	2	3	4	5
30 day Mortality %	0.7	3.2	13.0	17.0	41.5	57.0

In general, patients with CURB65 score of 0–1 are suitable for discharge with oral antibiotics, a score of two may be admitted or discharged, dependent on other clinical factors, but a score of three or above should be admitted to hospital. Patients presenting with CURB65 scores of four and five and who, therefore, have a predicted 30-day mortality of greater than 40%, should be considered for intensive therapy.

d Erythromycin is a macrolide antibiotic, frequently used to treat gram +ve infection in penicillin-allergic patients, and also where atypical pneumonia is suspected. However, it is not without side-effects, most commonly nausea, vomiting and diarrhoea but also cholestasis and arrhythmia (prolonged QT interval). In this patient, we must also warn that erythromycin may lower the efficacy of the oral contraceptive pill and barrier methods of contraception should be used for the duration of the antibiotic and for the next seven days.

e The GP letter should recommend review in seven days at termination of treatment, provision of smoking cessation advice and repeat X-ray in six weeks to ensure radiological resolution of the pneumonia. While it is not necessary to perform follow-up X-ray in every patient with pneumonia, it is advisable in those patients with persistent symptoms or signs, and those at risk of lung malignancy, such as smokers.

Further Reading

1. Corne J. (2002) *Chest X-ray made easy.* 2nd edn. Churchill Livingstone.
2. Williams AJ. (1998) Assessing and interpreting arterial blood gases and acid-base balance. *BMJ;* **317:** 1213–16.
3. British Thoracic Society (BTS) Emergency Oxygen Guideline Development Group, BTS guideline for emergency oxygen use in adult patients. (2008) *Thorax;* **63:** Suppl VI. Also online at www.brit-thoracic.org.uk
4. MacDuff A, Arnold T, Harvey J. Management of Spontaneous Pneumothorax British Thoracic Society Pleural Disease Guideline 2010. Found online at www.brit-thoracic.org.uk/clinical-information/pleural-disease/pleural-disease-guidelines-2010.aspx
5. The management of exacerbations of COPD. (2004) *Thorax;* **59:** i131–i156. Found online at thorax.bmj.com/cgi/reprint/59/suppl_1/i131
6. British Thoracic Society/Scottish Intercollegiate Guideline Network British guideline of the Management of Asthma. (2008) Found online at www.brit-thoracic.org.uk
7. Longmore M, Wilkinson I, Davidson E, *et al.* (2010). Oxford Handbook of Clinical Medicine, 8th edn. OUP; pp 736–39.
8. Hooper CY, Lee G, Maskell N. (2010) *Investigation of a unilateral pleural effusion in adults.* British Thoracic Society Pleural Disease Guideline. Found online at www.brit-thoracic.org.uk/clinical-information/pleural-disease/pleural-disease-guidelines-2010.aspx
9. NICE Guideline CG117. Tuberculosis: Clinical diagnosis and management of tuberculosis, and measures for its prevention and control. March 2011. Found at www.nice.org.uk/Guidance/CG117
10. The British Thoracic Society Standards of Care Committee, Pulmonary Embolism Guideline Development Group. BTS Guideline for the Management of Suspected Acute Pulmonary Embolism, 2003. *Thorax* (2009): **64:** Supplement III, pp iii1–iii64. Also online at www.brit-thoracic.org.uk
11. BTS guidelines for the management of community acquired pneumonia in adults: update 2009. *Thorax* (2004) **59:** i131-i156. Found at www.brit-thoracic.org.uk

12. Lim AS, *et al.* (2003) Defining community acquired pneumonia severity on presentation to hospital: an international derivation and validation study. Thorax; **58**: 377–82.

NEUROLOGICAL EMERGENCIES

Mathew Hall

Introduction

Core topics
- stroke
- transient ischaemic attack (TIA)
- central nervous system infection
- sub-arachnoid haemorrhage
- seizures (including status epilepticus)
- headache
- spinal cord compression
- Bell's palsy
- multiple sclerosis
- Parkinson's disease
- vertigo and ataxia
- peripheral neuropathy
- raised intracranial pressure, hydrocephalus and blocked shunts.

Core knowledge and data interpretation skills required for neurology SAQs might include:

- ROSIER stroke assessment tool
- ABCD^2 score for risk stratifying TIA patients
- the Glasgow coma score (GCS)
- interpretation of cerebrospinal fluid (CSF) results
- arterial and venous anatomy of the brain
- interpretation of CT brain scans and major abnormalities (ischaemic strokes and intracranial haemorrhage)
- knowledge of motor nerve roots, sensory dermatomes and reflexes.

Case 1

A 58-year-old woman presents to the emergency department (ED) with an episode of weakness of the left face and arm. Her husband says that, in addition, her speech was both slurred and jumbled. The symptoms lasted for around 40 minutes before resolving completely. She has a past medical history of mild COPD only. Her observations indicate that she is apyrexial, heart rate 76 bpm, blood pressure 135/85 mmHg, oxygen saturations of 96% on air and blood glucose 8.8 mmol/L.

a Define transient ischaemic attack (TIA).   [1]
b What is this patient's ABCD2 score and indicate the risk of stroke at seven days
   associated with the score you calculate?   [4]
c Aside from criteria relating to the ABCD2 score, give two other criteria for
   admission in patients with TIA.   [2]
d Your hospital policy indicates that discharge is appropriate for this patient.
   Give three essential management steps, including advice you would give,
   before discharge home.   [3]
                                                                                 [10]

Case 2

A 74-year-old man is brought to the ED by ambulance with acute onset weakness of the right side which began 90 minutes previously. He is alert but with marked weakness affecting the right face and arm, as well as difficulty speaking. He has only hypertension in his past medical history and takes amlodipine. His observations on arrival in the resuscitation room are temperature 37.2 °C, pulse 98 bpm regular, blood pressure 210/108 mmHg, oxygen saturations 96% on air. His CT brain scan is shown in Figure 5.1.

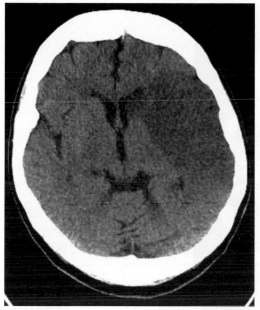

Figure 5.1

a The ambulance crew have phoned ahead to relay the patient's FAST score.
   What is the correct FAST score for this patient?   [2]
b What condition may mimic acute stroke and which needs urgently
   excluding at the bedside?   [1]
c List the six questions which make up the ROSIER score (part of the
   ROSIER Stroke Assessment Scale).   [3]
d Describe the abnormality in the CT brain image of this patient
   (Figure 5.1).   [2]
e Briefly summarize the main advantages and disadvantages of stroke
   thrombolysis.   [4]
                                                                          [12]

Case 3

A 68-year-old woman is brought to the ED with an occipital headache and
unsteadiness on her feet for the previous two hours. Her past medical history
includes asthma and type 1 diabetes. She is alert and the triage nurse records a pulse
of 66 bpm which is irregular, blood pressure 189/108 mmHg, oxygen saturations
91% on air and a blood glucose of 16.7. An image from her CT brain scan is shown
in Figure 5.2 below.

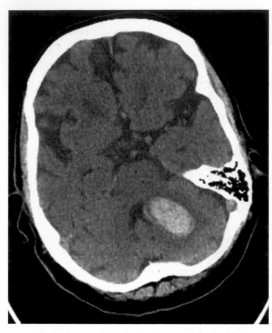

Figure 5.2

a Describe the abnormality in the CT scan (Figure 5.2). [2]
b Give four clinical signs you may also expect to see when examining this
   patient. [4]
c Give three further steps in your management of this patient. [3]
d You are called to review this patient. Her conscious level has dropped and
   she is now not eye opening at all, even to pain, moaning incomprehensibly
   but can just localize painful stimuli. What is her GCS? [1]
e Give two complications of this condition that could have caused her
   deterioration. [2]

[12]

Case 4

A 35-year-old woman has been advised to attend the ED by NHS direct. She has
been unwell for one day with severe headache and vomiting and the person she
spoke to on the phone was concerned it could be meningitis. She has a temperature
of 37.6 °C and although alert, feels lethargic with the headache.

a Give three organisms most commonly associated with bacterial meningitis
   in an adult. [3]
b List four clinical signs which would alert you to the presence of raised
   intracranial pressure such that a lumbar puncture is contra-indicated. [2]

c You organize a CT brain scan which is reported as normal by the radiologist. The patient is moved to the clinical decision unit where a lumbar puncture is performed and cerebrospinal fluid (CSF) sent for laboratory analysis. The following results are obtained from the patient's CSF.

White cell count	870/mm^3
Predominant cell type	lymphocytes
Organisms	None seen
Protein	0.8 g/dl
Glucose	3/4 plasma concentration

d Identify the abnormalities in the CSF obtained. What is the diagnosis based on this result? [4]
e What further test could be performed on CSF from this patient to investigate another possible cause of acute severe headache? [1]

[10]

Case 5

An 18-year-old female is brought in by ambulance having had three tonic-clonic seizures in close succession while in a department store, and then in the back of the ambulance. She has not recovered consciousness between seizures and, as she is wheeled into the resuscitation room, she begins to fit again. She has no past history of epilepsy.

a What is your immediate management before any tests or drugs? [3]
b Give two conditions which need to be urgently excluded at the bedside. [2]
c Outline in list or diagrammatic form, the drugs in the order you would use them to treat status epilepticus (with drugs, names, routes and doses). [4]
d Give three causes (other than those you give in answer to part b.) of status epilepticus in a previously well young person with no past history of epilepsy. [3]
e Once the seizure has been controlled, what further investigations should be performed in the ED to investigate the cause? [2]

[14]

Case 6

A 67-year-old man presents with lower thoracic back pain and progressive difficulty with walking. He is otherwise well with no significant past medical history.

a Give five 'red flag' symptoms which, if present, would indicate a sinister cause for back pain. [5]
b You suspect a spinal cord compression and perform a neurological examination. How would you distinguish an upper motor neuron (UMN) from a lower motor neuron (LMN) weakness of the lower limbs? [2]
c What, in particular, would you look for on sensory examination in this patient? [1]

d Your examination reveals power of only grade 2/5 on the medical research council (MRC) scale of grading muscle power. Define grade 2/5 on the MRC scale. [2]

e What urgent investigations should be requested for this patient given that your examination supports the diagnosis of spinal cord compression? [2]

[12]

Case 7

A staff nurse asks you to prescribe an anti-emetic for a patient with vertigo. You go and assess the patient and find a 48-year-old woman alert but lying still at 30 degrees on the bed clutching a vomit bowl. All her observations are normal.

a Describe the two features of true vertigo. [2]

b Give four clinical features of the history and examination which can be used to distinguish between a central and a peripheral cause of vertigo. [4]

c Name two conditions suggested where chronic hearing loss is associated with vertigo. [2]

d How may benign paroxysmal positional vertigo be clinically differentiated from vestibular neuronitis (labyrinthitis)? [1]

e How would you treat vestibular neuronitis (labyrinthitis)? In your answer give two classes of drugs you might prescribe with an example of each and briefly describe the advice you would give to the patient. [3]

[12]

Case 8

A 76-year-old man is referred to the ED by his GP with progressively decreasing mobility. The patient has been seen by one of the ED FY2 doctors who believes the patient may have Parkinson's disease and asks for your help in managing the case.

a What are the three cardinal features of parkinsonism? [3]

b Describe the gait abnormality that is commonly seen in this condition. [1]

c Other than idiopathic Parkinson's disease itself, give two other causes of parkinsonism to consider. [2]

d Give two drugs, briefly explaining their mode of action that may be used to improve mobility in Parkinson's disease patients. [4]

e Assuming he does not need acute admission to hospital, what further steps would you take in management of this patient. [3]

[13]

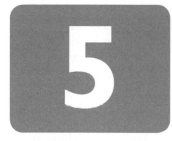

NEUROLOGICAL EMERGENCIES – ANSWERS

Case I

a Transient ischaemic attack (TIA) is defined as a sudden onset focal neurological deficit that resolves within 24 hours – the official answer. However, as TIA and stroke are really a continuum, separated by an arbitrary length of time, and that in at least half of TIA's lasting greater than 30–60 minutes some brain injury (though subclinical) has occurred, there is reason to redefine TIA as neurological deficit which resolves within 30–60 minutes.

b In patients with a clinical diagnosis of TIA, the ABCD2 score is a validated scoring system which identifies those with early high risk of stroke.[1] The ABCD2 score is calculated using the following clinical features of the patient and the event (Box 5.1):

Box 5.1 The ABCD2 score

Age > 60 years	1 point
Blood pressure at presentation >140/90 mmHg	1 point
Clinical features:	
Unilateral weakness	2 points
Speech disturbance without weakness	1 point
Duration of attack:	
10–60 minutes	1 point
>60 minutes	2 points
Diabetes	1 point

Thus, this patient therefore has an ABCD2 score of three (unilateral weakness = two points and duration 40 minutes = one point). The ABCD2 score then allows a prediction of the risk of stroke at two and seven days as follows:[1]

Table 5.1

ABCD2 score	Risk of stroke at two days (%)	Risk of stroke at seven days (%)
0–3	1.0	1.2
4–5	4.1	5.9
6–7	8.1	11.7

Thus, this patient with an ABCD2 score of 3 has a roughly 1% risk of stroke in the seven days following their presentation with TIA. Local protocols vary but the current NICE guidelines on stroke and TIA[2] divide patients into low risk (ABCD2 score one to three) and high risk (ABCD2 score >= four) and recommend that those at high risk of early stroke are either admitted immediately or are seen in a TIA clinic within 24 hours for urgent specialist assessment and investigation.

c Other factors which place patients with TIA at high risk of stroke include, those with more than one TIA in seven days (crescendo TIA), and those with a significant risk factor requiring intervention such as atrial fibrillation requiring immediate anticoagulation. These are therefore also indications for admission. Patients with TIA **and** significant headache, or who are on warfarin, might also be admitted for exclusion of intracerebral haemorrhage.

d The NICE guideline on stroke and TIA[2] recommend the following management of patients discharged with a clinical diagnosis of TIA:

- prescription of an anti-platelet regime immediately. First line is aspirin 300 mg: start immediately and continue for one week before reducing to 75 mg daily. Patients already on aspirin when they present with TIA can have dipyridamole added (e.g., persantin retard 200 mg bd). Those allergic or intolerant to aspirin should be started on clopidogrel instead
- referral to a specialist TIA clinic as soon as possible, and certainly within seven days
- patients should be advised to return to hospital **immediately**, if the symptoms recur
- finally, patients should be advised not to drive until assessed by a specialist (i.e. in TIA clinic).

Case 2

a The FAST (Face, Arm, Speech Test) is a stroke identification tool devised for pre-hospital healthcare personnel and involves answering three questions relating to the patients clinical condition:

Is there NEW onset facial weakness or asymmetry?
Is there a unilateral weakness of one or the other arm?
Is there a speech disturbance?

Affirmative answer to any of these questions gives a positive diagnosis of stroke and triggers urgent transfer to a hospital providing acute stroke services. In this question the patient's FAST score is three.

b Hypoglycaemia (BM <3.5) can complicate the diagnosis of acute stroke and requires urgent exclusion at the bedside with capillary blood glucose measurement.

c The most recent SIGN guideline on the Management of Patients with Stroke and TIA[3] recommend the use of the ROSIER Stroke Assessment Tool by ED personnel in order to increase the accuracy and speed with which stroke is diagnosed. Once hypoglycaemia has been excluded, six straightforward questions are asked about the history and neurological deficit (Box 5.2).

> **Box 5.2** ROSIER score as part of the ROSIER Stroke Assessment Tool
>
> | | | |
> |---|---|---|
> | Has there been loss of consciousness or syncope? | Y (-1) ☐ | N (0) |
> | Has there been seizure activity | Y (-1) ☐ | N (0) |
> | Is there a **NEW ACUTE** onset (or on awakening from sleep)? | | |
> | Asymmetric facial weakness | Y (+1) ☐ | N (0) |
> | Asymmetric arm weakness | Y (+1) ☐ | N (0) |
> | Asymmetric leg weakness | Y (+1) ☐ | N (0) |
> | Speech disturbance | Y (+1) ☐ | N (0) |
> | Visual field defect | Y (+1) ☐ | N (0) |
> | | Total Score__ | (-2 to +5) |

Where the total score for the patient is above zero (i.e., between 1 and 6) then stroke is likely[4] and if presentation is within 3 hours of symptom onset (some protocols four and a half to six hours) they should be immediately discussed with the stroke team for potential thrombolysis. Patients presenting outside the thrombolysis window should be transferred to an Acute Stroke Unit. ROSIER scores of 0, −1 or −2, indicate that acute stroke is unlikely, although not definitively excluded, and further medical assessment is required.

d   There is an area of low attenuation (density) in the left middle cranial fossa, likely to represent a cerebral infarct in the territory of the left middle cerebral artery (Figure 5.1).

e   A number of completed trials broadly agree that in stroke patients, with initially disabling neurological deficits, those treated with thrombolysis have a substantially better chance of living independently with little or no disability at three months after the event.[5] The disadvantage of stroke thrombolysis is the increase in post-thrombolysis intracranial bleeding which leads to increased morbidity in a small proportion of patients.

Case 3

a   There is an area of high attenuation in the left posterior fossa likely to represent an acute haemorrhage into the left cerebellum (Figure 5.2).

b   In addition to the symptoms of dizziness, vertigo and nausea, clinical signs of cerebellar injury in a conscious patient able to obey commands include:

- vomiting
- limb ataxia (past-pointing at finger-nose testing and clumsy dysdiadokinesia)
- truncal ataxia with wide based 'cerebellar' gait
- nystagmus (horizontal and vertical not improved with fixation)
- dysarthria (monotonous speech or 'scanning' dysarthria)
- neck stiffness may also be present.

c   There are several common steps in the emergency management of most patients with intracerebral haemorrhage.

- they should be placed nil by mouth until a formal swallow assessment has been performed

- routine blood tests should include a clotting screen to ensure no clotting abnormality is present which requires correction
- their case should be discussed as early as possible with, and their CT scan reviewed by, the neurosurgeon-on-call. Often, small bleeds in fully alert patients without significant neurological disability may be managed conservatively although close monitoring is required for any sign of deterioration
- ideally, the patient should be transferred to the care of the neurosurgeon but, if locally managed, they should be closely monitored in at least an HDU level environment
- good supportive care improves outcome and, in this case, should include non-sedative analgesia for the headache, oxygen where required to keep saturations 94–98% and tight glycaemic control with a sliding scale. Initially at least, the high blood pressure is probably left untreated as it will commonly normalize as the pain and stress of the acute episode subside.

d The GCS is now 8 (E=1, V=2, M=5).

e An expanding posterior fossa haematoma may cause two serious conditions: first, obstructive hydrocephalus from compression of the aquaduct and/or 4th ventricle; and second, compression of the brainstem itself (more often seen with larger midline cerebellar bleeds). Both complications cause neurological deterioration, coma and death, if untreated. Management would involve airway protection with early intubation and ventilation, repeat CT brain and urgent neurosurgical intervention.

Case 4

a The three organisms commonly causing childhood and adult bacterial meningitis are *Neisseria meningitides* (40%), *Streptococcus pneumoniae* (50%) and *Haemophilus influenza* (10%). Widespread uptake of the *H. influenza* type b (Hib) vaccination has led to a dramatic decline in meningitis from this organism and the consequent predominance of meningococcus and streptococcus as causes.

b Signs of raised intracranial pressure and, therefore, contraindications to lumbar puncture (LP) in suspected meningitis as outlined in NICE guidance 102[6] are:

- reduced or fluctuating level of consciousness
- focal neurological signs
- abnormal posturing
- pupillary signs (unequal, dilated or poorly responsive pupil(s))
- papilloedema
- abnormal 'doll's eye' movements (a sign of brain death!)
- relative bradycardia and hypotension (Cushing's reflex – a late sign).

Other contraindications to LP in this situation include suspected septicaemia (shock or spreading purpura), coagulation disorders and anticoagulants, seizures and respiratory insufficiency.

c The following table outlines the normal values for CSF, as well as the typical CSF pictures in bacterial, viral and tuberculosis meningitis.

Table 5.2

	Normal CSF	Bacterial meningitis	Viral meningitis	Tuberculous meningitis
Appearance	Clear	Cloudy	Clear	Classically 'fibrin web' or turbid
White cell count/mm³	<5	1000 +	50–1000	10–1000
Predominant cell type	Lymphocytes (no polymorphs)	Polymorphs	Lymphocytes	Lymphocytes
Organisms (at microscopy and culture)	-ve	+ve	-ve	-ve on microscopy (may be +ve after culture)
Protein (g/L)	<0.5	>1.5	1–5	<1
Glucose	Approximately 2/3 plasma glucose	<1/2 plasma	>1/2 plasma	<1/2 plasma

Thus, this patient has an abnormally high CSF lymphocyte count with no organisms present. In addition, the values for CSF protein and glucose are slightly elevated. This picture is consistent with a viral meningitis.

For completeness, treatment of uncomplicated viral meningitis is symptomatic with anti-pyretics, simple analgesia (NSAIDs), anti-emetics and observation in hospital until improving.

d Where sub-arachnoid haemorrhage (SAH) is suspected but the CT brain is normal, CSF may be obtained and tested for the presence of xanthochromia. Xanthochromia can be detected 12 hours after a sub-arachnoid bleed and is the yellow pigment arising from the breakdown of the haem component of haemoglobin. It is present in CSF only as a result of haemorrhage and is therefore diagnostic of SAH.

Case 5

a Immediate management of the patient with grand-mal seizure involves preventing further injury using pillows and blankets to shield flailing limbs and head; placing them into the recovery position to drain secretions from the oropharynx; and applying oxygen at 15 L/min via reservoir mask. A nasopharyngeal airway might be inserted as well but further airway management, although desirable, is often impeded by jaw spasm during the acute seizure.

b Hypoglycaemia should be excluded by checking the blood glucose level in all patients with a seizure. Blood glucose level below 4 mmol/L is considered low and should be corrected with glucagon 1 mg IV/IM and/or intravenous glucose (e.g., 250 ml 10% glucose). In women of childbearing age, think about eclampsia and look for a gravid uterus. If eclampsia is suspected, fast call for senior obstetric and anaesthetic help and give a bolus of 4 g magnesium sulphate IV over five minutes.

c Step 1

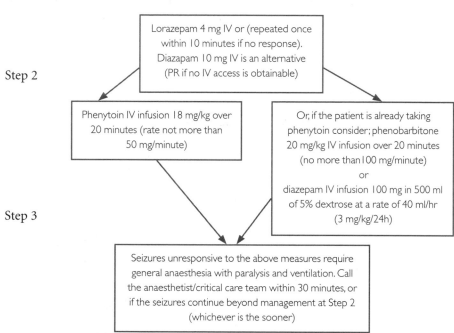

Step 2

Lorazepam 4 mg IV or (repeated once within 10 minutes if no response). Diazapam 10 mg IV is an alternative (PR if no IV access is obtainable)

Phenytoin IV infusion 18 mg/kg over 20 minutes (rate not more than 50 mg/minute)

Or, if the patient is already taking phenytoin consider; phenobarbitone 20 mg/kg IV infusion over 20 minutes (no more than 100 mg/minute) or diazepam IV infusion 100 mg in 500 ml of 5% dextrose at a rate of 40 ml/hr (3 mg/kg/24h)

Step 3

Seizures unresponsive to the above measures require general anaesthesia with paralysis and ventilation. Call the anaesthetist/critical care team within 30 minutes, or if the seizures continue beyond management at Step 2 (whichever is the sooner)

d While status epilepticus is most commonly seen in the context of a known epileptic, it is unusual as a presentation of newly diagnosed epilepsy in a young person. More common causes of status epilepticus in non-epileptics of this age are CNS infection (e.g., bacterial meningitis), a structural brain lesion (e.g., tumour or abscess) or an overdose of drugs causing seizure (e.g., tricyclic antidepressants). Other, much less common causes include cerebral malaria, cerebral tuberculosis, electrolyte disturbances, sub-arachnoid haemorrhage and other intracranial bleeds.

e Based on the likely causes above, urgent investigations to be initiated in the ED include:

- blood tests: electrolytes including calcium, WCC and CRP
- ECG for signs of tricyclic overdose (tachycardia, widened QRS, prolonged PR interval)
- toxicology screen
- CT brain
- lumbar puncture (provided there is no evidence of raised intracranial pressure)
- malaria screen if recent tropical travel.

Case 6

a Red flags are features of the patient history which might alert us to possible serious spinal pathology in an otherwise routine presentation of back pain. The following are common to most lists of the red flags and we should look for:

- age less than 20 or onset over age 55
- constant progressive pain
- non-mechanical pain (pain at rest and pain with any movement)
- persistent night pain
- thoracic pain
- systemically unwell, e.g., fever or weight loss
- bilateral leg weakness
- new onset bladder or bowel dysfunction or saddle anaesthesia
- significant past medical history of malignancy, HIV, drug abuse, long-term steroid use
- morning stiffness (ankylosing spondylitis)
- onset with significant trauma.

b Weakness is a feature of both upper motor neuron (UMN) and lower motor neuron (LMN) lesions but clinical examination can readily distinguish between the two using the following signs:

Table 5.3

Sign	UMN lesions	LMN lesions
Tone	Increased	Decreased or absent
Tendon reflexes	Increased	Decreased
Muscle wasting	Yes	No
Fasciculation	No	Yes
Plantar reflexes	Upgoing	Downgoing

c Spinal cord compression may give decreased sensation in the dermatomes below the level of the lesion and such a sensory level found on examination is highly predictive of serious spinal pathology. Remember that perineal (saddle) anaesthesia **on its own** is a feature of lumbosacral nerve root compression i.e., cauda equine syndrome, and not of cervical or thoracic cord compression.

d The Medical Research Council (MRC) grades power during a neurological examination as follows (Box 5.3).

Box 5.3 MRC grading of muscle power	
Grade	Description
0	no contraction
1	flicker of contraction only
2	active movement with gravity eliminated
3	active movement against gravity only
4	active movement against gravity and resistance
5	normal power (compared to the examiner)

e Acute cord compression is a neurosurgical emergency and the priority investigation is urgent MRI imaging of the spine to make the diagnosis, establish the cause, and give information on level and extent of disease.

In addition, patients may be investigated in the emergency room with the following:

- plain X-ray may show crush fractures or evidence of vertebral malignant disease
- inflammatory markers (WCC, CRP and ESR) looking for infection and inflammation
- PSA tumour marker where metastatic prostate malignancy is suspected
- bone profile for raised calcium and alkaline phosphatase in bone malignancy.

Case 7

a True vertigo is characterized by first, the illusion that the environment is moving in respect to the patient (or vice versa) and second, this sensation is made worse by movement of the patient themselves.

b Vertigo may result from disorders of the cerebellum and brainstem (central vertigo) or disorders of the VIIIth cranial nerve or inner ear (peripheral vertigo). It is important to distinguish between central and peripheral vertigo as the former is always due to serious pathology requiring urgent investigation. Features which may be of help include:

Table 5.4

Central vertigo	Peripheral vertigo
Rarely occurs in isolation	No accompanying neurological signs
Accompanying cerebellar or brainstem signs are usually present	Very intense sensation motion
	Aggravated by position
Less intense than peripheral	Hearing may be affected
Not positional	Tinnitus may be present
Hearing loss and tinnitus are rare	Nystagmus inhibited by ocular fixation
Nystagmus not inhibited by ocular fixation	

c Hearing loss is associated with vertigo in the following conditions:

- Ménière's disease is recognized from the triad of symptoms of vertigo, tinnitus and progressive deafness
- acoustic neuroma (schwannoma) or a meningioma at the cerebellopontin angle may compress the VIIIth nerve and cause a gradual loss of hearing which precedes the onset of vertigo
- suppurative labyrinthitis arising from chronic cholesteatoma or mastoiditis.

The above are all causes of peripheral vertigo and from an ED point of view, all have the same management – urgent referral for investigation by an ENT specialist.

d Benign paroxysmal positional vertigo (BPPV) is distinguished from vestibular neuronitis (labyrinthitis) by the duration of the vertiginous episodes. BPPV causes sudden bouts of intense vertigo lasting seconds and which occur after movements of the head. In contrast, the vertigo of vestibular neuronitis lasts days and is made worse by sitting up and standing.

In addition, the Dix-Hallpike test can be used to positively diagnose BPPV. Here, the patient begins sitting upright before the clinician grasps the head and rapidly lowers the patient to the supine position then rotates the head 45 degrees to the left, then right. A positive test indicative of BPPV occurs when, after a 2–20 second latency period, there is the onset of rotational nystagmus lasting less than one minute, followed by return to normal eye movements.

e Symptomatic vestibular neuronitis may be treated with:

- centrally acting anti-emetics (prochlorperazine most commonly but also promethazine or cyclizine can be used). Prochlorperazine has a buccal preparation (buccastem), particularly useful in vomiting patients
- certain anti-histamines also act as vestibular sedatives. Cinnarizine is commonly used for motion sickness and is used in the treatment of vertigo. Betahistine also treats vertigo, although in practice, is more often used in the treatment of Ménière's disease than vestibular neuronitis.

Patients should be told to lie flat during attacks of acute vertigo both to lessen symptoms and prevent falls. Symptoms may last for days before resolving and patients should avoid salt and alcohol. Most patients with vestibular neuronitis can be managed at home with GP review, but they should return to hospital if becoming dehydrated from persistent vomiting, or if they develop progressive symptoms.

Case 8

a Simply put, parkinsonism is a syndrome of tremor, rigidity and bradykinesia (slowness in movement).
b The parkinsonian gait is a short-stepped shuffle in the stooped position, sometimes called the festinant gait.
c There are a number of causes of parkinsonism, other than idiopathic Parkinson's disease itself, and these include, perhaps in order of relevance to exclude:

- drug-induced parkinsonism. Most commonly, the major antipsychotic medications are at fault but also prochloperazine and metaclopromide may be implicated
- stroke
- recurrent head trauma (boxers)
- Wilson's disease (copper overload)
- hydrocephalus
- for completeness, rarities include encephalitis, progressive supranuclear palsy and multiple systems atrophy.

d Parkinson's disease arises from loss of dopaminergic neurons of the substantia nigra and consequent low levels of the neurotransmitter dopamine in the brain.

Broadly speaking, there are three pharmacological approaches in use to help correct this:

- replace dopamine with dopaminergic drugs. L-dopa is the first-line medication and is converted into dopamine in the brain. It is administered in combination with a peripheral dopa-decarboxylase inhibitor to prevent conversion into dopamine outside the CNS thus prolonging the half-life of administered L-dopa and reducing peripheral side effects. Common drugs combining L-dopa and a dopa-carboxylase inhibitor are madopar and sinemet. Both may increase mobility in Parkinson's patients quite considerably but effects wear off over time
- dopamine receptor agonists such as pergolide and bromocriptine as well as more recent drugs such as ropinirole and pramipexole, stimulate dopamine receptors to mimic increased levels of dopamine. They are used when tolerance to L-dopa is developing or in younger patients where L-dopa therapy is delayed as far as possible
- anticholinergic/antimuscarinic agents such as benzhexol address the imbalance between dopamine and acetylcholine through inhibition of cholinergic and muscarinic receptors. Over 50% of Parkinson's' patients will see an improvement in motor function with benzhexol.

e Parkinson's disease is an progressive incurable condition which requires long-term specialist management in the community. Patient's with a new diagnosis of Parkinson's do not necessarily require admission; instead arrange urgent assessment by a neurologist with a view to starting medication, physiotherapy for their movement disorder and many hospitals now have a Parkinson's specialist nurse who can be contacted to provide support after discharge.

Further Reading

1. Johnston SC, Rothwell PM, Nguyen-Huynh MN, et al. (2007) Validation and refinement of scores to predict very early stroke risk after transient ischaemic attack. *Lancet.* Jan 27; 369(9558):283–92.
2. NICE/Royal College of Physicians guideline CG68. Stroke: The diagnosis and initial acute management of stroke and transient ischaemic attack (TIA) (2008) www.nice.org.uk/guidance/CG68
3. The Scottish Intercollegiate Network (SIGN) Guideline 108. The Management of patients with stroke or TIA: assessment, investigation, immediate management and secondary prevention. A National Clinical Guideline. Found at www.sign.ac.uk/pdf/sign108.pdf
4. Nor AM, Davis J, Sen B, et al. (2005) The Recognition of Stroke in the Emergency Room (ROSIER) scale: Development and validation of a stroke recognition instrument. *Lancet Neurology*; 4(11):727–34.
5. Wardlaw JM, Murray V, Sandercock PAG. (2008) Thrombolysis for acute ischaemic stroke: an update of the Cochrane thrombolysis meta-analysis. *Int J Stroke.* 3 (Suppl 1):50.
6. NICE Guideline CG102. (2010) Bacterial meningitis and meningococcal septicaemia. www.nice.org.uk/Guidance/CG102

6

GASTROENTEROLOGY

Malcolm Tunnicliff

Introduction

Core topics

- gastroenteritis (diarrhoea and vomiting)
- causes of upper gastrointestinal (GI) pain
- the jaundiced patient
- acute liver failure and hepatitis
- chronic liver disease and oesophageal varices
- upper and lower GI haemorrhage
- hepatic encephalopathy
- the ascitic patient (including spontaneous bacterial peritonitis)
- inflammatory bowel disease.

Specific data included in questions might be a set of liver function tests (LFTs) (know the various patterns of LFTs and their corresponding diagnosis), the INR (a gauge of liver failure) or some inflammatory markers (WCC, CRP and ESR). The interpretation of stool cultures results is fairly self-evident although do not forget to ask for microscopy for ova, oocytes and parasites in a travellers' diarrhoea! Be aware that the indications for abdominal X-ray in GI disease are few, and this investigation should only be requested where a specific pathology, such as toxic megacolon in acute colitis or a perforated duodenal ulcer, is being considered.

Gastroenterologists are also fond of scoring systems and we present three in the following questions: the Rockall score for acute upper GI haemorrhage,[1] the Truelove and Witt's criteria for severity of ulcerative colitis and the clinical grading of hepatic encephalopathy. Although not discussed here, the Blatchford score (Glasgow-Blatchford score)[2] for assessing the need for admission and emergency treatment for upper GI haemorrhage is being used in many Emergency Departments (EDs) as an alternative to Rockall.

Case 1

A 21-year-old Caucasian male presents to the ED with a 3-day history of bloody diarrhoea. He has no vomiting but complains that he has worsening gripping, intermittent lower abdominal pain. He has no significant past medical history, takes no routine medication and has no allergies. On examination, his abdomen is soft and bowel sounds are present. PR examination reveals fresh blood mixed into the semi-formed and watery stool. His observations are: heart rate 100 bpm, blood pressure 103/74 mmHg, temperature 37.7 °C and blood glucose 5.3 mmo/L.

a Give a differential diagnosis including three infective organisms that cause bloody diarrhoea and three non-infective causes of bloody stool. [3]
b What specific questions would you ask this patient to try to narrow the differential diagnosis (give four)? [4]
c Name three specific investigations you would carry out in the ED. [3]
d The young man reports having a chicken meal at a local restaurant one day before becoming ill and that two of his fellow diners are also unwell with similar symptoms. When would you prescribe antibiotics for this patient's diarrhoea and which antibiotic would you prescribe? [2]

[12]

Case 2

A 46-year-old male with a history of ulcerative colitis (UC) presents to the ED. He has developed abdominal pain and diarrhoea, with blood and mucus over the past two days, and has passed over eight watery stools in the previous 12 hours. He takes mesalazine 500 mg TDS for his chronic colitis. On examination, he looks pale and dehydrated, with pulse 100 bpm, blood pressure 115/68 mmHg and temperature 38.2 °C.

a What is the likely diagnosis in this patient? [1]
b Give three recognized markers of **severe** ulcerative colitis. [3]
c What serious abdominal complications may arise in this patient? [3]
d This man's colitis is severe and he needs admission for urgent treatment. What four treatments could you instigate in the ED? [4]
e Give three extra-intestinal signs of ulcerative colitis. [3]

[14]

Case 3

A 25-year-old female is brought to the ED by her college friends who say she has gone 'yellow' over the past two days. The woman has noticed that she has gone off her food, and has a mild ache in the right upper abdomen, but is otherwise well. On examination, you find she is markedly jaundiced and is tender over her right upper quadrant but without signs of peritonism. Her blood results are as follows:

Hb	10.4 g/dl	Bilirubin	98 µmol/L
WCC	15.6 × 10⁹/L	ALP	104 u/L
Platelets	213 × 10⁹/L	AST	1560 u/L
INR	1.1	ALT	780 u/L

a According to the most common method of classifying jaundice, what type of jaundice does this woman have? Explain your answer. [2]

b What questions is it important to ask, to help ascertain the cause of the jaundice in this woman (give four)? [4]

c Complete the following table giving the routes of transmission and availability of immunization for the following hepatitis viruses:

Table 6.1

Hepatitis virus	Route of transmission	Vaccine available (yes/no)
Hepatitis A		
Hepatitis B		
Hepatitis C		

[6]

[12]

Case 4

A 48-year-old man presents to the ED with confusion. He is a chronic alcoholic with numerous hospital admissions and failed detoxification programmes in the past. He also has hepatitis C, contracted from IV drug use. On examination, he has sweet smelling breath, is jaundiced, has gross ascites and is markedly confused and agitated. His observations are temperature 37.8 °C, pulse 98 bpm, blood pressure 100/70 mmHg and respiration rate 24/min.

Blood results are as follows.

WCC	14.0 × 10⁹/L	K⁺	3.8 mmol/L
Hb	11.9 g/dl	Creatinine	134 µmol/L
Platelets	209 × 10⁹/L	ALT	450 u/L
INR	1.9	ALP	85 u/L
Na⁺	132 mmol/L	Bilirubin	96 µmol/L

a What bedside test needs to be performed straight away? [1]

b Describe the abnormalities in this patient's blood tests and provide a brief interpretation. [3]

c Give two clinical features of grade III hepatic encephalopathy. [2]

d Give three possible precipitants of hepatic encephalopathy in this patient. [3]

e How would you treat this patient's agitation in the ED? [3]

[12]

Case 5

You are pre-alerted by the ambulance service that they are bringing in a 42-year-old male who has been vomiting bright red blood for the last hour. He is known to be a heavy drinker of alcohol and his past medical history includes a myocardial infarction one year ago, for which he takes an aspirin and a β-blocker daily. He has no previous attendances with gastrointestinal bleeding. On arrival in the ED, he is alert but showing signs of shock and you begin fluid resuscitation immediately.

a What is your differential diagnosis in this patient (give four)?   [4]
b List three drugs that may be used in the treatment of upper gastrointestinal haemorrhage in the ED.   [3]
c Briefly describe the mechanism of action of one of the drugs you list above.   [2]
d After adequate fluid replacement, a repeat set of observations show a heart rate of 120 bpm, blood pressure 95/60 mmHg and respiration rate 22/min. What is this patient's pre-endoscopy Rockall risk score?   [2]
e Name a non-pharmacological method of treating acute variceal haemorrhage in the ED.   [1]
                                                                                     [12]

GASTROENTEROLOGY –ANSWERS

Case 1

a Diarrhoea is defined as passing more than 300 g of stool over a 24 hour period, with likely change to the consistency and frequency of stool passage. Bloody diarrhoea is broadly divided into infective and non-infective causes, the most commonly considered given below:

Table 6.2

Infective Causes	Non infective Causes
Salmonella	Ulcerative colitis/Crohn's disease
Shigella	Ischaemic colitis
Campylobacter	Colonic polyps
E. coli	Colorectal carcinoma
Pseudomembraneous colitis (C. difficile)	
Entamoeba hystolica	

N.B. Irritable bowel syndrome **DOES NOT** cause bloody diarrhoea.

b The exact line of questioning differs slightly from the young person with an acute onset illness (likely infective colitis) and an older person with more chronic symptoms (likely a more sinister cause) but, in any patient with bloody diarrhoea, it is important to ask about:

- recent travel abroad (dysentery). Ask what drinking water was used (entamoeba)
- recent meals, especially if fellow diners are similarly unwell (food poisoning)
- recent hospitalization or use of broad spectrum antibiotics (pseudomembraneous colitis)
- previous episodes or chronicity of diarrhoea (inflammatory bowel syndrome – could also ask about joint and eye problems)
- preceding change in bowel habits, weight loss or family history (bowel carcinoma).

c Important investigations to perform in the ED, include electrolytes and renal function to check for dehydration and electrolyte imbalance. LFTs may reveal hepatitis, sometimes seen with *E. coli* or amoeba. A FBC count will demonstrate a leucocytosis with a likely neutrophilia, but more importantly, will check haemoglobin levels in heavy or prolonged bleeding. Essential in diagnosing bloody diarrhoea is a stool sample sent for both culture and microscopy (ova, oocytes and parasites). If inflammatory bowel syndrome is suspected, and the patient has abdominal signs or symptoms, an abdominal X-ray is indicated looking for megacolon (the abdominal X-ray is of no use in suspected infective colitis).

d In general, it is best to avoid blind antibiotic therapy when treating diarrhoea to avoid promoting antibiotic resistance. However, the following situations may require treatment with antibiotics:

- systemically unwell patients who require admission
- when a causative organism is identified from culture or on microscopy of faecal smear
- more than two weeks of bloody diarrhoea strongly suspected to be infective.

Ciprofloxacin treats salmonella, campylobacter and shigella and is a good place to start. Oral metronidazole treats amoebic dysentery (less likely in the UK). Both may be used in severe cases of travellers' diarrhoea.

For completeness, remember the mainstay of the treatment of diarrhoea is fluid hydration and electrolyte replacement, as required by clinical circumstance. Avoid anti-diarrhoeals in bloody diarrhoea. Finally, food poisoning is a notifiable disease. Advice on when to return to work is also important, especially with workers handling food.

Case 2

a This patient has an acute flare-up his ulcerative colitis (UC). If you had been asked for a differential diagnosis then all the infective causes of bloody diarrhoea (see above), diverticular disease, ischaemic colitis and Crohn's colitis could all be included.

b When presented with a patient with acute colitis, it is important to assess severity. The Truelove and Witt's criteria were developed to assess the severity of ulcerative colitis (UC) as follows (Box 6.1).

Box 6.1. Truelove and Witt's definition of severe Ulcerative Colitis

More than 6 stools per day **AND** one or more systemic features below
- heavy rectal bleeding
- haemoglobin <10.5 g/dL
- temperature >37.8 °C
- pulse > 90 bpm
- ESR > 30 mm/h

---

c Acute severe colitis may give rise to the following life-threatening complications:

- GI haemorrhage
- bowel perforation
- toxic megacolon (dilatation colon >6 cm on the plain abdominal X-ray).

Colon cancer is, of course, another serious complication of UC but is not related to the acute flare-ups.

d Patients with severe acute colitis, regardless of whether it is a flare up of known disease or a new presentation of UC, should be admitted and jointly reviewed by the medical and surgical teams. They should have blood taken for FBC, clotting studies, U&Es, LFTs, ESR and CRP and glucose. Stool microscopy, culture and sensitivities (MC&S) should also be sent looking for infective causes and an erect chest and abdominal X-ray performed to look for perforation or megacolon. It is reasonable to start treatment in the ED with:

- IV fluid rehydration (with electrolyte replacement, as indicated by U&E results)
- steroids are the acute treatment. Give 100 mg hydrocortisone IV qds.
- PR steroids (100 mg hydrocortisone in 100 mL N saline instilled rectally by Foley catheter over 30 minutes)
- consider blood transfusion where the Hb <10 g/dL with on-going rectal bleeding
- antibiotics (metronidazole and ciprofloxacin) for systemically unwell patients (temp >38 °C).

e The extra-intestinal manifestations of ulcerative colitis are many, and a favourite of examiners:

Table 6.3

System	Feature
Musculoskeletal	Ankylosing spondylitis, arthritis, sacroiliitis
Skin/mucosa	Erythema nodosum, pyoderma gangrenosum, clubbing, apthous ulcers
Eyes	Episcleritis, iritis
Biliary	Cholangiocarcinoma, primary sclerosing cholangitis
Kidney	Renal stones
Metabolic	Osteomalacia, amyloidosis

Case 3

a It is not uncommon for patients with jaundice to present to the ED. As in this case, it is often relatives or friends who first notice changes in the skin pigmentation. Jaundice is caused by an increase in plasma bilirubin. It normally becomes apparent when bilirubin level exceeds 40 µmol/L, but can be quite a subtle sign to pick up. Most commonly, jaundice is divided into pre-hepatic, hepatocellular or post-hepatic (obstructive). The table below summarizes the different types, their biochemical profile and their common causes:

Table 6.4

Jaundice	Aetiology	Biochemistry	Common causes
Pre-hepatic	Excess of bilirubin production or reduced liver uptake of bilirubin	$\uparrow$ unconjugated bilirubin, Also $\uparrow$ LDH and elevated reticulocytes with haemolysis	RBC haemolysis (sickle cell, malaria, G6PD deficiency) Neonatal jaundice Abnormal bilirubin metabolism (e.g. Gilbert's syndrome)

Hepatocellular (intra-hepatic)	Hepatocyte damage with or without cholestasis	Normal or ↑ unconjugated bilirubin ↑↑ aminotransferases (AST/ALT) ↑ alkaline phosphatase	Viral hepatitis Drug-induced (paracetamol, anti-TB drugs, halothane) Alcoholic hepatitis Liver cirrhosis Hepatic vein obstruction (Budd-Chiari syndrome) Right heart failure Autoimmune hepatitis Haemochromotosis Amanita phalloides mushrooms
Post-hepatic (obstructive)	Blockage of bilirubin excretion from the liver	↑conjugated bilirubin ↑↑ alkaline phosphatase ↑ aminotrantferases (AST/ALT)	Gallstones Cholangitis Cholangiocarcinoma Primary biliary cirrhosis Cholestasis of pregnancy

Thus, the woman in the question has massively elevated liver aminotransferases with only moderate rise in alkaline phosphatase indicating that she has hepatocellular jaundice.

b A detailed history is essential for diagnosing the cause of hepatocellular jaundice and important questions to ask include:

● any recent travel abroad (hep A)
● contacts with other jaundiced persons (hep A)
● ask about recent sexual activity (hep B/C)
● intravenous drug use (hep B/C)
● any tattoos or piercings? (hep B/C)
● have you ever had a blood transfusion? (hep B/C)
● ask about recent alcohol use (alcoholic hepatitis)
● chronic alcohol abuse (cirrhosis)
● detailed drug history (including over the counter and herbal medications) and cross-reference with the BNF, those which may cause liver damage – there are many!
● family history of liver disease (haemochromotosis).

The table should have been completed as follows, indicating the routes of transmission and availability of vaccination for the three main causes of viral hepatitis.

Hepatitis virus	Route of transmission	Vaccine available
Hepatitis A	Faecal/oral	Yes
Hepatitis B	IV drug use, unprotected sexual intercourse, blood products	Yes
Hepatitis C	IV drug use, unprotected sexual intercourse, blood products	No

Case 4

a Any patient presenting with confusion and/or agitation, should have a bedside blood glucose test done as soon as possible. This is particularly important in alcoholics and patients with liver failure, who are prone to hypoglycaemia. Blood glucose below 4 mm/L should be treated.

b The blood tests demonstrate hepatocellular jaundice (bilirubin above 40 μmol/L with raised AST and normal ALP). The patient also has an elevated INR, indicating that as well as hepatocyte damage, the normal synthetic function of the liver is affected (remember vitamin K is produced by the liver). However, the degree of liver failure (look at the degree of jaundice and coagulation abnormality) is out of proportion with the degree of hepatocyte damage (look at the AST). This is the typical picture of acute on chronic liver failure (also called decompensated chronic liver disease) where a new insult to the liver comes on top of longstanding impairment due to cirrhosis.

c Hepatic encephalopathy is abnormal mental function arising from liver failure. Toxic metabolites normally cleared by the liver accumulate causing a spectrum of neurological features and ultimately cerebral oedema. Hepatic encephalopathy is graded by severity as follows:

Table 6.5

Grade of Hepatic Encephalopathy	Features
Grade I	Altered mood, sleep disturbance, mild dis-orientation, inability to draw a five-pointed star
Grade II	Drowsy, slurred speech, mild confusion, impairment complex mental tasks
Grade III	Incoherent speech, very confused, agitated, restless, stupor
Grade IV	Obtunded/comatose

d Acute chronic liver failure and hepatic encephalopathy arise from a further physiological insult on an already chronically impaired liver. High on the list for this patient would be:

- alcohol binge
- infection (including bacterial peritonitis in the patient with ascites)
- GI haemorrhage (increased nitrogen load)
- myocardial infarction
- hepatotoxic drug ingestion.

e Agitated patients with hepatic encephalopathy are more unwell than they may look. Avoid opiates and benzodiazapines which exacerbate encephalopathy. Use haloperidol under close observation, and with experienced help, if the need for sedation is unavoidable. Importantly, be aware that patients with grade III or IV encephalopathy require HDU/ITU care and often sedation with invasive ventilation to control severe neuropsychiatric features.

Case 5

a   Gastrointestinal haemorrhage proximal to the third part of the duodenum can present with fresh haematemesis and may be due to:

- peptic ulcers
- oesophageal varices
- Mallory-Weiss tear
- gastroduodenal erosions
- oesophageal or gastric malignancy
- vascular malformations of the upper GI tract
- aorto-enteric fistula in patients with aortic grafts
- swallowed blood from epistaxis!

Remember anticoagulants such as warfarin are themselves not a **cause** of bleeding but a risk factor for substantially heavier bleeding, once bleeding occurs.

b   The following table gives drugs which may be used in patients presenting with upper GI bleeding along with their mechanism of action:

Table 6.6

Drug	Mechanism of action
Omeprazole (and other proton pump inhibitors)	Inhibits gastric acid production in the stomach by blocking the hydrogen – potassium – ATPase (the proton pump) of the gastric parietal cell
Terlipressin	Terlipressin is a derivative of the posterior pituitary hormone vasopressin. It is used to reduce hepatic portal pressures, and is effective in controlling haemorrhage from oesophageal varices
Ocreotide	Reduces gastric mucosal blood flow in both normal and portal hypertension helping to control variceal haemorrhage
Ranitidine	Ranitidine reduces gastric acid production by blocking the histamine H2 receptor on the surface of the gastric parietal cells. This reduces the stimulus to the parietal cell to produce gastric acid
Vitamin K	Vitamin K is a fat-soluble vitamin that is necessary for the production of blood clotting factors. Patients who have problems with fat malabsorption, especially those with hepatic disease, will therefore be deficient and more prone to bleeding

c   The Rockall score[1] risk stratifies patients with upper GI bleeding by predicting mortality, based on patient age and co-morbidities, the degree of shock **after** adequate fluid resuscitation and the findings at endoscopy. For ED practice, a pre-endoscopic Rockall score can be calculated (see table below), and is useful in guiding the urgency of clinical response.

Table 6.7

	0 points	1 point	2 points	3 points
Age	<60 years	60 – 79	80 +	
Shock (systolic BP, pulse rate)	BP >100 mmHg Pulse <100	BP >100mm Hg Pulse >100	BP <100 mmHg	
Co-morbidities	None	Cardiac failure, Ischaemic heart disease	Renal failure, liver failure	Metastases

By using the table, this patient's Rockall score is three (his BP is less than 100 mmHg systolic (two points) and he has ischaemic heart disease (one point). A score of two or less corresponds to a mortality of below 1%, while a score of six or greater is taken to be an indicator for HDU care and urgent endoscopy.

d In experienced hands, a Sengstaken-Blakemore tube may be lifesaving for patients with torrential upper GI haemorrhage due to variceal haemorrhage. It uses inflatable balloons to compress both oesophageal and gastric varices. The tube is inserted into the ocsophagus and the gastric balloon inflated, then pulled back to impact and compress the gastro-oesophageal junction. The oesophageal balloon is inflated to compress bleeding oesophageal vessels. Associated risks of using this device are oesophageal necrosis or rupture.

Further Reading

1. Rockall TA, Logan RF, Devlin HB, *et al.* (1996) Risk assessment following acute gastrointestinal haemorrhage. *Gut*; **38**:316–21.
2. Blatchford O, Murray W and Blatchford M. (2000) A risk score to predict need for treatment of upper gastrointestinal haemorrhage. *Lancet*; **356**:1318–21.

7

RENAL AND ELECTROLYTE EMERGENCIES

Emma Townsend

Introduction

Core topics
- renal failure (acute, chronic and acute on chronic)
- renal failure (pre-renal, renal and post-renal)
- urinary tract infection
- renal calculi
- the dialysis patient
- rhabdomyolysis
- haemolytic uraemic syndrome
- fluid compartments and fluid therapy
- hypo/hypernatraemia
- hyperkalaemia
- hypo/hypercalcaemia.

The interpretation of blood biochemistry, in relation to renal disease, is obviously important for renal and electrolyte SAQs. Urine biochemistry can also crop up (for example, urine sodium and osmolality in hyponatraemia) as well as the use of dipstick urinalysis (knowing the sensitivity and specificity for UTI is useful). Furthermore, renal tract imaging – the plain X-ray (KUB for renal stones) and the intravenous urethrogram (IVU) in renal obstruction[1] – has featured in previous exams and their interpretation is a skill worth having in the ED. Finally, the ECG changes of the various electrolyte abnormalities, (particularly hyperkalaemia) is always an exam favourite!

Case 1

A 32-year-old female has been brought into the emergency department (ED) having been found collapsed and unconscious on the floor of a concrete stairwell. She is a known intravenous drug user, and had not been seen since the previous day. There is no evidence of head injury, although she does have a notably swollen left arm and thigh, on which she was lying when found. A trial of naloxone by the ambulance crew transiently improved her conscious level. On arrival in the ED, she is placed on a monitor in the resuscitation room and a naloxone infusion begun. Her blood results are phoned down urgently from the laboratory:

Na^+	144 mmol/L
K^+	5.8 mmol/L
Urea	25 mmol/L
Creatinine	601 μmol/L
Ca^{2+}	1.6 mmol/L
CK	3766 u/L
Glucose	4.2 mmol/L

a What is the likely cause of her renal impairment? [1]
b Outline the main steps in your treatment of this diagnosis (drug doses not required). [4]
c What would you expect on urine dipstick, and then on subsequent urine microscopy? [2]
d Give three different causes of this diagnosis other than prolonged immobilization. [3]
e Name two complications of this condition (other than those relating to renal impairment). [2]

[12]

Case 2

A 30-year-old female presents to the ED, complaining of urinary frequency and burning on passing urine for the past two days. Today, she has worsened with rigors, vomiting and pain in her left flank area. She has no prior medical history, and does not normally suffer from cystitis. Her observations are temperature 37.8 °C, pulse 90 bpm and regular and blood pressure 110/70 mmHg.

She has supplied a specimen of urine which shows the following on dipstick testing: leucocytes 2+, nitrites 2+, and blood 1+. The urinary pregnancy test is negative.

a What is the approximate sensitivity and specificity of dipstick nitrite testing for urinary tract infection (UTI)? [2]
b Give three reasons why a UTI may be classified as 'complicated' [3]
c Which four organisms most commonly cause uncomplicated lower urinary tract infection in adults? [2]

d Give four steps in the ED management of this patient (include the doses
of any drugs you would give)? [4]
e Give three non-pharmacological measures which may be advised for
women with UTI. [3]

[14]

Case 3

A 61-year-old male has been asked by his GP to attend the ED urgently because
of abnormal blood tests. The GP's letter also states he has known mild renal
impairment and hypertension which is poorly controlled on multiple medications.
A section of his ECG taken in the ED is shown in Figure 7.1.

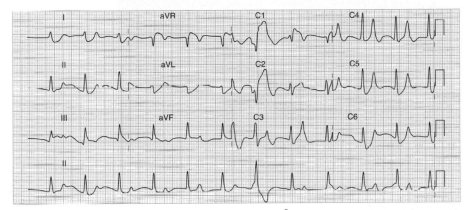

Figure 7.1

a Give three abnormalities of this patient's ECG (Figure 7.1). What is the
diagnosis? [4]
b List three commonly encountered drugs which may cause this diagnosis. [3]
c Give three clinical features of this diagnosis. [3]
d Give four drugs, with doses and routes of administration, which you would
use in the emergency treatment of this patient. [4]

[14]

Case 4

A 58-year-old male with diet controlled diabetes attends your ED with sudden
onset severe loin pain. An FY2 doctor working in the ED has seen the patient and
suspects renal colic. She has asked for your help in managing the case.

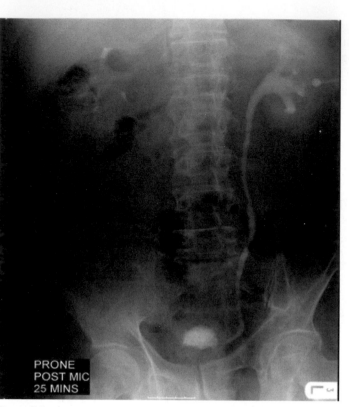

PRONE
POST MIC
25 MINS

Figure 7.2

a What advice would you give to the FY2 doctor on managing this patient's
   pain? [2]
b The FY2 asks if she should request an intravenous urethrogram (IVU).
   Give three simple investigations you would recommend be done **before**
   requesting an IVU. [3]
c Interpret this patient's IVU in Figure 7.2. [2]
d You are satisfied the diagnosis of renal colic is correct in this patient and
   your discussion with the FY2 now turns to whether or not the patient needs
   admission. Give three indications for admission in patients with a diagnosis
   of renal colic. [3]
e Give two circumstances (other than local policy) where CT-KUB is more
   appropriate than IVU for the ED investigation of suspected renal colic [2]
   [12]

Case 5

A 79-year-old man presents to the ED reporting that he cannot pass urine and has
worsening lower abdominal pain. He has a distended bladder on examination.

a Give four causes of urinary retention commonly seen in the ED. [4]

b Several attempts at urethral catheterization fail and the patient is becoming distressed with pain. You decide to pass a supra-pubic catheter. What anatomical structures must be traversed during insertion of a supra-pubic catheter? [3]

c The same patient returns to the ED two months later still with a supra-pubic catheter in situ but now with supra-pubic discomfort and a mild fever. His urinary dipstick is shown below:

protein +
blood ++
nitrites +ve
leucocytes ++
glucose –ve

What bacterial organisms commonly colonize long term urinary catheters (give two)? [2]

d How would you treat him now? [3]

[12]

Case 6

A normally healthy three-year-old girl is brought to the ED by her parents with diarrhoea for the past two days, which has now turned bloody. The child is alert, afebrile and has no clinical signs of shock. The only positive findings, on examination, are a marked pallor and a few petechiae around the foot and ankle. Her blood tests are as follows:

Na$^+$	134 mmol/L
K$^+$	3.7 mmol/L
Urea	17.8 mmol/L
Creatinine	346 μmol/L
Hb	6.7 g/dL
Platelets	35 × 10^9/L
WCC	13.6 × 10^9/L
INR	1.1
APTT	0.9

a Describe the abnormalities present in the blood tests. [3]

b What is the likely diagnosis in this child and give two common causative organisms? [3]

c Give two further laboratory investigations you would expect to be abnormal in this diagnosis. [2]

d Describe three key elements in the management of this condition. [3]

e A related condition is found in adults, where it produces a significantly more severe illness. What is the name of this condition and give two further clinical features that would point to this diagnosis in an adult? [3]

[14]

Case 7

A 64-year-old man attends the ED on the Monday morning, after having suffered with acute diarrhoea over the weekend, and is now worried he is passing little urine. His past history includes type II diabetes and heart failure. He cannot remember all his medications but does tell you he takes metformin 1 g BD and that two weeks ago, he was started on a medication for a painful big toe by his GP. On examination, he is fully alert, afebrile and has a pulse of 98 bpm and a blood pressure of 105/70 mmHg. His bloods were taken earlier by the ED nurse and are available for you to review:

Na^+	153 mmol/L
K^+	4.6 mmol/L
Urea	36 mmol/L
Creatinine	673 μmol/L

You look up his last blood tests on the computer and discover his creatinine two months ago was 143.

a Give three nephrotoxic drugs this patient may be taking, based on the past history given. [3]
b Describe how you would initiate treatment for this man's renal failure in the ED. [5]
c Define oliguria. [1]
d What are the indications for dialysis in acute renal failure (give three)? [3]
e What serious side-effect of metformin therapy may occur in this patient? [2]
[14]

Case 8

A 76-year-old man has arrived at hospital by blue light ambulance. He is very confused and the ambulance crew report that he had a tonic-clonic seizure in the back of the ambulance en route to hospital. He is known to have end-stage lung cancer but has not had any fits previously, according to the relative accompanying him. After initially stabilizing the patient, and protecting his airway, you turn to consideration of the cause of the confusion and seizures. His blood tests come back as follows:

Na^+	106 mmol/L
K^+	3.8 mmol/L
Urea	6.8 mmol/L
Creatinine	98 μmol/L

a Briefly describe why severe hyponatraemia causes neurological dysfunction? [2]
b How will you assess this patient's fluid status? Include in your answer, clinical signs you would look for, and how you would interpret them to help identify the cause of hyponatraemia. [4]

c The patient appears clinically euvolaemic. Next, you send a urine sample for biochemical analysis and the lab returns the following values:

| Urinary sodium | 45 mmol/L | (normal range 25–200 mmol/L) |
| Urinary osmolality | 760 mosm/kg | (normal range 300–1200 mosm/kg) |

Interpret the results of the urine biochemistry and give the likely cause of this man's severe hyponatraemia based on these results. [3]

d Outline your approach to treating hyponatraemia in this patient. [4]

e What serious consequence may arise from over rapid correction of a low sodium? [1]

[14]

Case 1

a Massively elevated creatinine kinase (CK) enzyme and a story of prolonged immobilization indicate rhabdomyolysis is the likely cause of renal failure in this young woman. Muscle tissue necrosis from prolonged pressure leads to massive cell lysis and release of the intracellular contents, particularly myoglobin and CK. A rise in CK of more than 10 times normal (often much greater) is the characteristic laboratory finding of rhabdomyolysis, while it is the circulating myoglobin that is nephrotoxic in large quantity, and causes myoglobinuric renal failure.

Further electrolyte abnormalities are common in rhabdomyolysis – hyperkalaemia, hyperphosphataemia, hypocalcaemia and metabolic acidosis can be present. It remains a serious condition with a mortality of approximately 5%.

b Aims of treatment in rhabdomyolysis are two-fold: promoting myoglobin clearance and supporting the kidneys through the period of insult.

- initiate prompt fluid resuscitation with large volumes of normal saline, up to 400 ml/hour if tolerated, aiming for a urine output of 200–300 ml/hour. There is the danger of fluid overloading in susceptible patients and central venous pressure monitoring is often required
- intravenous diuretics, for example, mannitol, are used to maintain volume status and promote urine output (furosemide should be avoided as it tends to acidify the urine)
- urinary alkalinisation, with 1.24% sodium bicarbonate enhances the solubility of myoglobin and aids clearance: aim to keep the urinary pH >6.0 and blood pH >7.5
- treat any underlying cause (see below)
- patients need cardiac monitoring (risk of arrhythmia due to electrolyte disturbance) and frequent checks of electrolytes and renal function
- worsening renal failure, acidosis, hyperkalaemia or fluid overload indicates the need for haemodialysis or haemofiltration.

Note that patients with a more moderate rise in CK but history suggestive of rhabdomyolysis, may be spared renal injury if aggressive fluid replacement and forced alkaline dieresis are started early.

c   Dipstick urinalysis is positive for blood – a false positive due to the haem
    contained in myoglobin. Microscopy, therefore, reveals no red cells.
    Myoglobinuria is pathognomonic for rhabdomyolysis; also causing the urine to
    be red-brown (coca-cola colour) in appearance.

d   Trauma, primarily crush injuries, and prolonged immobilization are the most
    common causes of rhabdomyolysis, but there is a much broader range of causes
    including the following more common ones:

    ● substance abuse (cocaine, heroin, amphetamines, ecstasy) is now probably the
      second most common cause
    ● other drugs with direct muscle toxicity such as statins
    ● high voltage electrical burns and third-degree burns
    ● epileptic fits
    ● muscle overactivity (marathon runners)
    ● infections (e.g., Influenza virus A&B, legionella)
    ● malignant hyperthermia
    ● hypothermia.

e   Although death in rhabdomyolysis is most often the result of renal failure and
    hyperkalaemia, other serious complications of muscle necrosis are compartment
    syndromes and disseminated intravascular coagulation (DIC). Compression
    neuropathies may also complicate this diagnosis.

Case 2

a   Most gram–ve urinary pathogens produce enzymes which reduce urinary
    nitrates to nitrite. Nitrites as detected by dipstick testing are quite specific
    (>90%) but not very sensitive (~50%) for the presence of urinary tract infection
    (UTI). One reason for low sensitivity is that it takes the bacterial enzymes at least
    6 hours to convert nitrates to nitrites in sufficient quantity for detection.

b   For both males and females, UTI can be usefully classified as upper or lower; in
    addition, as either complicated or uncomplicated. Urosepsis is a further category
    of UTI.[2]

    Lower UTI are those affecting the bladder and urethra (cystitis and urethritis),
    upper UTI involve the ureters (ascending UTI) or kidneys (pyelonephritis).
    Complicated UTI occurs in patients with culture +ve UTI and risk factors
    for complications or treatment failure, such as structural and functional
    abnormalities of the genitourinary tract, or underlying disease which increases
    the risk of acquiring UTI, suffering complications or failing treatment. More
    specifically, these risk factors include:

    ● hospital acquired UTI
    ● recent urinary tract intervention/instrumentation
    ● indwelling urinary catheter
    ● functional or anatomical abnormality of the urinary tract (e.g., incomplete
      voiding, vesico-ureteric reflux etc.)
    ● recent use of antibiotics

- symptomatic for more than seven days at presentation
- pregnancy
- diabetes mellitus
- immmunosuppression.

Uncomplicated UTIs occur in otherwise healthy patients who lack any of these risk factors.

Although the question does not directly ask, this patient would have an uncomplicated upper urinary tract infection (uncomplicated pyelonephritis).

c The most common pathogens in uncomplicated UTI are *E. coli* (80–90%) and *Staphylococcus saprophyticus*. Others include klebsiella, proteus, enterococcus and chlamyidia. Complicated UTI are characterized by antibiotic resistant forms of *E. coli*, pseudomonas, *Staph. aureaus,* enterobacter and serratia species.

d Uncomplicated upper UTI may be treated as an inpatient or outpatient, depending on the individual circumstance. The woman in this question appears to have marked systemic upset with fever and rigors, and her vomiting precludes oral treatment, at least initially. Thus:

- admit to a short stay ward
- symptomatic treatment with analgesia (codeine phosphate 30–60 mg PO/ IM), antipyretic (paracetamol 1 g PO/PR) and anti-emetic (metaclopromide 10 mg IV)
- IV fluids three litres a day until drinking well
- send urine for culture. If available, and the patient is acutely unwell, urine microscopy can confirm the diagnosis and give a gram stain result within hours, to guide initial therapy. Baseline electrolytes, renal function and inflammatory markers. Blood cultures where there is pyrexia or evidence of sepsis
- IV antibiotics. Previous recommendations have included the flouroquinolones (ciprofloxacin 500 mg IV BD) or a cephalosporin. But with increasing concern over antibiotic associated diarrhoea, many hospitals have moved to narrow spectrum regime of gentamycin (dose according to weight and renal function) and trimethoprim 200 mg BD
- early investigation with ultrasound of the renal tract, especially if renal function is impaired or there is any suggestion of renal obstruction as the cause.

General advice for women with UTI whether admitted or not should be to maintain a good fluid intake, to practice double voiding, and voiding after intercourse. Cranberry juice is reported a good treatment and preventative measure.[3]

Case 3

a The ECG (Figure 7.1) shows tall T waves, widened QRS complexes and flattened/ absent P waves; all consistent with a diagnosis of hyperkalaemia. Where P waves can be made out, the PR interval is long. As serum potassium further increases the PR interval lengthens and the QRS widens such that the ECG ultimately takes on a sinusoidal appearance. Once ECG changes of hyperkalaemia are apparent, the myocardium is electrically unstable and at risk of arrhythmia (VT/VF) and sudden death.

b Commonly encountered drugs which cause raised potassium include:

- K^+ sparing diuretics e.g., spironolactone, amiloride
- NSAIDs
- ACE I inhibitors (angiotensin receptor antagonists to a lesser degree)
- cyclosporin
- also, potassium supplements used overenthusiastically or without proper monitoring!

For completeness, common non-drug causes of hyperkalaemia are:

- renal impairment (usually severe or acute deterioration of)
- Addison's disease (mineraocorticoid deficiency gives high K^+, low Na^+)
- burns or rhabdomyolysis (K^+ release from cell necrosis)
- massive transfusion (K^+ leakage from ageing RBCs)
- metabolic acidosis (K^+ and H^+ are co-transported across cell membranes)
- don't forget artefact from haemolysis during venepuncture.

c A good proportion of patients with hyperkalaemia are asymptomatic, especially if it has developed over time. However, it is worth asking about tiredness, lethargy and palpitations, as well as about muscle weakness and paraesthesia, all of which are symptoms of raised potassium. Clinical signs are mostly neurological: decreased reflexes, weakness and even focal deficit. Patients with cardiac dysrhythmia may be haemodynamically unstable.

d Plasma potassium greater than 6.5 mmol/L and/or ECG changes of hyperkalaemia indicate the need for immediate treatment. Give:

- 10 mL of 10% calcium gluconate IV slowly. This acts within one to three minutes to stabilize myocardial cell membrane and can be repeated every 10–20 minutes until ECG abnormalities improve
- 10 IU of short-acting human soluble insulin with 50 mL of 50% dextrose IV infusion over 10–20 minutes. An insulin-dextrose infusion acts within 15–30 minutes to lower serum potassium by stimulating its intracellular uptake (though has no effect on total body K^+)
- nebulized salbutamol (2.5–5 mg) also promotes intracellular potassium uptake. Repeat doses can be given, though use with caution in patients with ischaemic heart disease
- calcium resonium binds potassium in the gut and reduces whole body potassium. It is given orally (15 g calcium resonium TDS) or as an enema (30 g PR).

Having treated hyperkalaemia emergently, we can now address any underlying cause such as renal impairment, Addison's disease or rhabdomyolysis. Always review medications and remove likely causative drugs (see above). It may also be worth giving dietary advice to reduce potassium intake – give up bananas! Persistently raised potassium despite the above treatment requires haemodialysis or haemofiltration on HDU/ITU.

Case 4

a Diclofenac 100 mg PR has been shown to be most effective in colicky pain and
   is the initial analgesic of choice in renal colic. A proportion remain with severe
   pain despite PR diclofenac and an intravenous opiate titrated to effect should
   then be used.

b Prior to having an intravenous urethrogram (IVU) patients with suspected renal
   calculi should have the following investigations:

   ● urinalysis reveals haematuria in 80–90% of patients with acute renal colic.
     The absence of even microscopic traces of blood in the urine does not rule
     out renal colic but should at least raise suspicion of an alternative diagnosis,
     especially if the presentation is not entirely typical of a renal stone
   ● urea, creatinine and electrolytes should be obtained routinely, prior to the
     administration of contrast medium, to avoid giving a nephrotoxic agent to
     already impaired kidneys
   ● an abdominal X-ray of the kidneys-ureter – bladder (KUB) is obtained
     before an IVU to visualize a calculus which would otherwise be obscured
     by the contrast of an IVU. Around 80% of renal calculi contain calcium
     and are radio opaque (2/3 calcium oxalate, 1/3 calcium phosphate) while
     cystine containing stones are semi-opaque and urate and xanthine stones are
     radiolucent). The utereopelvic junction, the pelvic brim (where the ureter
     crosses the iliac vessels) and the ureterovesical junction (narrowest point of
     ureter) are the most common sites of stone impaction.

   Further investigation of importance, but which do not need to be carried out
   prior to requesting an IVU are:

   ● urine for microscopy and culture looking for signs of infection
   ● the white cell count, again for any sign of infection
   ● serum calcium and urate.

c There is slow draining of contrast from the left kidney, consistent with partial
   renal obstruction and hydronephrosis throughout the length of the ureter, which
   suggests a stone in the ureterovesical junction.

d Indications for admission in a patient with suspected or confirmed renal colic
   include:

   ● evidence of renal tract infection; fever, high WCC, positive urine dipstick for
     infection
   ● severe pain refractory to appropriate analgesics
   ● calculi greater than six mm are unlikely to pass spontaneously
   ● abnormal renal function
   ● structural abnormalities of the renal tract, including solitary kidney or a
     transplanted kidney
   ● intractable vomiting
   ● complete obstruction of the kidney.

Approximately 75–80% of all stones will pass spontaneously (half of these within 24 hours) and only a small proportion require in-patient intervention. However, all patients allowed home with suspected or proven renal calculi, should be given urology follow up, ideally within a month.

e Abdominal CT (CT-KUB) is an alternative diagnostic modality to IVU in suspected renal colic. CT-KUB does not use contrast and so is preferable in patients with contrast allergy and those with significant renal impairment (remember contrast medium is nephrotoxic). In many hospitals, CT-KUB has superseded IVU as the first line investigation for renal colic due to speed, absence of nephrotoxicity and improved diagnostic accuracy (the radiation dose being roughly equivalent to the series of abdominal X-rays required for an IVU anyway!).

Case 5

a Urinary retention is a frequent problem presenting to the ED. Common causes are:

- prostatic enlargement (benign hyperplasia, carcinoma or infection – prostatitis)
- post-operative retention
- faecal impaction
- urethral stricture
- drugs: (anticholinergics, tricyclic antidepressants, antihistamines, alcohol)
- neurological (cauda equina syndrome).

In females, urinary retention may also be caused by multiple sclerosis, pregnancy in a retroverted uterus and atrophic urethritis.

b The usual site for insertion of a supra-pubic catheter is in the midline 2.5 cm above the pubic symphysis. Structures traversed are the skin, subcutaneous fat, rectus sheath containing the rectus abdominis muscle either side of the midline, the transversalis fascia, and finally the smooth muscle of the bladder wall. As the overfilled bladder distends upwards, it pushes the abdominal peritoneum out of the way of the trochar or aspirating needle thus, reducing the risk of bowel perforation.

c Supra-pubic catheters are generally cleaner than urethral catheters and easier to maintain. However, both types of indwelling catheter over time become chronically colonized. Many of the same urinary pathogens seen in non-catheter associated infection are found – E.coli and entrococcus species – but, in addition, candida, pseudomonas and gram +ve staphylococcus species often colonize indwelling catheters.

d Chronic catheter colonization leads to bladder bacteriuria and pyuria and frequently gives positive urinalysis, and urine culture, even in the absence of symptomatic urinary tract infection (UTI). Thus, in patients with chronic bacteriuria, symptoms are a better guide to the need for treatment than are urinalysis or even urine culture.

Table 7.1

Bacturia + the following symptoms	Treatment
Asymptomatic	No treatment is usually required
Symptomatic of UTI	Culture urine Change catheter Give a single dose of gentamycin
Systemically unwell/urosepsis	Admit and resuscitate as required IV aminoglycoside Trimethoprim BD orally If recently in hospital, think of resistant organisms (e.g. vancomycin-resistant enterococcus)

Case 6

a The blood tests demonstrate moderate renal failure as well as anaemia with thrombocytopenia. The WCC is also slightly elevated.

b The clinical picture and blood tests are typical of the haemolytic uraemic syndrome (HUS). HUS is a common cause of acute renal failure in younger children (three months to five years of age) and is characterized by the triad of:

- microangiopathic haemolytic anaemia
- thrombocytopenia, and
- renal failure.

It most commonly follows an acute gastroenteritis caused by either *E.coli 0157* or *Shigella. dysenteriae* and hence the association with bloody diarrhoea.

Damage to the endothelial wall of the renal vessels caused by bacterial exotoxin, triggers an abnormal coagulation cascade ending with platelet-fibrin microthrombi throughout the renal microvasculature. These microthrombi are the key event in HUS, as they cleave passing red blood cells generating the microangiopathic haemolytic anaemia, consume platelets leading to thrombocytopaenia and reduce renal perfusion, causing the acute renal failure characteristic of the disease. Importantly, these microthrombi do not use up clotting factors and HUS, therefore, does not lead to disseminated intravascular coagulation (DIC); in HUS the INR and APTT are within normal range.

Around 10% of cases are not associated with diarrhoea and, in these, the trigger may have been a respiratory illness or drugs such as penicillin or a sulphonamide.

c Other laboratory investigations we may expect to be abnormal in a microangiopathic haemolytic anaemia are:

- the diagnosis is pretty much confirmed by finding fragmented RBCs (schistocytes and helmet cells) in the peripheral blood film
- unconjugated biliribinaemia caused by intravascular haemolysis
- raised lactate dehydrogenase (LDH)
- urinalysis will show positive for blood (haemoglobin released from damaged RBCs) and protein
- urine microscopy will reveal red cell casts (a sign of renal tubulular insult).

d Most cases of HUS in young children are self-limiting and only good supportive care is required. From an ED point of view we would:

- admit the child
- treat dehydration with fluid replacement as required
- treat profound anaemia with blood transfusion
- treat bleeding with FFP (not platelets as this simply worsens microthrombi formation)
- involve specialist paediatricians, renal physicians and haematologists early in the patient's care
- steroids may be used under expert guidance
- avoid blindly treating the dysentery with antibiotics as this may promote *E.coli* verotoxin production
- In the smaller number of children with severe disease (20%) plasma exchange and dialysis may be used on the paediatric intensive care unit.

e Adults suffer a closely related illness to HUS called thrombotic thrombocytopaenic purpura (TTP). TTP differs from HUS in that endothelial damage and microthrombi formation is not limited to the kidneys and occurs throughout the body, causing multiple organ failure. Particularly affected, is the CNS where seizures, reduced consciousness and focal deficits are prominent. Fever, florid purpura and acute internal bleeding all occur in TTP but not HUS. TTP requires ITU care and urgent plasma exchange to avert death.

Case 7

a The patient in this question has acute-on-chronic renal failure. Remember that a creatinine even slightly above the normal range, indicates already substantial compromise of renal function as measured by glomerular filtration rate (GFR) and means the patient is highly susceptible to further renal insult from nephrotoxic drugs and/or acute illness. We are told this patient has heart failure and so is likely to be taking diuretics (furosemide or a thiazide), as well as an ACE I inhibitor or angiotensin receptor antagonist; all drugs which can impair renal function. Furthermore, he has recently been placed on a medication for what sounds like acute gout – probably a nephrotoxic NSAID. The question makes the point that it is essential to review the medications of any patient with a deterioration in renal function.

b Prompt initiation of treatment for acute or acute-on-chronic renal failure at presentation is essential to prevent further deterioration of function and shorten time to recovery. Thus, although patients with renal failure are admitted and typically require treatment spanning several days, the initial ED management is of considerable importance (just ask any renal consultant):

- consider post-renal obstruction; catheterize if in any doubt
- rehydrate with IV fluids (normal saline) at a rate appropriate to the degree of fluid deficit
- **STOP** all nephrotoxic drugs
- aggressively treat precipitants e.g., sepsis, diarrhoea and vomiting, CCF
- monitor urine output and start a fluid balance chart

- patients with this degree of acute renal impairment and/or oliguria require aggressive fluid rehydration, and should also have central venous pressure monitoring, to avoid fluid overload cardiac failure. This is especially important in patients with known pre-existing cardiac disease
- initiate appropriate investigation of the underlying cause: urinalysis, renal tract ultrasound and vasculitic markers
- refer early to the medical team and HDU/ITU team.

c The consensus seems to be that oliguria means urine output of less than 400 ml/day in adults or less than 0.5 ml/kg/hour in children.

d Indications for dialysis in acute renal failure are:

- pulmonary oedema
- dangerous hyperkalaemia despite medical therapy (K^+ >7.0)
- persistent metabolic acidosis of renal cause (pH <7.2)
- severe complications of uraemia (e.g., encephalopathy or pericarditis).

e Metformin is 90% renal excreted, and so accumulates in oliguric renal failure. Metformin associated lactic acidosis is a rare but serious side-effect of metformin excess and still today carries a high mortality.

Case 8

a Low plasma sodium leads to a relative hyposmolarity of the extracellular space and water moves into cells to compensate. This causes swelling and tissue oedema which, in most tissues, is of little importance but in the restricted volume of the skull, the resulting cerebral oedema causes rising intracranial pressure and neurological dysfunction, even death through cerebral herniation. Symptoms depend on the degree of hyponatraemia as well as the rate of plasma sodium reduction, though whether acute or chronic, a plasma sodium of below 110 mmol/L makes serious neurological sequelae likely.

b The first step in diagnosis of the cause of hyponatraemia is to assess the patient's fluid balance clinically.[4]

Table 7.2

Fluid status	Clinical signs	Interpretation	Causes
Hypovolaemic (dehydrated)	Dry skin and/or mucous membranes Reduced skin turgor tachycardia postural hypotension	Sodium and water are being lost together, either through the kidneys or via another route	**Renal loss** – diuretic therapy, Addison's disease, diuretic phase of renal failure. **Loss elsewhere** – burns, diarrhoea, high output fistulas, excess sweating from heat exposure or over-exercise
Euvoleamic	The absence of signs of hypo- or hypervoleamia	There is too much water in the body, relative to sodium	SIADH polydipsia
Hypervoleamic (fluid overloaded)	Peripheral oedema Raised JVP Ascites	Sodium and water are both in excess but with proportionately more sodium	Nephritic syndrome Liver cirrhosis Congestive heart failure

c We are told the patient is clinically euvolaemic and so, the cause of their low sodium is an excess of body water. Looking at the urine biochemistry, a urine sodium level greater than 20 mmol/L indicates the urine is concentrated and the urinary osmolality above 500 mosm/kg confirms this (remember the greater the osmolality, the more concentrated the urine). Thus, the urine is being concentrated, despite an excess of body water, indicating dysfunction of water homeostasis in the kidney – the diagnosis is a syndrome of inappropriate anti-diuretic hormone secretion (SIADH). SIADH has many causes including malignancy, lung disease, trauma, cerebral injury and neuroleptic drugs, but we know this patient has lung cancer and SIADH has a well-known association with small cell lung carcinoma.

d Hyponatraemia-induced seizures or coma require urgent treatment:

- give either 0.9% normal saline or 1.8% hypertonic saline IVI depending on hydration status and risk of fluid overload
- remember, 0.9% normal saline contains 154 mmol/L sodium and 1.8% saline double that. Whichever fluid is given, the rate of administration should not exceed 70 mmol Na+/hour and the initial aim is to raise plasma sodium by around 4–6 mmol, sufficient to reverse serious neurological sequelae. In a 70 kg adult one litre of 1.8% saline over six to eight hours will achieve this
- once out of danger, slow the rate of sodium administration and aim for a total correction of not more than 12 mmol/L in plasma sodium over 24 hours. Use frequent electrolyte checks to guide therapy. Continue until the plasma sodium is above 120 mmol/L and the patient is asymptomatic
- once asymptomatic patients with SIADH are treated by oral fluid restriction and treatment of the underlying cause, in this case malignancy.

e The danger in over-rapid correction particularly of a chronic hyponatraemia, is central pontine myelinosis, an osmotically induced demyelination syndrome affecting the pons. Central pontine myelinosis results in motor deficits of the limbs, speech and swallow. One-third of patients die, one-third have irreversible serious neurological disability and the final third recover – not good odds, so avoid in the first place!

Further Reading

1. Dawson C and Whitfield H. (1997) *ABC of Urology*. Wiley-Blackwell.
2. European Association of Urologists (EAU) Guidelines on urological Infections. (2010). Summary version found at www.uroweb.org/gls/pockets/english/ Urological Infections 2010.pdf
3. Scottish Intercollegiate Guidelines Network (SIGN). Management of Suspected Urinary Tract infection in Adults: A National Clinical Guideline. (2006) Found at www.sign.ac.uk/pdf/sign88.pdf
4. Longmore M, Wilkinson I, Davidson E, *et al.* (2010) *Oxford Handbook of Clinical Medicine*, 8th edn. OUP; pp 686–87.

8

ENDOCRINE EMERGENCIES

Chet R Trivedy

Introduction

Core topics

- thyroid disorder, including thyrotoxicosis
- diabetic ketoacidosis (DKA)
- addisonian crisis
- hyperosmolar hyperglycaemic state (HSS)
- hypoglycaemia
- acute pituitary apoplexy
- new onset diabetes.

Diabetic emergencies are common; other endocrine crisis less so. Be able to interpret the various metabolic abnormalities, on routine chemistry and arterial blood gas analysis, associated with each emergency, and be able to calculate the serum osmolality. Also be familiar with the changes in thyroid function tests with thyroid disease.

Case I

A 56-year-old female presents to the Emergency Department (ED) with a two-month history of a swelling in her neck (Figure 8.1), weight loss and exertional dyspnoea. Her observations are heart rate 120 bpm (irregular), blood pressure 136/90 mmHg, oxygen saturations 96% on air, temperature 37.8 °C.

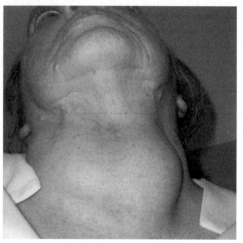

Figure 8.1 (see colour plate.)

a   Describe the abnormality in the picture (Figure 8.1).   [2]
b   Given her symptoms what biochemical abnormality is present and what is
    the most likely diagnosis?   [2]
c   If this lady became acutely unwell with high fever, tachycardia, raised blood
    pressure and confusion what serious complication of her chronic condition
    may have arisen?   [2]
d   How would you treat this complication (give four key steps. Doses of drugs
    used are not required)?   [4]
                                                                          [10]

Case 2

A 50-year-old female presents to the ED with a two day history of vomiting, diarrhoea and finally an episode of collapse at home. She looks unwell and is confused with low-grade fever and hypotension. The ED nurse shows you a medic alert bracelet indicating the patient has Addison's disease.

a   Apart from a medic alert bracelet, what clinical **signs** are associated with
    chronic adrenal insufficiency (give two)?   [2]
b   Outline the disturbances you expect to find on **routine** biochemistry in this
    patient.   [3]

c What additional non-routine blood tests might be requested when the patient is first seen. [2]

d Outline your management of this patient giving doses and routes, where appropriate. [5]

[12]

Case 3

A female 23-year-old insulin-dependent diabetic arrives in the ED by ambulance after 2 days of gastroenteritis where she has been unable to eat and has consequently stopped her normal insulin regime for two days in fear of going 'hypo'. She is dehydrated and quite lethargic. The following observations were handed over by the ambulance crew: pulse 118 bpm, blood pressure 100/70 mmHg and temperature 37.8 °C, respiratory rate 28/min and oxygen saturations of 98% on air.

a Give two immediate investigations you would perform? [2]

b Give three criteria for the diagnosis of diabetic ketoacidosis (with values). [3]

c Outline the ED management of this patient. [4]

d List six signs of poor prognosis in diabetic ketoacidosis (when referral to the ITU is indicated). [3]

[12]

ENDOCRINE EMERGENCIES – ANSWERS

Case 1

a The photograph (Figure 8.1) shows large diffuse lobulated swelling of the lateral neck. In this case it is almost unmistakably a goitre of the thyroid gland. However, it is always worth having in mind a differential diagnosis for neck swellings by location:

Table 8.1

	Midline neck swelling	Lateral neck swelling
Congenital	Thyroglossal cyst Dermoid cyst	Branchial cyst Dermoid cyst Cystic hygroma
Acquired	Pharyngeal pouch Plunging ranula Laryngoceole Sublingual dermoid cyst Laryngeal carcinoma	Thyroid mass Lymphadonapthy Carotid body tumour Carotid artery aneurysm Arterio-venous fistula (pulsatile)

b This woman has a diffuse goitre and is symptomatic – weight loss, breathlessness, tachycardia with low grade fever – which together suggest thyrotoxicosis, itself a hypermetabolic syndrome caused by elevated levels of triiodothyronine (T3) and free thyroxine (T4). Greater than 50% are due to Graves' disease (diffuse toxic goitre), an autoimmune condition where rogue IgG antibodies stimulate TSH receptors to cause thyroid overactivity and tissue growth within the gland.

c Thyroid storm is a serious complication of thyrotoxicosis which still carries a 10% mortality, if untreated. It arises acutely where excess physiological stress is applied to an already thyrotoxic state. Common precipitants are predictable:

- recent surgery
- infection
- manipulating the thyroid
- trauma or emotional stress
- contrast dye containing iodine
- withdrawal of anti-thyroid drugs
- thyroxine overdose.

The diagnosis of thyroid storm is sometimes difficult as many conditions – e.g., severe sepsis, meningitis, delirium tremens – can mimic. The Burch and Wartofsky scale is a validated scoring system that is used to predict the severity of the thyroid storm. It uses indices including arrythmia, heart failure, hepatic dysfunction, temperature, central nervous system dysfunction, as well as features in the clinical history to create a composite score. A score of more than 25 makes thyroid storm possible whereas a score greater than 45 makes thyroid storm likely.[1]

d Once recognized, early intervention in thyroid storm is critical and medical treatment is based on three key principles:

- first; counteract the peripheral effects of T3 and T4 to reduce the adrenergic symptoms of tachycardia and hyperthermia – (anti-pyretics, peripheral cooling, β-blockers, plasmapheresis). Propranolol is often favoured as it also inhibits peripheral conversion of T4 to the more active T3
- second; inhibit the release of further thyroid hormone (hydrocortisone, anti-thyroid drugs (propythiouracil/carbimazole)
- third; treat any ensuing systemic complications (treat underlying cause, shock and heart failure)
- finally, if medical treatment does not result in a clinical improvement within 12–24 hours then thyroidectomy should be considered.

Case 2

a Chronic adrenal insufficiency describes inadequate cortisol and mineralocorticoid production by the adrenal glands. It may be divided into primary adrenal insufficiency (Addison's disease), where the adrenals themselves are diseased or damaged, or secondary where the pituitary gland secretes too little ACTH, the hormone which stimulates cortisol production from the adrenals. Secondary adrenal insufficiency is more common by far, for example, in patients where long-term glucocorticoid therapy has suppressed the hypothalamic-pituitary-adrenal axis, and is mostly a deficiency of cortisol alone.

Primary adrenal insufficiency (Addison's disease) affects all ages, both sexes and has a number of clinical symptoms and signs:

Table 8.2

Symptoms	Signs
• Weakness/fatigue • Muscle aches/cramps • Weight loss • Abdominal pain • Mood disturbance • Craving for salt • Syncope	• Hyperpigmentation of the skin (particularly palmer creases, nipples and buccal mucosa) is present in 95% of patients with Addison's disease. This results from increased ACTH production by pituitary in an attempt to stimulate a defective adrenal gland; ACTH chemically mimics melatonin. • Postural hypotension • Low-grade fever • Reduced pubic hair in women

b Primary adrenal insufficiency also causes a number of characteristic biochemical abnormalities which may be exacerbated in adrenal crisis:

- hyponatraemia (aldosterone deficiency)
- hyperkalaemia (aldosterone deficiency)
- low blood sugar (cortisol deficiency – remember **gluco**corticoids have glucogenic effects)
- hypercalcaemia
- metabolic acidosis (multifactorial)
- in addition, this patient is dehydrated from enteral fluid loss and may have raised urea and creatinine.

c Request a random serum cortisol and ACTH level. Look for a low cortisol (<170 nmol/L) in conjunction with a raised serum ACTH level (>80 ngl/L) to support a diagnosis of primary adrenal insufficiency. The synacthan test, while required for the formal diagnosis of Addison's disease, is not so useful in the emergency setting.

d Acute physiological stress on a background of either primary or secondary adrenal insufficiency can provoke a potentially life-threatening adrenal crisis (acute adrenocortical insufficiency or Addisonian crisis). Features include diarrhoea and vomiting, cardiovascular collapse – postural syncope to frank shock – as well as altered mental status, confusion and coma. Precipitants include infection, trauma, surgery, dehydration and do not forget acute withdrawal from long term steroid use.

Key steps for managing Addisonian crisis in the ED include:

- replace missing cortisol with hydrocortisone 100 mg either IV or IM (most important)
- support the circulation with IV fluid resuscitation (1L normal saline : stat)
- monitor blood glucose and correct hypoglycaemia urgently (10% glucose IVI)
- correct serious electrolyte disturbances
- treat any possible triggers. Perform a septic screen (blood cultures, MSU, chest X-ray) and give broad spectrum IV antibiotics where there is any sign of infection.

For completeness: once the patient is stable, switch to oral steroids (prednisolone titrated to effect) and for primary adrenal insufficiency, add fluococortisone as a long-term mineralocortcoid replacement therapy (50–300 mcg daily). Patients should also be given counselling on how to prevent further crisis and written advice on receiving extra steroid cover prior to surgical procedures.

Case 3

a Unwell insulin-dependent diabetics should have the following tests straight away in the ED:

- capillary blood glucose measurement
- **venous** blood pH and bicarbonate measured using a blood gas analyser

- blood ketones (bedside ketone meters are increasingly available which can measure 3-β-hydroxbutyrate)
- urinalysis for ketonuria.

b Diabetic ketoacidosis (DKA) is the triad of ketonaemia, hyperglycaemia and acidaemia. Specific criteria for diagnosis exist using the bedside tests above[2] (Box 8.1).

Box 8.1 Criteria for diagnosis of diabetic ketoacidosis in an adult	
venous pH	<7.3
bicarbonate (HCO₃⁻)	<15 mEq/L
blood glucose	>11 mmol/L (or known diabetes mellitus)
ketonaemia	>3 mmol/L (or more than 2+ ketones on urine dipstick analysis)

c Treat DKA in **adults** quickly and aggressively. Give:

- IV fluids. Regimes differ but 1 L normal saline STAT followed by further bags over one, two and four hours is typical. Caution in the elderly and those with cardiac failure (central line required)
- serum potassium may be normal, low or high at presentation, but whole body potassium is always depleted. Unless measured serum potassium is high, supplement the second and further bags of fluid with 20–40 mmol K+ as indicated by hourly electrolyte checks aiming for 4.5–5.5 mmol/L
- start insulin therapy with a continuous insulin infusion at 0.1 unit/kg/hour (typically 7 ml/hour of the standard 50 ml actrapid in 50 ml 0.9% saline solution for a 70 kg adult). Aim for blood ketones to fall by at least 0.5 mmol/L/hour or venous bicarbonate to rise by 3 mmol/L/hour
- DKA is a hypercoagulable state – even in the young – give DVT prophylaxis (e.g. heparin 5000 units BD)
- central venous access and urinary catheter may be required to monitor fluid status
- look for, and treat, the precipitating cause. Perform a septic screen (blood cultures, MSU and chest X-ray) and give antibiotics where there is any sign of infection.

d Signs of severity and markers of poorer outcome in DKA, and indicating the likely need for HDU/ITU level care, include:

Table 8.3

Biochemical markers of severity	Patient factors indicating severe DKA
Venous pH <7.1	Reduced level of consciousness
Bicarbonate level below 5 mmol/L	Hypotension
Blood ketones over 6mmol/L	Hypoxia
Serum osmolality >320 mosm/L	Age >65 years
Hypokalaemia on admission (K+<3.5)	Significant cardiac or renal co-morbidity

NB: the treatment of DKA differs in important respects between adults and children. Refer to Question 8 in the Paediatric Emergencies Chapter for a question regarding the management of DKA in the child.

Further Reading

1. Burch HB, Wartofsky L. Life-threatening thyrotoxicosis. (1993) Thyroid storm. *Endocrinol Metab Clin North Am* Jun 22(2):263–77.
2. Joint British Diabetes Societies Inpatient Care Group. The management of Diabetic Ketoacidosis in Adults. (March 2010). Found at www.diabetes.org.uk/About_us/Our_Views/Care_recommendations/The-Management-of-Diabetic-Ketoacidosis-in-Adults/

HAEMATOLOGY AND ONCOLOGY

Mitesh Davda

Introduction

Core topics

- massive transfusion
- transfusion reaction
- sickle cell crisis
- common haemoglobinopathies
- haematological malignancy
- macrocytic anaemias
- pancytopaenia
- complications of anticoagulation (high INR)
- disseminated intravascular coagulation (DIC)
- neutropenic sepsis
- hypercalcaemia of malignancy
- complications of local tumour progression (superior vena cava syndrome, effusions, acute cord compression, raised ICP)
- symptom control/palliative care in advanced cancer.

Data for SAQs in haematology and oncology will involve interpretation of the full blood count (FBC) and clotting studies in relation to disease, along with understanding the significance of certain more specific investigations, such as the differential blood cell count, haematinics, B12, folate, reticulocytes, fibrinogen and FDPs. Also be familiar with the ABO blood groups, the key points of the clotting cascade and the common biochemical markers of malignancy. *The Oxford Handbook of Medicine* Chapter on haematology[1] is a good place to start, as is the *ABC of Clinical Haematology*[2]. Your hospital will also have policies for many haematological and oncological emergencies such as neutropaenic sepsis, managing excess anticoagulation, treatment of bleeding in haemophiliacs and massive blood transfusion, which will cover all the important points where national guidelines are scarce.

Case 1

A 28-year-old man presents to the Emergency Department (ED) with a 2-day history of malaise. He is currently being treated for acute lymphoblastic leukaemia. His observations at triage are temperature of 38.7 °C, heart rate 110 bpm, blood pressure 100/40 mmHg, oxygen saturations 99% on room air. Examination is unremarkable, except for the presence of a Hickman line. His full blood count result is below:

Hb	8.9 g/dL	Lymphocytes	0.3×10^9/L
WCC	1.0×10^9/L	Neutrophils	0.4×10^9/L
MCV	71 fL	Monocytes	0.1×10^9/L
Platelets	67×10^9/L		

a Describe the blood picture above. [3]
b In light of the clinical picture, what is the ED diagnosis? [1]
c What other relevant ED investigations are required? [5]
d Outline a suitable antibiotic regime and rationale for your choice assuming no drug allergies. [3]

[12]

Case 2

A 75-year-old man with known multiple myeloma presents with vomiting and thirst. On examination, he appears lethargic, has a pulse rate of 110 bpm, blood pressure 90/60 mmHg, dry mucous membranes, but no other specific findings. Blood tests reveal the following biochemical profile:

Na^+	142 mmol/L	Albumin	32 g/L
K^+	3.7 mmol/L	Calcium	3.35 mmol/L
Urea	9.6 mmol/L	Phosphate	1.32 mmol/L
Creatinine	140 mmol/L	ALP	97 u/L

a Describe two abnormalities in the blood picture given above. [2]
b What is the corrected calcium? [1]
c What ECG abnormality may be seen with this patient's corrected calcium? [1]
d Apart from lethargy, vomiting and thirst, give three other clinical features that may be seen with this patient's biochemical abnormality. [3]
e Outline your management of this patient. [5]

[12]

Case 3

A 26-year-old female, originally from Nigeria, presents with severe and worsening pain in her knees, hands and chest. She has a past history of homozygous sickle cell disease (Hb SS) and her only medication is hydroxyurea. Observations are temperature of 37.3 °C, pulse rate 100 bpm and blood pressure 125/80 mmHg. Her FBC is given below:

WCC	16.8×10^9/L
Hb	7.6 g/dL
MCV	105 fl
Platelets	670×10^9/L
Reticulocytes	16%

a What is the cause of the raised MCV? [1]
b How would you initially manage this patient? (Give four key steps) [4]
c Give two indications for blood transfusion in sickle cell disease. [2]
d On review, the woman is complaining of worsening pleuritic chest pain. Her respiratory rate is 24/min and oxygen saturations are now 93% on room air. You request a chest X-ray which shows a left lower zone infiltrate. What complication of sickle cell disease is likely to be present and what additional management is indicated? [4]
e Name three other complications of sickle cell disease related to vaso-occlusion. [3]

[14]

Case 4

A 58-year old man taking warfarin for atrial fibrillation is brought by blue light ambulance to the ED with three episodes of coffee ground vomiting and epigastric pain. Observations include a pulse of 120 bpm, BP 92/46 mmHg, respiratory rate 24/min. Examination reveals clinical shock with mild epigastric tenderness and meleana on digital rectal examination. His blood picture is given below:

Hb	6.2 g/dL
WCC	13.1×10^9/L
Platelets	440×10^9/L
INR	6.3
APTT	56 secs

a What is the diagnosis and complicating/contributing factor? [2]
b Why is the APTT also affected? [1]
c Give three treatments aimed specifically at reversing the effects of warfarin in an emergency (doses not required). [3]
d While carrying out your initial assessment your patient passes a large amount of dark red blood PR, drops his blood pressure further and his pulse becomes thready and difficult to palpate. Outline your approach to emergency massive blood transfusion in the ED. [6]
e During the course of resuscitation the patient required 10 units of packed cells before haemodynamic stability was obtained. Give four complications of massive transfusion. [2]

[14]

Case 5

A 16-year-old boy known to have haemophilia A presents to the ED minors area with an acutely swollen and painful left knee. He is well informed about his condition and reports several minor bleeding episodes needing brief hospital treatment since a toddler.

a Give two further questions you would ask this patient to further understand his clotting disorder and guide therapy. [2]

b What will the clotting screen show in this young man in terms of PT, APTT and platelet count? Is the intrinsic or extrinsic clotting pathway primarily affected in haemophilia A? [4]

c Outline your management of this patient. [5]

d What further treatment should be given for life threatening bleeds in haemophilia? [1]

[12]

Case 6

A 72-year-old man presents with a three day history of worsening pain down both of his legs, difficulty walking and faecal incontinence. On examination, he has reduced sensation around his perianal region and absent ankle reflexes.

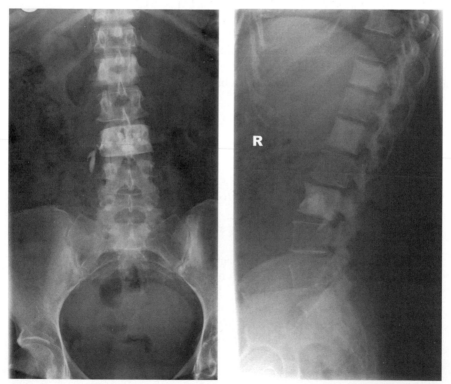

Figure 9.1

a What emergency does this man present with? Give a differential diagnosis
   of causes.   [4]
b Give four non-radiological investigations you could perform to help
   establish the cause.   [4]
c You obtain a plain X-ray of the lumbar spine (Figure 9.1). Describe the
   abnormalities on the X-ray.   [2]
d How would you manage this man now and what specialized treatment
   options exist for which you might refer him urgently?   [4]
                                                                        [14]

Case 7

A 25-year-old female presents to the ED with a three-day history of a swollen
red and tender left calf. She complains of no chest pain, shortness of breath or
haemoptysis. She has a past medical history of a previous deep vein thrombosis
(DVT) in the right leg two years ago, for which she was treated with warfarin for six
months. She is currently on no medication.

a List five components of the Well's clinical score for risk stratifying patients
   with suspected DVT.   [5]
b Outline the test characteristics of the ELISA d-dimer test with regard to the
   diagnosis of DVT in low and intermediate risk patients.   [2]
c What is the test of choice for diagnosing DVT in this woman?   [2]
d Name three **inherited** causes of thrombophilia which, when present,
   predispose patients to recurrent DVT.   [3]
                                                                        [12]

HAEMATOLOGY AND ONCOLOGY – ANSWERS

Case 1

a Abnormalities of the full blood count in this patient are:

- microcytic anaemia
- thrombocytopenia
- leucopenia with severe neutropenia (leucopenia is WCC $<1.0 \times 10^9$/L and severe neutropenia, neutrophils $<0.5 \times 10^9$/L).

b The working diagnosis is neutropenic sepsis of unknown source. This diagnosis is made where the neutrophil count is less than 0.5×10^9/L **and** there is either fever >38.5 °C, or >38.0 °C on two occasions one hour apart, or clear clinical evidence of sepsis.

A patient with neutropenic sepsis is at danger of rapid deterioration even if they present appearing quite well. The possibility of neutropenic sepsis should have been raised at triage and the patient placed in a sideroom for barrier nursing and prioritized for an ED doctor to see.

c At presentation, the cause of fever in a neutropenic patient is often not obvious. A detailed examination including chest, abdomen, CNS, skin and all IV access sites is required. This is followed promptly by baseline bloods and comprehensive septic screen performed in the ED. All culture samples should be obtained before antibiotics are given. In this patient, ED investigations include:

- clotting screen
- peripheral blood culture
- Hickman line culture
- swab throat, nose and any sites of skin or IV line infections
- urine culture
- chest X-ray.

d Bloods and a septic screen should be performed as soon as possible and once the diagnosis confirmed and appropriate cultures obtained, broad spectrum antibiotics started immediately – and ideally within one hour of presentation. Local policy dictates but typically a combination therapy of:

- gentamicin (5 mg/kg IV) for Gram negative cover
- tazocin® (4.5 gms IV) or ceftazidime (2 gms IV) which provides good Gram positive and anti-pseudomonal coverage
- If Hickman line sepsis or MRSA is likely then include vancomycin (1 gm IV)

Case 2

a The two biochemical abnormalities are hypercalcaemia (normal range calcium 2.15–2.65 mmol/L) and mild renal impairment. This blood picture is typical of multiple myeloma where proliferation of plasma cells in the bone marrow causes osteolytic lesions and raised calcium but normal alkaline phosphatase. In addition, the overproduction of immunoglobulins sludge in the renal tubules causing varying degrees of renal dysfunction from mild impairment to end-stage renal failure requiring dialysis.

b Roughly 40% of plasma calcium is bound to albumin. However, it is the unbound calcium which is physiologically active and this fraction varies with albumin concentration. Thus, the measured calcium is corrected for albumin concentration to give a better idea of how much physiologically active calcium is present in the plasma:

Corrected calcium (mmol/L) = measured Ca^{2+} (mmol/L) + 0.02 (40 – serum albumin [g/L]), where 40 g/L is normal albumin concentration.

An alternative approximate method is to add or subtract 0.1 mmol/L to the measured calcium for every 4 g/L that albumin varies from 40 g/L.

Thus, in this patient, the corrected calcium would be 3.51 mmol/L by the former method and 3.55 mmol/L by the latter method.

c Elevated serum calcium characteristically gives a short QT interval on the resting ECG.

d The features of hypercalcaemia are often taught as 'bones, stones , groans and psychic moans'.[1] To expand:

- bone pain
- renal calculi
- gastrointestinal symptoms are prominent – abdominal pain, nausea and vomiting, constipation
- confusion and in severe hypercalcaemia, coma
- depression and psychosis
- tiredness and lethargy
- polyuria
- dehydration and thirst.

e Corrected calcium of greater than 3.5 or symptomatic hypercalceamia requires urgent treatment.

- IV access and cardiac monitoring
- IV crystalloid bolus (500 ml normal saline to treat shock. Repeat until clinical improvement then follow with a regime of 3–4 L/day IV fluids
- diuretic therapy with furosemide (40 mg IV) lowers calcium
- bisphosphonate therapy (e.g., pamidronate, 60–90 mg IV, or zoledronic acid 4 mg IV)
- admission under Haematology for continued management

Case 3

a Reticulocytes are immature red blood cells (RBCs) and are produced in greater number in sickle cell disease to compensate for the shortened lifespan of the sickle RBC. Reticulocytes are significantly larger than mature RBCs and so when present in large numbers (10–20% as is typical in sickle cell disease compared to <1% in non-sickle patients) the MCV, an average of the volumes of all the RBCs in the blood, is consequently increased. Hydroxyurea also increases the MCV.

b This patient is having a vaso-occlusive crisis where increased numbers of sickled RBCs occlude the small vessels giving pain from tissue ischaemia. Initial treatment is aimed at treating symptoms and reversing the sickling process.

- oxygen to maintain saturations 94–98%
- prompt analgesia according to severity of pain. Use a pain ladder and use opiates where clearly appropriate
- ensure the patient is warm (cold is a precipitant of sickling)
- ensure adequate hydration with oral or IV fluid, as appropriate
- cross-match blood in case transfusion becomes required
- perform an infection screen with blood cultures, MSU and chest X-ray
- empirical antibiotics if infection is likely.

c Sickle cell patients routinely have a haemoglobin of between 6–8 g/dL and transfusion is not normally required at these levels and indeed may be counterproductive. However, there are two broad situations where blood transfusion is beneficial:

- where there is a sudden exacerbation of anaemia (Hb <5 g/dL) or cessation of reticulocyte production, blood transfusion is indicated and may be lifesaving. This may occur in aplastic crisis (switching off of RBC production by parvovirus infection causes rapidly plummeting Hb) or in sequestration crisis (RBCs lodge in the spleen and liver causing sudden reduction in circulating RBCs and Hb falling as low as 2–3 g/dL)
- where there is a need to dilute out the sickle RBCs with normal red cells to improve oxygenation and reverse severe vaso-occlusive crisis, such as the acute chest crisis, stroke or priapism. A HbS level below 30% is usually the target.

d The chest symptoms, signs of respiratory compromise, and chest X-ray appearance of pulmonary infiltrates point to the acute chest crisis in sickle cell disease. The acute chest crisis carries a 10% mortality, even with treatment and requires aggressive management. In addition to our initial measures in the ED, we should:

- correct hypoxia (15L via reservoir mask if required)
- give IV antibiotics with cover for atypical pneumonia (chlamydia and mycoplasma are common)
- give inhaled bronchodilators (nebulized salbutamol and atravent) if there is wheeze
- involve the most senior haematologist from the outset

- significantly hypoxic patients should be cared for on ITU. Deterioration requiring ventilation is common
- consider blood transfusion as guided by the haematologist.

e Further complications of vaso-occlusion in sickle cell are cerebral infarction, splenic sequestration and subsequent hyposplenism, dactylitis (swollen painful fingers), avascular necrosis of the femoral head and priapism.

Case 4

a The diagnosis is acute upper gastrointestinal bleeding complicated by excess anticoagulation.
b As well as affecting the extrinsic pathway of blood clotting, warfarin inhibits factors II and IX, which are measured by the APTT assay.
c Three treatments which may be given in an emergency to correct the INR in a patient taking warfarin are:[4]

- vitamin k (10 mg IV)
- fresh frozen plasma (15 ml/kg IV)
- prothrombin complex concentrates (e.g., Beriplex® 25–50 IU/kg IV).

Warfarin inhibits the vitamin K-dependent synthesis of active forms of calcium-dependent clotting factors II, VII, IX and X. Administering vitamin K overcomes this inhibition but requires time (24 hours or longer) for the synthesis of these clotting factors to recover. Fresh frozen plasma (FFP) contains all the clotting factors normally present in plasma while prothrombin complex concentrate (PCC) contains clotting factors II, VII, IX and X in a more concentrated form than FFP. PCC reverses the effects of anticoagulation immediately and is used for life-threatening bleeding in anticoagulated patients. It is expensive and in most UK Trusts requires approval from a haematologist.

d This patient is in hypovolaemic shock and peri-arrest; he needs blood urgently. Start with cross-matching for 10 units although this will take 40 minutes at least to arrive. In the meantime:

- you can give two units of O negative blood immediately from the ED fridge

⬇

- follow this with two units of group specific blood. Group specific blood has been matched for major ABO blood groups but not for minor antigens; however, it has the advantage of being available in 15 minutes

⬇

- fifth and subsequent units should be fully cross-matched and given as required

⬇

- massive transfusion causes coagulopathy as transfused red cells do not contain clotting factors. Thus as a rule of thumb give two to four units FFP for every four units of blood or packed cells. The haematologist may give further advice once contacted

⇧

- platelets are also diluted during massive transfusion and should be replaced as indicated by platelet counts. Again, the haematologist will advise regarding this and other blood products.

Many EDs have a massive transfusion protocol which once activated spells out the relative amounts of blood product to be requested as well as alerting the haematologist on call to give direct input. Guidelines also exist[6].

e Complications of massive transfusion include:

- worsening coagulopathy
- hypothermia
- thrombocytopenia
- hypocalcaemia
- transfusion reactions
- TRALI (transfusion related acute lung injury)
- infection with blood borne diseases.

Case 5

a In a patient with inherited clotting disorder, it is first important to establish the type of disorder present and therefore the clotting factor deficiency:

haemophilia A	(factor VIII deficiency)
haemophilia B	(factor IX deficiency)
von Willebrand's disease	(deficiency of von Willebrand's factor)

You are told this patient has haemophilia A already, so to answer the question, ask about the degree of factor VIII deficiency, this being divided into mild, moderate and severe as follows:

Table 9.1

Type of haemophilia A	% factor VIII activity
Mild	>5%
Moderate	1–5%
Severe	< 1%

The history given suggests he has a mild or moderate form of haemophilia as his disease began when he was a toddler (>1 year old) and he has had only minor complications to date. In patients with mild to moderate disease, it is useful to know their responsiveness to desmopressin (DDAVP) during previous haemorrhagic events.

b The clotting screen in haemophilia (A or B) demonstrates a raised APTT with a normal PT (INR) and normal platelets. Thus, the intrinsic clotting pathway is primarily affected. It is worth remembering the clotting abnormalities of the various coagulation disorders:[2]

Table 9.2

Disorder	Deficiency	INR/PT	aPTT	Bleeding time	Platelets
Haemophilia A	Factor VIII	N	↑	N	N
Haemophilia B	Factor IX	N	↑	N	N
Von Wille-Brands disease	vWF (required for platelet adhesion)	N	N	↑	N
Warfarin/Vit K deficiency	Vit K dependant clotting factors (II, VII, IX and X)	↑	N/↑	N	N
DIC	Clotting factors and fibrinogen	↑	↑	↑	↓

c Bleeding in haemophilia A patients may be seen as minor, major or potentially life-threatening. An acute haemarthrosis is considered a major bleed and is managed as follows:

- give symptomatic treatment in the form of appropriate analgesia early
- major haemorrhage in haemophiliacs requires administration of recombinant factor VIII concentrate aiming to give factor VIII levels >50% of normal
- involve the haematologist early in any significant bleed in a patient with clotting disorder (it is likely you will have to contact them to authorize factor VIII concentrate anyhow)
- pressure bandage and elevation may also help, but haemarthrosis in haemophiliacs are not aspirated as this merely promotes further bleeding.

For completeness, minor bleeds such as small cuts and peripheral bruises are treated with aggressive but standard measures: pressure and elevation. Intranasal desmopressin (DDAVP) increases factor VIII levels by up to four fold and may be sufficient to give haemostasis in mild to moderate haemophilia A. Potentially life-threatening bleeding is dealt with below.

d Potentially life-threatening bleeds such as after major trauma, intracranial haemorrhage, gastrointestinal haemorrhage and severe epistaxis requires factor VIII replacement therapy to 100% normal in addition to emergency measures to halt the bleeding.

Case 6

a This patient has cauda equina syndrome (CES), a neurosurgical emergency. CES describes the amalgam of features caused by mechanical compression of the lumbosacral nerve roots (the cauda equina) in the spinal canal below the level of the spinal cord. The most common of these features are:

- low back pain
- sciatica pain in one or both legs
- bowel and bladder dysfunction
- saddle anaesthesia (loss of sensation around the anus, central buttock and genitalia due to compression of the S3, S4 and S5 nerve roots)
- weakness and sensory loss in one or both legs

- lower motor neuron signs in the lower limbs (reduced tone and decreased or absent deep tendon reflexes).

A brief differential diagnosis of common causes of CES would include lumbar disc prolapse, vertebral collapse, multiple myeloma, lymphoma metastatic malignancy (e.g., from the prostate), primary tumour, abscesses, ankylosing spondylosis.

b Blood tests of value in distinguishing between the above, list of causes include a FBC and blood film (lymphoma and leukaemia), calcium and ALP (malignancy primary or metastatic) and PSA (raised hundredfold in prostate metastasis to the lumbar spine). Abnormal immunoglobulin bands on serum protein electrophoresis and urinary Bence-Jones protein are diagnostic of multiple myeloma.

c There is abnormal sclerosis of the bodies of T11, L1 and L3 consistent with metastatic disease of the lumbar spine (Figure 9.1).

d ED management of this patient with CES due to metastatic disease includes:

- symptomatic relief with analgesia as indicated by pain score, either oral or intravenous opioid titrated to response
- urgent imaging in the form of MRI of the lumbar spine is required to confirm the diagnosis of CES and demonstrate the causative lesion
- dexamethasone (16 mg/day) to reduce oedema around lesions and buy time
- once a more specific diagnosis is made from MRI imaging, specific therapy for CES caused by malignancy includes radiotherapy, chemotherapy or surgical decompression via laminectomy and requires referral to appropriate specialists – oncologist and neurosurgeon respectively.[7]

Case 7

a The Well's score[5] is used to determine the clinical probability of deep vein thrombosis (DVT) and involves scoring the patient using the following features:

- active cancer (treatment on-going, or within six months or palliative)	+1
- paralysis or recent plaster immobilization of the lower extremities	+1
- recently bedridden for >three days or major surgery <four weeks	+1
- localized tenderness along the distribution of the deep venous system	+1
- entire leg swollen	+1
- calf swelling >3 cm compared with the asymptomatic leg	+1
- pitting oedema (greater in the symptomatic leg)	+1
- previous proven DVT	+1
- collateral superficial veins (non-varicose)	+1
- alternative diagnosis (as likely or greater than that of DVT).	-2

Adding up the points, a score of three or more = high probability, one to two = intermediate, zero or less = low probability. Alternatively, a score of >two indicates DVT is likely and <two unlikely.

b D-dimer is a breakdown product of cross-linked fibrin in blood clots and may be measured quantitatively using an enzyme-linked immunoabsorbent assay (ELISA). The ELISA D-Dimer test has high sensitivity and negative predictive value for venous thromboembolism but poor specificity and positive predictive value. This test cannot, therefore, be used to diagnose DVT but is useful in ruling out DVT in patients of appropriate pre-test probability. Thus, patients with low or intermediate risk of and a negative ELISA D-dimer can have DVT safely ruled out, but high-risk patients should go straight to have definitive investigation for DVT with no role for D-Dimer testing.

c Compression Doppler ultrasound scanning of the deep veins of the leg.

d The most common inherited thrombophilic conditions include:

- factor V Leiden
- prothrombin mutation
- activated protein C resistance
- protein C
- protein S deficiency
- antithrombin deficiency.

Further Reading

1. Longmore M, Wilkinson I, Davidson E, *et al.* (2010) *Oxford Handbook of Clinical Medicine*, 8th edn. OUP.
2. Provan D. (2007) *ABC of Clinical Haematology*, 3rd edn. Blackwell Publishing.
3. Provan D, Singer C, *et al.* (2009) *Oxford Handbook of Clinical Haematology*, 3rd edn. OUP.
4. Hanley JP. (2004) Warfarin reversal. *J Clin Pathol.* **57**: 1132–9.
5. Scarvelis D and Wells PS. (2006) Diagnosis and treatment of deep-vein thrombosis. *Canadian Medical Assoc J.* **9**: 175.
6. British Committee for Standards in Haematology, Stansby D, *et al.* (2006) Guidelines on the management of massive blood loss. *Br J Haematol* **135**: 634–41.
7. NICE Clinical Guideline CG75 (2008) Metastatic Spinal Cord Compression.

INFECTIOUS DISEASE AND SEPSIS

Arif Ahmed

Introduction

Core topics

- sepsis (SIRS, sepsis and septic shock)
- fever in the returning traveller
- pyrexia of unknown origin
- infectious disease and the immunocompromised patient
- the UK immunization schedule
- tetanus and tetanus prophylaxis
- hospital acquired infection (MRSA, *C. difficile*)
- needlestick injury and blood borne viruses
- gastroenteritis and dysentery
- HIV and AIDS
- infective hepatitis
- malaria
- tuberculosis
- chickenpox
- sexually transmitted diseases.

From a data point of view, be familiar with requesting and interpreting the key diagnostic tests for different infectious diseases.

Case I

A 62-year-old man is brought into the resuscitation room having collapsed at home. He is confused with a GCS of 13. Other observations include temperature 34.7 °C, heart rate 128 bpm regular and blood pressure 77/47 mmHg. He has cool and cyanosed peripheries. You place him on oxygen, initiate fluid resuscitation and obtain an arterial gas sample, as well as requesting an urgent plasma lactate level and full blood count. The results of these investigations are shown below:

pH	7.21	Hb	11.7 g/dL
pCO_2	3.1 kPa	WCC	2.1×10^9/L
pO_2	10.8 kPa	Platelets	110×10^9/L
BE	−13.3	Plasma lactate	6.9 mmol/L
HCO_3^-	14.9 mEq/L		

a What are the four systemic inflammatory response syndrome (SIRS) criteria? Does this patient have SIRS?   [5]
b What is the normal range for plasma lactate?   [1]
c Define **severe** sepsis?   [2]
d Give three treatment 'goals' which are aimed for in the early treatment of severe sepsis.   [3]
e Which vasopressor drug is most suitable for use in hypotension associated with severe sepsis unresponsive to fluid therapy?   [1]
                                                                              [12]

Case 2

A 38-year-old zoo-keeper presents to the Emergency Department (ED) with a painful, red and hot patch of skin around a small oozing scratch-mark on the dorsum of his left hand. Otherwise, he feels well. He states that he was bitten by a bat at the zoo whilst cleaning a cage three days ago. He is not sure of his tetanus vaccination status. His observations are all within normal limits and he can move all his fingers normally.

a Name three common pathogens which can complicate animal bites in the UK.   [3]
b Give four steps in the management of this man's infected bite wound.   [4]
c How would you treat this man for tetanus prevention?   [2]
d Aside from tetanus, what other potentially fatal infection is this man at risk of having contracted from the bite?   [1]
e Give four factors which may place a patient with cellulitis at higher risk of treatment failure.   [4]
                                                                              [14]

Case 3

An 82-year-old woman is sent to the ED by her GP, with a two-day history of severe diarrhoea and crampy abdominal pains. She had been discharged home from the surgical ward four days earlier, following prolonged treatment for a post-operative wound infection, with broad spectrum antibiotics. She was discharged with, and is still taking, an oral cephalosporin.

a What organism is most likely responsible for this woman's diarrhoea?   [1]
b Other than a cephalosporin, give two further antibiotics most commonly
   associated with this diagnosis.   [2]
c Give two antibiotics with routes of administration that are effective in
   treating severe forms of this illness.   [2]
d What are the complications of this condition? (give three)   [3]
e Briefly describe how you would prevent cross-infection in the ED and
   reduce spread of this condition within the hospital.   [4]
                                                                              [12]

Case 4

A 32-year-old man who is known to have acquired immunodeficiency syndrome (AIDS), presents to the ED unwell with shortness of breath. Clinical examination reveals a respiratory rate of 30/min and bilateral fine crepitations on chest auscultation. You place the patient on oxygen and request a chest X-ray which shows the following: (Figure 10.1).

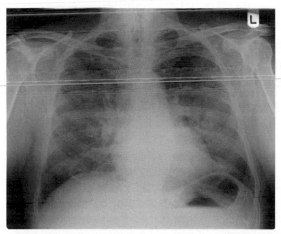

Figure 10.1

a Describe the findings on the chest X-ray (Figure 10.1). What is the likely
   diagnosis in this patient?   [3]
b Give the **three** typical clinical features of your diagnosis in **a.** above.   [3]
c What antibiotics do you know that are used to treat this condition (give two)?   [2]
d List four of the **most common** AIDS defining illnesses.   [4]
                                                                              [12]

Case 5

A GP refers a 40-year-old man to the ED for a malaria screen. The man has recently returned from missionary work on the Thai-Burma border and has become unwell with fever and lethargy. You arrange blood tests and place the man on the observation ward to await the results.

a What is the incubation period of *P. falciparum*?   [1]
b Give two abnormalities of the full blood count that you would expect to
   see in a patient with malaria.   [2]
c The malaria screen comes back positive in this patient with a parasitaemia
   of 3%. Aside from parasitaemia, what other clinical features or abnormal
   investigations indicate that a patient with *Falciparum* malaria requires
   inpatient care?   [5]
d When you return to review the patient, and inform him of the diagnosis,
   you find he has become drowsy and confused. What is your diagnosis now
   and give three key steps in your management of this condition?   [4]
                                                                                        [12]

Case 6

A 27-year-old backpacker is brought to the ED from a nearby airport, having become unwell while on stopover in a flight from Africa back home to Australia. She is drowsy but can answer questions when seen at triage, and has a temperature of 38.3 °C, a pulse of 128 bpm and blood pressure 100/55 mmHg.

a Give four questions that you would ask as part of a travel history.   [4]
b Give four common causes of fever that should be considered in a traveller
   returning from a tropical region.   [4]
c What immediate action should be taken when any seriously unwell patient
   recently returned from a tropical area presents to the ED?   [2]
d Give two clinical features on further examination that would raise suspicion
   of viral haemorrhagic fever in this patient?   [2]
                                                                                        [12]

Case 7

A staff nurse from one of the wards attends A&E out-of-hours having suffered a needlestick injury whilst taking blood from a 48-year-old patient on the ward who, according to the notes, is being treated for pneumonia.

a What features of the needlestick itself increase the risk of the transmission
   of blood borne viruses (BBV)?   [4]
b What relevant questions should you ask the staff nurse about her
   vaccinations?   [2]
c Give key steps in the management of the needlestick injury in this patient.   [5]

d The staff nurse asks you what the risk is of her contracting HIV from the
needlestick if the donor patient is HIV positive. [1]

[12]

Case 8

You are asked by the ED Sister to see a 31-year-old woman who has presented with
48 hours of violent diarrhoea and vomiting. She has not been abroad recently but
reports her partner had a milder form of the illness, and they both think it came
from eating a reheated chicken and rice dish the night before the illness began. She
is alert but appears dehydrated and continues to vomit into a bowl at triage. Triage
observations show she is afebrile but tachycardic with a pulse of 110 bpm and blood
pressure 110/65 mmHg. Her blood gas analysis and electrolytes are shown below:

pH	7.58
pCO_2	4.9 kPa
pO_2	12.9 kPa
HCO_3^-	34.5 mEq/L
BE	+13.4
Na^+	136 mmol/L
K^+	2.9 mmol/L
CL^-	76 mEq/L

a Give three causes of gastroenteritis which have incubation times less than
12 hours. [3]
b Interpret and explain the cause of the blood gas and electrolyte
abnormalities in this patient. [4]
c Give three signs on clinical examination which indicate severe dehydration. [2]
d How would you manage this patient? [3]
e Give two indications for antibiotic treatment in a patient with gastroenteritis. [2]

[14]

Case 9

A pregnant mother brings her four-year-old child to the ED with a rash. She thinks
it is chickenpox and knows there is nothing to be done, but is worried because she is
pregnant, and has heard about the dangers of chickenpox in pregnancy. The mother
herself remembers having had chickenpox as a child.

a Give three features of the rash seen in chickenpox. [3]
b What is the incubation time of chickenpox? [1]
c Give two serious potential complications of varicella-zoster virus (VZV)
infection. [2]
d Give five causes of immunocompromise that you would recognize as
placing a patient with VZV at higher risk of complications. [5]
e What advice will you give to this woman regarding being exposed to
chickenpox whilst pregnant? [2]

[13]

Case 10

The local out-of-hours GP service has urgently referred a six-year-old child to the paediatric ED with possible meningococcal disease. The child has had a febrile illness for the past day but this afternoon has become more unwell, is uninterested in food and drink and has developed a petechial rash over the lower legs. The paediatric triage nurse calls you immediately to see the child.

a What is the current immunization schedule for meningococcal disease
   in the UK?   [2]
b Your examination confirms a petechial rash over the child's feet and shins.
   Give four indications for **immediate** intravenous antibiotics in this child
   presenting with a petechial rash.   [4]
c What antibiotic should be administered (include routes and doses/kg)?   [1]
d A neighbour of the child in the question brings her daughter to the ED the
   next day worried that they might also contract meningococcal disease since
   the two children attended the same nursery the previous week. Outline how
   you would risk stratify and manage potential contacts of a confirmed case of
   meningococcal disease.   [3]
                                                                                [10]

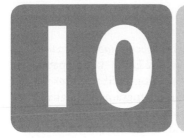

INFECTIOUS DISEASE AND SEPSIS – ANSWERS

Case 1

a The four systemic inflammatory response syndrome (SIRS) criteria are shown in Box 10.1.

Box 10.1 SIRS criteria	
Temperature	<36 °C or >38 °C
Heart rate	>90 bpm
Respiratory rate	>20 breaths/min **or** $PaCO_2$ <4.3 kPa
White blood cell count	>12,000 **or** <4,000 cells/mm^3

To be diagnosed with SIRS two out of the four criteria must be met. This patient meets all four criteria and so has SIRS.

b The normal level of serum lactate is below 2.0 mmol/L. Above 4–5 mmol/L is considered lactic acidosis and, when accompanied by metabolic acidosis, is evidence of septic shock.

c Sepsis is the presence of a presumed or known site of infection plus two out of four of the SIRS criteria (see above). **Severe** sepsis is sepsis with evidence of organ dysfunction.

d Goal-directed therapy is the recognition and aggressive early treatment of severe sepsis with specific attention to obtaining the following 'goals' within the first 4 hours of treatment:

- central venous pressure (CVP) ≥8 mmHg, (≥12 mmHg, if mechanically ventilated)
- mean arterial pressure (MAP) between 65 and 90 mmHg
- urine output ≥0.5 ml/kg/hr
- central venous oxygen ($ScvO_2$) >70%.

This involves central line placement and fluid boluses to gain a CVP >8 mmHg then vasopressors to obtain a MAP >65 mmHg, if this was not obtained by fluid therapy alone. Blood transfusion to obtain a haematocrit >30%, where the $ScvO_2$ was <70%, and further vasopressor therapy if the $ScvO_2$ remains <70% despite an adequate haematocrit and fluid resuscitation.

e Noradrenaline is the most often used vasopressor in septic patients. It increases peripheral resistance (vasoconstricts) through alpha-adrenergic stimulation.

Case 2

a Commonly complicating animal bites are the usual suspects, *Staphylococcus aureus* and *Streptococcus* sp. but, in addition, we have the gram −ve oral pathogens of the various animals: *Pasteurella multicoda* (cats and dogs), *Eikenella corrodens* (human bites), *Streptobacillus* sp. (rat bite fever) and other gram −ve bugs such as *Klebsiella*, *Bacteroides* and anaerobics like *Clostridium tetani*. Most often, a mixture of aerobic and anaerobic bacteria are found in infected bite wounds.

b Localized cellulitis from an animal bite in a systemically well patient can be managed as follows:

- swab the wound
- elevate in high arm sling to prevent swelling
- oral antibiotics with gram −ve cover (co-amoxiclav 625 mg TDS)
- review in clinic in 36 hours
- instructions to return if the infection is spreading or they feel unwell or feverish
- it is probably too late to wash out a three-day old wound.

c Tetanus vaccinations in the UK are given at two, three and four months followed by a pre-school booster, three years later and finally a 'school leaver' booster given between 13−18 years old. Persons who have received all five vaccinations have lifelong immunity. Where tetanus immunization status is unclear, or the patient is known not to be vaccinated, the following table sets out how to proceed:

Table 10.1

	Clean wound	Tetanus prone wound	*High risk* tetanus prone wound
Fully immunized (5 doses vaccine)	No action	No action	Human tetanus immunoglobulin (HTIG)
Incomplete vaccination or uncertain	Give booster now and refer to GP to check vaccination record and complete a course of tetanus vaccination, as appropriate	Human tetanus immunoglobulin (HTIG)	Human tetanus immunoglobulin (HTIG)
Non-immune or uncertain	Give booster now and refer to the GP for a complete course of tetanus vaccination	Human tetanus immunoglobulin (HTIG)	Human tetanus immunoglobulin (HTIG)

Note that tetanus-prone wounds are considered to be those requiring surgical treatment delayed by six hours, those involving devitalized tissue, those arising from puncture wounds, those with foreign bodies in situ, those caused by compound fractures and those contaminated with soil or manure. High-risk tetanus prone wounds are those with extensive devitalized tissue and/or heavily contaminated with soil, manure.

Mammalian mouths are colonized with *Clostridium tetani* and thus animal bites should be considered as tetanus-prone wounds, particularly puncture wounds from long teeth, although unless the bite has caused extensive devitalized tissue it should not be considered high risk. Ensuring adequate tetanus immunization is part of the routine care of bite wounds and the man in this question, who is unsure of his vaccination status, should be given both tetanus toxoid (booster) and human tetanus immunoglobulin (HTIG) 250–500 units IM, then referred to his GP to check his vaccination record, and complete his course of vaccination as required.

d Although rare in the UK, there is a potential risk of contracting rabies with recent evidence that some bats in the UK may carry a rabies-like virus, the European bat Lyssavirus. Workers handling bats should be fully immunized against rabies, but if not, you would need to administer rabies vaccine and human rabies immunoglobulin, half given IM and half infiltrated around the wound.

e A number of factors may place patients with cellulitis at risk of treatment failure and indicate the need for more aggressive treatment: admission, IV antibiotics and strict elevation. They include:

- swelling of the affected limb
- subcutaneous pus collection
- extremes of age
- diabetes mellitus
- immunosuppressive illness (HIV, leukaemia)
- immunosuppressive drugs (steroids, cytotoxic chemotherapeutics)
- poor diet/malnutrition.

Case 3

a Broad-spectrum antibiotics such as cephalosporins disrupt the normal intestinal flora leading to opportunistic infection with *Clostridium difficile* and resulting in antibiotic associated colitis. Elderly hospitalized patients are most at risk of *C. difficile* infection and symptoms are profuse watery diarrhoea, sometimes mixed with blood.

Diagnosis is by assaying for *C. difficile* toxin in the stool, either by looking for direct cytotoxicity of cultured cells or through immunoassay. Stool culture is of little value as non-cytopathic strains of *C. difficile* are often present.

b The most common antibiotics to cause *C. difficile* diarrhoea are:

- cephalosporins
- broad-spectrum penicillins – amoxicillin, ampicillin, co-amoxiclav
- clindamycin
- quinolones – ciprofloxacin, norfloxacin

c Most *C. difficile* diarrhoea will resolve with just stopping the offending antibiotics, but where symptoms are severe or prolonged, treatment is with metronidazole or vancomycin. Both metronidazole and vancomycin have high bioavailability in the stool when given orally, although for reasons of cost, metronidazole is first-line therapy. Metronidazole (but not vancomycin) can also be given IV where the oral route is not possible.

d Complications of *C. difficile* colitis include dehydration and shock, intestinal haemorrhage from pseudomembrane formation (pseudomembraneous colitis), toxic megacolon and perforation of the intestine causing peritonitis.

e Manage suspected *C. difficile* infection within the ED and hospital as follows:

- isolate patients in a sideroom immediately (do not wait for laboratory confirmation)
- initiate barrier nursing of suspected cases – use gloves and aprons at all times within the sideroom, especially when dealing with bed pans/faecal matter
- enforce strict hand-washing throughout the department or ward (alcohol gel alone does not kill *C. difficile* spores)
- minimize patient movements within the ED or ward and around the hospital between wards
- make sure all staff are aware, and that appropriate precautions are being taken by the ward, prior to patient transfer from the ED
- make sure all rooms and locations exposed to *C. difficile* are 'deep' cleaned (chlorine containing disinfectants reduce spore contamination) before re-use
- at all times, employ prudent antibiotic prescribing to reduce the use of broad-spectrum antibiotics and liaising closely with microbiologists whenever advice is required to do this.

Case 4

a The chest X-ray (Figure 10.1) shows bilateral perihilar pulmonary shadowing, the classical appearance of pneumocystis pneumonia (PCP). PCP is caused by the unicellular organism *Pneumocystis jiroveci* (previously known as *Pneumocystis carinii*).

b PCP typically presents with the triad of:

- fever
- dry cough
- exertional dyspnoea.

c Patients with severe PCP are treated with high dose IV co-trimoxozole (trimethaprim-sulphamethoxazole) as first line or with IV pentamidine if co-trimoxazole is not tolerated.

Milder disease can be treated with inhaled pentamidine, with combination therapy of trimethoprim and dapsone, or clindamycin and primaquine. Atovaquone may also be used in mild cases.

d A patient infected with HIV is considered to have clinical AIDS when their CD4+ cell count falls below 200 cells/microlitre and/or they acquire one of the so-called AIDS-defining illnesses. Patients with an AIDS-defining illness, should have prompt HIV testing (if they are not already known to be HIV +ve), although all of these illnesses **can** present in the absence of HIV. There are almost 30 AIDS-defining illnesses of which the most common are listed below.

- oesophageal candidiasis
- candida infection of the respiratory tract
- pneumocystis pneumonia (PCP)
- disseminated tuberculosis
- cytomegalovirus retinitis
- cerebral toxoplasmosis
- AIDS encephalopathy
- Kaposi's sarcoma
- cryptococcal meningitis
- Burkett's lymphoma
- invasive cervical cancer
- wasting syndrome.

Case 5

a The average incubation period of *Falciparum malaria* is 7–12 days but in some individuals it may be several weeks.

b Anaemia and thrombocytopaenia are common findings in the full blood count of a patient with malaria. The white cell count is rarely raised in malaria alone. Other blood test abnormalities include evidence of haemolysis – raised reticulocyte count, raised LDH and bilirubinaemia.

c Firstly, the following groups of patients are more at risk of the complications of severe malaria and should therefore be admitted:

- children under six years of age are particularly prone to cerebral malaria and seizures
- pregnant women are at high-risk of severe complications
- immunosuppressed patients.

Then, those with any signs of the complications of severe malaria should be admitted for aggressive treatment.

- cerebral malaria – reduced GCS, seizures, papilloedema
- acute renal failure – raised creatinine and/or discoloured urine (blackwater fever)
- pulmonary oedema – respiratory distress, hypoxia
- severe anaemia – haemoglobin <5 g/dL
- shock (known as algid malaria) – hypotension, acidosis, DIC.

In addition, the following are markers of poor prognosis in malaria and should prompt admission:

- hyperparasitaemia (>5% RBCs)
- hypoglycaemia (blood glucose <2 mmol/L)
- HCO_3^- <15 mEq/L
- elevated plasma lactate.

Finally, vomiting patients must also be admitted for IV anti-malarials until the oral route can be used.

d It is likely that this patient now has cerebral malaria, a serious complication of malaria with high mortality. Key steps in the management of this patient would be:

- check the blood glucose as hypoglycaemia is also a complication of severe malaria!
- CT brain to look for cerebral oedema and exclude other causes of reduced consciousness such as intracranial bleeding
- urgent IV anti-malarial treatment. Start therapy with 20 mg/kg quinine salt by intravenous infusion over four hours. Artesunate or artemether are as effective as quinine but may not be as readily available. Remember most *P. falciparum* is now resistant to chloroquine
- advice from the microbiologist or better, from a tropical diseases specialist, should be sought
- the patient should be cared for on the intensive therapy unit (ITU).

Case 6

a Important questions to ask a febrile or unwell patient who has recently returned from abroad include:

- which geographical regions and countries have been visited particularly in the previous six weeks? Did they visit rural, as well as urban centres, and be sure to ask about any stopovers en route, no matter how brief? Try to relate the onset of symptoms to the dates of travel to and from particular areas
- ask about previous immunizations, including those not routinely part of the UK vaccination schedule, such as hepatitis A&B, typhoid, yellow fever and rabies
- ask about malaria prophylaxis. Was the drug taken appropriate for the area visited? Was the patient 100% compliant with the regime? Did they also use mosquito netting and repellent
- ask about sexual contacts whilst travelling. Think of hepatitis B&C, as well as HIV seroconversion illness, and other sexually transmitted diseases in those with new or multiple partners whilst abroad
- explore the hygiene arrangements in the places they visited. Were they exposed to unsanitary conditions? If so, think of disease spread by the faecal-oral route
- ask about food and drink. Did they drink only bottled water or drink local water; eat local food or only self-cooked food; wash food before eating?
- any animal or insect bites sustained?
- were there any specific health warnings issued for the areas visited (e.g., for SARS, cholera)?

b A large proportion of returning travellers will have cosmopolitan infections such as viral upper respiratory infections, influenza, infectious mononucleosis, pneumonia or urinary tract infections.

However, of the illnesses imported into the UK from the tropics, the most common are the infective diarrhoeas including *E. coli* (known as Travellers' diarrhoea), shigella, giardia, campylobacter and amoebiasis. Also in this group, remember cholera still occurs in epidemics caused by poor sanitation and cramped conditions.

After the infective diarrhoeas, malaria is the next most common tropical illness, and should certainly be suspected and excluded in any febrile patient returning from a malarious area. Ninety per cent of *P. falciparum* malaria presents within two months although the benign malarias (*P. ovale*, *P. malariae* and *P. vivax*) may present over a year after infection.

Less common but should always be considered are the other tropical diseases causing systemic illness such as dengue fever, typhoid and amoebic liver abscess. Hepatitis A may be contracted via the faecal-oral route, virtually anywhere on the globe, whilst hepatitis B&C and HIV are contracted through sexual intercourse, sharing used needles or contaminated blood products. Where respiratory symptoms predominate, think of legionella or tuberculosis. Ricksettial illness such as typhus still occurs throughout Europe, the Middle East and Africa.

c Severely unwell travellers returning from tropical regions should be isolated in a negative pressure sideroom and barrier-nursed with full precautions (gloves, apron and facemasks) as soon as the situation is realized and until the diagnosis is established. Local isolation policies should be followed and the Health Protection Agency/local tropical diseases centre consulted immediately for advice.

d The viral haemorrhagic fevers (VHFs) include dengue haemorrhagic fever (tropical Australia, Asia, India and South America), Lassa fever (West Africa), yellow fever (Africa and South America) and ebola (sub-Saharan Africa). They are highly infectious viral illnesses which cause acute and rapidly progressing systemic illness, often ending in death. Key clinical features common to the VHFs include high fever, headache, pronounced rash, clinical shock and, as the name suggests, a bleeding diathesis.

Case 7

a Features of a needlestick injury itself which increase the risk of blood-borne virus transmission are:

- visibly contaminated needle
- hollow needle
- the recipient not wearing gloves
- deep skin penetration or penetration of a blood vessel in the recipient
- minimal time, from contamination of the needle, to needlestick injury.

b You should enquire of any needlestick recipient, about their hepatitis B vaccination record, and also when and what was the result of their last hepatitis B antibody titre. Ensure also that they are up-to-date with tetanus prophylaxis.

c Manage a needlestick injury as follows:

- immediately after the stick, expel blood from the stick site and wash thoroughly
- take a clotted serum sample from the recipient, and send to the lab for serum saving
- arrange for the ward doctor to consent and take blood from the donor patient and send it to the lab for Hepatitis B, hepatitis C and HIV testing
- if the recipient nurse is not adequately immunized against hepatitis B, give both hepatitis B immunoglobulin and a hepatitis B booster vaccination. If they are adequately vaccinated, no action is necessary on this front
- on the whole, post-exposure prophylaxis (PEP) for HIV is only recommended where the donor is known to be HIV positive or is at high-risk of being HIV positive. Where the donor is HIV negative, or their status is unknown, but they are considered low-risk for HIV, PEP is not generally indicated
- refer the staff nurse to the hospitals occupational health department the next day
- advise her that she should not carry out any exposure prone procedures until cleared by occupational health to do so
- encourage the staff nurse to fill out an incident report.

d The risk of HIV seroconversion from a hollow needlestick from a patient known to be HIV positive is approximately 1 in 300 (0.3%).

Case 8

a We can divide up the causes of acute infective gastroenteritis by their approximate incubation time as follows.

Table 10.2

Short (<12 hours)	Medium (12–48 hours)	Long (>48 hours)
Scromboid poisoning (occurs within an hour of eating toxin contaminated fish)	Salmonella food poisoning	Giardia lamblia (giardiasis)
	Clostridium botulinum (botulism)	Shigella food poisoning
Bacillus cereus food poisoning	E. coli 0157 food poisoning	Entamoeba histolytica (amoebic dysentery)
Staph aureus food poisoning	Yersinia enterocolitica	
		Campylobacter food poisoning
Vibrio cholera (cholera from contaminated water)	Viral gastroenteritis, including rotavirus and norovirus	Some viruses have long incubations (e.g., rotavirus)

b The blood gas abnormalities are a high pH with raised HCO_3^- and excess base indicating that a metabolic alkalosis is present. The pO_2 and pCO_2 are within normal limits. Causes of a metabolic alkalosis are given in Box 10.2.

Box 10.2 Causes of metabolic alkalosis

Loss of H+ ions through the gut	Vomiting, laxative abuse
Excess base ingestion	Hydrogen carbonate administration, excess antacids
Loss of H+ ions through the kidney	Diuretics, hyperaldosteronism
Severe hypokalaemia	H+ moves out of cells with K+ to compensate

The electrolytes abnormalities are a low potassium and a very low chloride (normal range of plasma chloride is 95–105 mEq/L). Hypochloraemia most commonly results from chloride loss from the gut in profuse vomiting; postassium is also lost in this way.

Thus, the blood gas and electrolytes demonstrate a hypochloraemic, hypokalaemic metabolic alkalosis caused in this patient by excess loss of gastric acid (HCL) from the gut in severe vomiting. It is the classic picture seen in neonatal pyloric stenosis, but can also occur in older children and adults, where vomiting is profuse and prolonged.

c We often talk about the signs of dehydration to look for in children but the same clinical signs also occur in the dehydrated adult and, are a good guide to the severity of fluid loss. Dry mucous membranes and postural hypotension are signs of mild to moderate dehydration. In addition, signs of more severe dehydration are:

- lethargy
- sunken eyes
- reduced skin turgor
- tachycardia
- mildly prolonged capillary refill time (CRT)
- reduced urine output.

As the degree of fluid loss progresses to frank shock, we see cold cyanosed peripheries, markedly prolonged CRT, weak or absent peripheral pulses, oligouria and changes in consciousness level.

d Key steps in the management of this patient are:

- isolate in a sideroom with barrier nursing
- initiate IV fluid therapy with normal saline. Severely dehydrated adults may have lost 10% or more of their total body fluid (i.e., five to eight litres). Aim to replace this over 48 hours
- set up a fluid input/output chart so that on-going losses can be calculated and replaced daily
- send a stool culture to the laboratory asking for culture as well as microscopy for ova and oocytes
- anti-emetics are beneficial in vomiting caused by gastroenteritis (metaclopromide 10 mg IV)
- cautious use of anti-diarrhoeals can slow stool fluid loss but are **contraindicated** in bloody diarrhoea, where salmonella or *E.coli* are suspected as the cause or where systemic symptoms are prominent. Use codeine phosphate IM/PO or oral loperamide
- admit under the medical team.

e Antibiotics are indicated where either a susceptible pathogen is isolated from stool culture, in patients with severe bloody diarrhoea such that treatable cause is suspected, and in the systemically very unwell or immunocompromised patient. Ciprofloxacin treats salmonella, shigella and campylobacter, while metronidazole treats amoebic dysentery; they can be used in combination if necessary.

Case 9

a Chickenpox is caused by the varicella-zoster virus (VZV). The typical rash of chickenpox starts as small papules which develop into fluid-filled vesicles over a flat erythematous base. The vesicles burst after 12 hours or so, releasing high numbers of VZV particles, then crust over. Successive waves of spots appear every 12–24 hours so that one characteristic of chickenpox is the presence of crops of lesions of different ages. Remember, it is a centripetal rash, meaning it starts on the trunk, and spreads to the limbs and face.

b Chickenpox is highly infectious with an incubation time typically around two weeks (8–21 days range). Transmission occurs by either contact with vesicular fluid of more commonly from respiratory droplets. It is generally considered that once all the spots are dry, and have scabbed over, the sufferer is no longer infectious.

c The vast majority of chickenpox occurs as a self-limiting illness of children, often with minimal systemic upset. However, there are a number of serious complications of VZV infection which are seen from time to time, particularly in susceptible groups (see answers to part d and e). These complications include:

● varicella pneumonia (approx. 1 in 500 adults with chickenpox. Carries 20% mortality)
● varicella encephalitis (approx. 1 in 4000 children with chickenpox. 15% mortality)
● disseminated varicella infection and sepsis (neonates and the immunocompromised)
● bacterial superinfection of chickenpox lesions (most commonly with *Staphylococcus aureus* and *Streptococcus pyogenes*) causing erysipilis, cellulitis, and impetigo
● shingles (herpes zoster). Dermatomal reactivation of VZV causes recurrence of rash and, in a proportion, a painful post-herpetic neuralgia, as well as the more serious complications of corneal ulceration from ocular involvement, and facial palsy with the Ramsey–Hunt Syndrome (50% do not resolve).

d Ever increasing numbers of patients with various forms of immunodeficiency present to the ED, and it is essential to recognize those with potential for more serious complications so as not to under treat. Think of immunodeficiency as either primary (inherited) or secondary (acquired):
   Secondary (acquired) causes are by far the commonest and include:

● diabetes mellitus
● cytotoxic chemotherapy (neutropenia)

- haematological malignancies
- immunosuppressant drugs (e.g., long-term steroids, methotrexate, tacrolimus)
- HIV and AIDS
- asplenic individuals (susceptibility to encapsulated organisms)
- severe debilitating disease (end-stage cancer, liver failure)
- malnutrition
- alcoholism
- extremes of age.

Primary or **inherited** causes are rare in the ED, and mainly due to deficiency of T and B cell function, such as IgA deficiency, X-linked agammaglobulinaemia, DiGeorge anomaly, complement deficiencies and severe combined immunodeficiency.

e Previous chickenpox infection or immunization confers lifelong immunity in healthy people from further infection. Antibodies to VZV pass across the placenta and so similarly protect the unborn baby. Thus, your advice to the woman in this question should be that neither they, nor their unborn baby, are at risk from being exposed to chickenpox during pregnancy.

However, chickenpox does complicate around 1 in 5000 pregnancies where the mother is not immune to VZV, and carries a number of serious implications: firstly, pregnant woman are at much greater risk of potentially life-threatening varicella pneumonia; secondly, VZV infection in the first trimester can lead to birth defects (foetal varicellar syndrome); and thirdly, mothers acquiring VZV in the days around the time of birth risk their newborn also becoming infected and consequent risk of neonatal disseminated varicella (25% mortality). Thus, chickenpox in pregnancy is taken seriously. Pregnant women with chickenpox should be treated with anti-virals (zovirax), whilst non-immune pregnant women, who are exposed to chickenpox, should be given varicella-zoster immunoglobulin (VZIG) to avert active infection. Newborns to non-immune mothers exposed to chickenpox in the seven days after birth, should also be given VZIG and, if they become actively infected, should be admitted for treatment with IV acyclovir due to the risk of disseminated disease.[2]

Case 10

a The meningitis vaccine (MenC) is administered at 3, 4 and 12 months in UK and is effective against the meningitis C serotype. The meningitis B serotype is more common in the UK but currently has no vaccine.

b NICE guidance on bacterial meningitis and meningococcal septicaemia[3] give five indications for immediate IV antibiotics in a child with a petechial rash:

- petechiae start to spread
- the rash becomes purpuric
- there are signs of meningitis
- there are signs of septicaemia
- the child appears ill to a healthcare professional.

c Intravenous ceftriaxone 80 mg/kg is the antibiotic of choice in a child with suspected meningococcal disease (cefotaxime 50 mg/kg IV is an alternative).[3] The question asks for the antibiotic treatment only, but for completeness, the wider management of a child with suspected meningococcal septicaemia would involve oxygen, IV fluid boluses to treat shock, and an early call for the most senior paediatric help available, together with a paediatric anaesthetist and/or retrieval team. A child with meningococcal septicaemia will get worse and is going to the PICU.

d The following should be offered antibiotic prophylaxis after contact with a confirmed (index) case of meningococcal disease:

- close contacts **residing** in the same house
- nursery contacts in the seven days prior to disease onset (high chance contact with respiratory secretions)
- kissing contacts
- healthcare staff that came into contact with respiratory secretions from the index case. Most others do not require prophylaxis, unless under specific advice from an informed microbiologist, or the Health Protection Agency due to a wider outbreak.

Rifampicin, ciprofloxacin and ceftriaxone can all be used for prophylaxis but only rifampicin (600 mg BD for two days in adults or 10 mg/kg BD in children over one year), is licensed for this purpose in the UK.

Further Reading

1. Immunization against Infectious Disease – 'The Green Book'. Department of Health. Chapter 30. Table 30.1. Found online at www.dh.gov.uk/greenbook
2. British National Formulary 55. (March 2008). Section 14.5. Page 661.
3. NICE Guideline CG102. (2010) Bacterial meningitis and meningococcal septicaemia. www.nice.org.uk/Guidance/CG102

PAEDIATRIC EMERGENCIES

Sam Thenabadu

Introduction

Core topics

- the floppy baby
- the child with stridor
- the septic child
- the febrile child
- the wheezy child
- croup
- bronchiolitis
- gastroenteritis
- urinary tract infections
- diabetic ketoacidosis in the child
- purpura and bruising in the child
- meningitis
- febrile convulsions
- the viral exanthems (measles, scarlet fever, rubella/german measles, erythema infectiosum/parvovirus B19 infection and roseola infantum)
- Kawasaki's disease
- scarlet fever
- the painful hip
- non-accidental injury.

In covering the whole of paediatric emergencies, a large variety of data types can form part of question stems. Laboratory blood results, capillary gases, X-rays, urine dip testing results, lumbar puncture findings and pictures of rashes, are all likely data stems considering the range of clinical scenarios given above.

Multiple national guidelines exist around which paediatric MCEM questions could be framed, and it is important to keep abreast of the latest guidelines pertaining to each topic, where appropriate. Finally, it is essential to be aware of the national resuscitation guidelines for children.[1]

Case 1

A four-year-old Asian boy presents to the emergency department (ED), with a 1-week history of abrupt onset fevers, despite antipyretics. His parents are worried that over the last 24 hours, the skin on his palms has begun to 'peel' off and that his lips look 'raw'. His observations at triage are: heart rate 160 bpm, capillary refill time (CRT) <2 sec, respiratory rate 24/min and oxygen saturations 97% on air.

a What is the likely diagnosis?   [1]
b Give five defining features of the diagnosis you give above.   [5]
c Specify four blood tests that may be deranged with this condition.   [2]
d Name the most significant cause of mortality with this condition and the
   investigations used to monitor it?   [2]
e Name one drug that can be initiated in the ED and one further drug that
   can be considered by the specialist team?   [2]
                                                                                    [12]

Case 2

A six-year-old boy comes to your ED with two days of a sore throat and painful neck. His parents are concerned that despite him drinking considerable amounts of fluid his tongue is still 'red raw' and that, over the last 12 hours, a very red sandpaper-like rash has appeared, spreading from his face down to his chest. He is pyrexial at 38.4 °C but all other observations are within normal limits.

a What is the likely diagnosis and causative organism in this boy?   [2]
b Describe two characteristic features of this diagnosis.   [2]
c Give two diagnostic tests that may be performed to confirm this diagnosis?   [2]
d What treatment should be started in this boy and how long should it be
   prescribed for?   [2]
e Give two early and two late complications which may arise from this illness.   [4]
                                                                                    [12]

Case 3

A two-year-old boy is brought to the ED by his mother having experienced three days of unrelenting fever, despite antipyretics. He appears pale to his mother, but has no other specific symptoms. He has no past medical history and is up-to-date with his immunizations. He is sleepy in his mother's arms, but wakes on stimulation. He is irritable when examined, has obvious nasal flaring and cries without tears.

Observations taken by the paediatric nurse indicate temp 38.4 °C, heart rate 165 bpm, CRT 3 sec, oxygen saturations 91% on air and respiratory rate 40/min. The child weighs 12 kg. His capillary blood glucose is 4.1.

a You consult the NICE guidelines for feverish illness in children to guide your assessment of this child. Give four components of the clinical assessment required by these guidelines, in order to risk stratify this child into either low-, medium- or high-risk. [2]

b Following your assessment, which risk category (low-, medium- or high-) does this child fall into? Give four clinical features from the scenario above to justify your answer. [3]

c According to the NICE guidelines, what investigations should be carried out for a child assessed to have the risk category you give in answer to part **b.** above? [2]

d The child becomes increasingly drowsy with a worsening tachycardia, capillary refill time (CRT) of greater than three seconds and rising temperature. You decide to give a fluid bolus and start maintenance fluids. What volume of fluid would you give as an initial bolus and what volume of maintenance fluid would you prescribe over 24 hours? [5]

e In addition to fluid management, give two further steps in your management of this child in the ED. [2]

[14]

Case 4

A mother brings her six-week-old baby daughter to the ED, complaining that she has been crying inconsolably for the last 24 hours, has had minimal bottle feeds and has felt very hot. She was born at 39/40, by uncomplicated spontaneous vaginal delivery, and went home the following day. She is yet to have her first immunizations. On examination, she has a weak, high-pitched cry, is mottled peripherally, but has no obvious rash. You cannot pinpoint a focus on examination.

Her observations are: heart rate 190 bpm, CRT three sec, respiratory rate 65/min and oxygen saturations 93% on air. Her temperature is 38.4 °C.

a Roughly what weight would you expect for a six-week-old child? [1]

b Given the clinical information above, which risk category, as defined by the NICE guidelines for feverish children does this child fall into? Give two clinical features of this baby's presentation that support your answer. [3]

c What mandatory investigations should be performed in the ED? [4]

d Give two indications for lumbar puncture in the ED? [2]

e The paediatric team ask you 'to cover this child for meningitis'. What antibiotics would you prescribe (doses not required)? [2]

[12]

Case 5

You are asked to see a five-year-old girl with a two-day history of worsening breathlessness and wheeze. She has been using her salbutamol inhaler via spacer, every four hours, but continues to worsen. Her father has given her ten puffs of salbutamol with no improvement. She has a past medical history of eczema and asthma for which she has never previously been admitted to hospital. She is mildly febrile with a temperature of 37.9 °C, heart rate 156 bpm, respiratory rate 38/min and oxygen saturations 92% on air.

a What are the indications for giving supplemental oxygen to children with exacerbation of asthma?   [2]
b Describe two clinical signs of acute severe, and two signs of life-threatening, asthma you will examine for in this child.   [4]
c List three medications (with doses and routes) you would give.   [3]
d On review, there is no improvement with your initial treatment. What is your next line treatment in the ED for unresponsive or worsening asthma in a young child?   [2]
e You perform a capillary blood gas on this patient as you are concerned she is deteriorating.

pH	7.02
pO_2	6.2 kPa
pCO_2	10.8 kPa
HCO_3	21.0 mEq/L
BE	−1.8
K^+	2.3 mmol/L

Interpret these findings and state your next management step   [3]
                                                                        [14]

Case 6

A five-month-old boy is brought to the paediatric ED by his parents with concerns that he appears breathless and is 'off his feeds'. His mother states that he is taking less than half his normal milk, and that his nappies are barely wet. On examination, he is alert, has a mild clear rhinorrhoea, a dry cough and some subcostal and intercostal recession. Auscultation demonstrates fine bi-basal inspiratory crepitations only. He is recorded to have a temperature of 38.1 °C and respiratory rate of 65/min by the paediatric ED nurse.

a What is the likely diagnosis in this child? Give a definition of this condition. [3]
b Name the most common organism to cause this illness.   [1]
c Give three clinical features which would indicate the child is suffering a severe episode of this illness and should be admitted.   [3]
d Name three treatments that could be initiated in the ED.   [3]
e This illness is highly contagious. Give two methods which may be undertaken in hospital to reduce transmission.   [2]
                                                                        [12]

Case 7

A three-year-old boy presents at two am with his parents who are worried about his cough. He has had a low-grade fever and rhinorrhoea for the last two days but has now developed a 'seal-like' or 'barking' cough. In front of you in the ED, he is alert and playing with his sister, but has an audible stridor. He is normally fit and well and up-to-date with his immunizations. You immediately think he has croup.

a Give three differential diagnoses of stridor in a young child (other than croup)? [3]
b What organism most commonly causes croup? [1]
c List the five clinical parameters of the Westley croup scoring system used to assess the severity of croup. [5]
d What is the first-line treatment (with dose and route) for croup in young children? [2]
e How would you respond if this child becomes more unwell with worsening stridor and significant respiratory distress (give any medications you would give and other actions you would take)? [2]
[13]

Case 8

A GP refers a six-year-old boy with suspected diabetic ketoacidosis to hospital by blue light ambulance. The boy was diagnosed six months ago with type I diabetes.

You meet the ambulance and, noting that the child is dehydrated and drowsy, record the following observations: heart rate 160 bpm, blood pressure 70/50 mmHg with CRT of 4 seconds centrally, respiratory rate 30/min and oxygen saturations 99% on oxygen. He scores a V on the AVPU score of conscious level. The capillary blood glucose is 18.8.

a Give three clinical **signs** of diabetic ketoacidosis in a child. [3]
b What are the normal pulse, blood pressure and respiratory rate for a child of this age? [3]
c What **initial** fluid resuscitation will you give? [2]
d After appropriate fluid resuscitation, outline the major **difference** between treating DKA in a child versus an adult. [2]
e Despite appearing better hydrated, the boy's mental state deteriorates and he is now responding only to pain. Other than airway measures, name two treatment options to address this deterioration. [2]
[12]

Case 9

A four-year-old girl is 'blued in' by the ambulance service to your ED after five minutes of violent shaking, which spontaneously resolved, before the paramedics arrive. Over the last two days, she has had a sore throat and persistent high fever. She has had no previous fits and only has a past medical history of eczema. On arrival to the ED she has stopped fitting and appears drowsy but cries normally when roused. Her temperature is 38.9 °C. Apart from scoring a V on the AVPU consciousness score, all other observations are normal.

a What is the likely aetiology of this child's seizure? [1]
b Between what ages is this type of seizure most commonly seen? [2]
c Assuming that the airway, breathing and circulation are stable, what two immediate bedside tests will you perform? [2]
d Which children with this diagnosis should be admitted under the paediatric team? [3]
e Assuming the child makes a full recovery in the department and discharge is considered appropriate, what advice will you give to the parents? [4]
[12]

Case 10

A 15-year-old boy presents himself to the ED with five days of sore throat, pain when opening his mouth to swallow, and over the previous day, a painful swollen scrotum. He has lived in the UK for three years but was born in Eastern Europe and is uncertain of his childhood immunizations. His casualty card indicates he is pyrexial and that a urine dipstick test shows only 2^+ of proteinurea.

a What is the likely diagnosis in this young man and give the underlying organism? [2]
b According to the UK vaccination schedule, at what ages should children be immunized against this condition? [2]
c Give a differential diagnosis for acute testicular pain and swelling. [2]
d Name four possible complications of this diagnosis. [4]
e Outline your management plan for this young man. [2]
[12]

Case 11

A 12-year-old boy attends the ED complaining that for three days he has had difficulty walking which began after a minor slip on a wet pavement. On questioning, however, his mother feels he has been limping on and off for nearly six months, despite regular painkillers. A colleague has requested an X-ray of the boy's pelvis (Figure 11.1) which you now review:

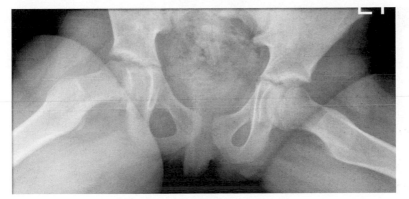

Figure 11.1

a What is the differential diagnosis of hip pain and difficulty walking in a child? [4]
b Looking at the X-ray above (Figure 11.1), what is the radiological diagnosis
   in this boy?   [1]
c Give three risk factors associated with this condition.   [3]
d What might you expect to find on examination of the affected hip?   [3]
e What is the management of this condition from the ED perspective?   [3]
                                                                                  [14]

Case 12

You are called to the paediatric area to see an eight-week-old boy with bruising
to the left side of his forehead. His father tells you he rolled from the bed onto
the floor whilst having his nappy changed twelve hours ago. The baby appears
alert but has a 5 cm boggy swelling on his forehead. His initial observations in
the department are all stable and the father, having been told the child appears
medically stable, is now keen to take the baby home.

a What do you suspect is the underlying cause for this presentation?   [1]
b List six potential factors which may put a child at risk of this underlying
   diagnosis.   [3]
c Name four types of fractures strongly associated with this underlying
   diagnosis?   [4]
d Name four professionals you would need to inform and involve in the
   management of this case?   [4]
                                                                                  [12]

PAEDIATRIC EMERGENCIES – ANSWERS

Case 1

a This child likely has Kawasaki's disease (KD), a systemic vasculitis that most commonly affects children of ages ranging from <u>six months to five ye</u>ars.

b It is important to be aware of the five defining features of Kawasaki's disease. Patients will have experienced a fever of abrupt onset for a minimum of five days and have at least four of the five following.[2]

- cervical lymphadenopathy >1.5 cm
- bilateral non-purulent conjunctivitis
- erythema +/- desquamation of the palms and soles
- oral changes including crusting of lips and 'strawberry tongue'
- widespread non-vesicular rash.

c Children with Kawasaki's disease may have the following abnormal blood tests, which, together with the typical clinical features above, help make the diagnosis:

Table 11.1

Blood test	Abnormality
Hb	Normochromic normocytic anaemia
WBC	Leftward shift
Platelets	Thrombocythaemia
CRP & ESR	Elevated
Bilirubin & LFT	Elevated

d Myocardial inflammation and coronary artery aneurysms are the most common causes of mortality following the acute episode of illness in Kawasaki's disease. ECG, echocardiography and CT angiography can all provide evidence of aneurysm formation, and regular follow-up by paediatric cardiologists is essential.

e Aspirin should be started in the ED. It will initially be at high doses for its anti-inflammatory properties then reduced to low dose for the anti-platelet effect. The paediatric team will then consider the use of intravenous Immunoglobulin.

Case 2

a The clinical vignette describes scarlet fever, an exotoxin-mediated bacterial illness caused by group A β-haemolytic streptococcus.

b Scarlet fever begins with abrupt onset fever and a focal bacterial tonsillitis or pharyngitis – 'strep throat'. After one to two days a white exudate appears on the tonsils and tongue giving the white furry tongue that then progresses to a red-raw 'strawberry tongue'. Local illness progresses to the systemic rash in around 10% of cases of strep throat where the infecting streptococci are of the exotoxin-releasing variety. The rash, beginning after around 48 hours, spreads from the face and neck to the chest wall and trunk, and is bright red or scarlet in appearance, hence the name scarlet fever. After one week, the rash subsides but the skin peels in a generalized desquamation.

c It is important to confirm the presence of group A β-haemolytic streptococcal infection in both a patient with scarlet fever and in suspected strep throat as this influences the duration of treatment; longer treatment of 10 days being required to prevent complications in confirmed cases. The two most commonly used investigations are:

- laboratory culture of throat swabs. These are 90% sensitive for group A β-haemolytic streptococcal infection of the throat and are generally most useful in acute illness
- antibodies specific to group A β-haemolytic streptococcus in the blood are detected with the anti-streptolysin O test (ASO titres) which is high in both acute illness and for weeks or months afterwards
- streptococcal antigen detection tests are also available. These are financially more costly.

d Scarlet fever (and streptococcal throat infection) is treated with a 10-day course of penicillin V (or erythromycin, if penicillin allergic). It is of paramount importance that if a streptococcal infection is strongly suspected, or at a later stage confirmed on culture, the full 10 days of penicillin is prescribed to prevent complications (see below).

e Well-recognized complications of group A β-haemolytic streptococcus infection include:

Table 11.2

Early complications	Late complications
Peritonsillar abscess	Rheumatic fever
Systemic sepsis	Post-streptococcal glomerulonephritis (main cause of
Toxic shock syndrome (toxin mediated life-threatening illness)	nephritic syndrome particularly in children)

Case 3

a The NICE guidelines for feverish illness in children under the age of five[3] recommend clinical assessment of the child's **colour**, **activity level**, **respiratory system** and **hydration status** in order to identify the likelihood of serious disease and allow categorization of the child as low-, medium- or high-risk. In addition, a series of '**other**' clinical features should be sought and which also influence risk stratification of the febrile child.

b The traffic light system – where low-, medium- and high-risk are given colour labels green, amber and red respectively – for identifying likelihood of serious illness is reproduced below.[3]

Table II.3

	GREEN – Low-Risk	AMBER – Medium-Risk	Red – High-Risk
Colour	Normal colour skin, lips and tongue	Pallor reported by carer	Pale/mottled/ashen/blue
Activity	Responds normally to interaction Smiles Awakens quickly Strong cry	Not responding to normal interaction Decreased activity No smile Wakes only with prolonged stimulation	Appears ill to healthcare professional No response to social cues Unable to rouse or maintain awake Weak high-pitched cry
Respiratory		Nasal flaring Tachypnoea: RR >50 6–12 months RR >40 12+ months Crackles on chest O_2 sats <95%	Grunting Tachypnoea: RR >60 Chest indrawing
Hydration	Moist mucus membranes	Dry mucus membranes CRT ≥3 secs Reduced urine output	Reduced skin turgor
Other		Fever > 5 days	Fever >38° <3 months Fever >39° 3–6 months
		Swelling of limb or joint Non-weight bearing	Non-blanching rash Neck stiffness Bulging fontanelle Focal neurology or seizures
		New lump >2 cm	Bile stained vomit

From this table the child in the question falls into the medium- or amber-risk category as they have decreased activity, nasal flaring, oxygen saturations of less than 95% and a CRT of three seconds.

c The table below outlines the initial investigations recommended for a febrile child over the age of three months in each of the risk categories defined by the NICE guidelines:[3]

Table 11.4

	GREEN – Low-Risk	AMBER – Medium-Risk	Red – High-Risk
Perform	Urine test for UTI	Urine test for UTI FBC CRP Blood culture Chest X-ray, if fever >39 °C **and** WCC >20 × 10⁹/L	Urine test for UTI FBC CRP Blood culture
Consider as guided by clinical assessment		Lumbar puncture, if child under 1 year of age	Lumbar puncture in any age child Chest X-ray Serum electrolytes Blood gas

d The question is alerting you to the deterioration in the child's clinical condition; he now appears in shock with cerebral dysfunction. An immediate fluid bolus of 20 ml/kg of 0.9% normal saline is required and following reassessment, repeated as necessary. The child in this questions weighs 12 kg and so the initial fluid bolus should be 12 kg × 20 mL/kg = 240 ml normal saline. If the child's exact weight is not available, remember it can always be estimated using the formulae (age+4) × 2. (Note that exceptions to this rule are paediatric trauma and diabetic ketoacidosis where fluid boluses of 10 ml/kg are used).

Once clinical signs of shock have improved, the child should be placed on paediatric maintenance fluids with the amount to be given over 24 hours is calculated as follows (Box 11.1).

Box 11.1. Calculating maintenance fluid requirements for children

100 mL/kg for the first 10 kg of the child's weight plus
50 mL/kg for the next 10 kg of weight plus
20 mL/kg for all subsequent kg weight

Thus, in this 12 kg child (10 kg × 100mL/kg) + (2 kg × 50 mL/kg) = 1100 mL IV fluid over 24 hours should be prescribed.
A common paediatric maintenance fluid is 0.45% NaCl + 5% dextrose.

---

e In addition to fluid management, a shocked child should receive oxygen and parenteral antibiotics (third generation cephalosporin – cefotaxime or ceftriaxone), acyclovir cover if there is any suspicion of herpes simplex virus infection, and urgent assessment by a senior paediatrician along with involvement of paediatric intensive care.

Case 4

a The formula weight = (age + 4 × 2) only works after the first year and so, when calculating the weight of children below the age of one, it is useful to have an idea of the following: typical weight at birth is 3–4 kg, at six months 6–7 kg and at one year 10 kg.

b This baby falls into the high risk RED category due to multiple concerning features (see answer to Case 3 above) including:

- mottled skin
- fever over 38 °C at age below three months
- respiration rate > 60/min
- weak high pitched cry.

c The NICE guidelines indicate that the mandatory septic screen in a febrile child under three months of age includes:[3]

- urine testing for UTI
- blood tests including FBC, CRP
- blood cultures
- a chest X-ray if respiratory signs are present (as in this case)
- stool sample if there is diarrhoea.

d Lumbar puncture should be performed in all babies under one month with a fever, and in babies of one to three months old who appear unwell or have a white cell count (WCC) $<5 \times 10^9$/L or $>15 \times 10^9$/L[3,4].

e Antibiotic guidelines for the treatment of suspected meningitis in children will of course vary from institution to institution, however, NICE recommends in the first instance use of a third generation cephalosporin (cefotaxime or ceftriaxone) along with the use of ampicillin or amoxicillin to cover Listeria in the under 3 month age group.[4]

Case 5

a Any child with oxygen saturations <92% on air, or signs of life-threatening asthma requires oxygen administered by either a face-mask or nasal cannulae and at a flow rate to achieve adequate oxygenation.

b Acute exacerbation of asthma is a common childhood presentation to the ED and thus an often encountered question. Asthma in children is managed according to the combined BTS/SIGN guidelines[5] which details protocols for the assessment and treatment of children below two years of age and those over two years. As with adults, assessment of the five-year-old girl in this question begins with looking for clinical features of severity and placing the attack into one of three categories; moderate, acute severe or life-threatening asthma using the table below.[5]

Table 11.5

Moderate exacerbation asthma	Acute severe asthma	Life-threatening asthma
SpO$_2$ > 92%	SpO$_2$<92%	As for acute severe asthma plus any one of :
Resp rate <40/min (2–5 yrs) <30/min (>5 yrs)	Resp rate >40/min (2–5 yrs) or >30/min (>5 yrs)	• Cyanosis
Heart rate <140 (2–5 yrs) or <125 (>5 yrs)	Heart rate >140 (2–5 yrs) or >125 (>5 yrs)	• Silent chest • Hypotension • Poor respiratory effort ($\downarrow$RR)
Able to talk in sentences	Unable to complete sentence in one breath or too breathless to talk or feed	• Exhaustion • Confusion or coma
Not using accessory muscles	Using accessory muscles	

If the child is old enough to perform a peak flow, PEF >50% best or predicted correlates with moderate asthma exacerbation, PEF 33–50% with acute severe asthma and <33% with potentially life-threatening asthma. Remember that a child's predicted peak flow is calculated using the child's height not their age or weight.

c To decide on appropriate treatment, you must first use the clinical information to decide into which category the child in the question falls: moderate, acute severe or life-threatening asthma. In this case, the information given indicates acute severe asthma without life-threatening features and initial treatment should be:

- salbutamol nebulizers – 2.5–5 mg repeated every 20–30 minutes
- ipratropium bromide nebulizers 250 mcg repeated every 20–30 minutes for the first two hours of treatment
- oral prednisolone 2 mg/kg (up to 40 mg) stat dose.

d Intravenous salbutamol, 15 mcg/kg given as a single bolus over 10 minutes, is second-line treatment in a child who has on-going severe asthma despite first-line treatments.

A continuous infusion of salbutamol may be given for further refractory asthma although this requires HDU/PICU level monitoring and care. As in adults, magnesium sulphate is increasingly being used to bronchodilate in children with acute asthma. However, at present IV salbutamol still remains the second-line treatment for children with asthma unresponsive to initial nebulizer therapy.

e A capillary or venous blood gas in severe asthma can give a clear indication of severity. The blood gas in the question shows significant respiratory acidosis with hypercapnia. This is likely to be secondary to a tiring child with a failing respiratory rate – they are exhausted and peri-arrest. Urgent senior paediatric and anaesthetic assessment is required with consideration of intubation and ventilation.

Case 6

a This patient is by far most likely to have bronchiolitis. Bronchiolitis is defined as 'a seasonal viral illness characterized by fever, nasal discharge and fine inspiratory crepitations and/or expiratory wheeze'. Fever is common in bronchiolitis but a high-grade fever should alert you to consider alternative diagnoses such as a bacterial pneumonia. Bronchiolitis mainly affects the 'under twos' with the peak incidence being between three to six months and a seasonal prevalence during the winter months of November to March.

b Respiratory Synctial Virus (RSV) accounts for 75% of the cases, however other common organisms include adenovirus, parainfluenza virus, enterovirus, followed by the bacteria mycoplasma pneumonia and *Chlamydia psitticai*. Nasopharyngeal aspirates (NPA) are performed for RSV immunofluorescence.

c Severe features of bronchiolitis which suggest admission as defined by the SIGN guidelines[6] are:

● poor feeding <50% of normal feeds
● history of apnoea from parents
● respiratory rate >70
● oxygen saturations <94% on air
● cyanosis
● severe chest wall recession.

Coryza is generally present for a few days before the lower respiratory symptoms of bronchiolitis appear. Bronchiolitis itself lasts a minimum of 72 hours before clinical improvement and the stage of illness should, therefore, be considered when deciding upon admission.

d The key symptoms to address in bronchiolitis are hypoxia and poor feeding due to breathlessness. Simple measures that can be readily initiated are supplemental oxygen by face-mask or nasal cannulae, nasogastric feeding for infants who cannot maintain adequate oral intake and IV fluids if there are signs of dehydration.

Despite frequent trials, there is no actual evidence for the use of nebulized bronchodilators such as salbutamol, ipratropium bromide or adrenaline and also no evidence for empirical antibiotics or systemic steroids in bronchiolitis.

e Bronchiolitis from RSV is highly contagious, transmitted by droplet infection and able to survive on surfaces for 6–12 hours. Healthcare professionals should wear gloves and aprons and fully decontaminate their hands with soap and alcohol gel washes. Patients with suspected bronchiolitis should ideally be isolated in the ED and, while on the ward, placed in cohorts of RSV proven bronchiolitis to reduce transmission to others.

Case 7

a Although croup (laryngotracheobronchitis) is indeed the most likely diagnosis in this patient, it is always important to consider the wider differential diagnoses of stridor in a young child, and exclude other causes by a thorough history and examination. Other causes of stridor include:

- inhaled foreign body
- epiglottitis
- bacterial tracheitis
- anaphylaxis
- laryngomalacia
- quinsy
- diphtheria.

b Croup is precipitated by para-influenza virus in 80% of cases and most cases occur below age six with peak incidence in the second year of life. The virus infects the upper airway respiratory mucosa causing swelling and airway narrowing. Most common is the 'barking' or 'seal-like' cough where the narrow airway is only evident at moments of particularly high airflow, but more serious airway compromise can occur with audible stridor during normal respiration and in a small number, progressing to respiratory distress and threatened life.

c The most commonly used croup scoring system is the Westley score (Box 11.2):

Box 11.2. Westley croup score		
Parameter	Grade	Score
Stridor	None	0
	audible with stethoscope	1
	audible without stethoscope	2
Retractions	None	0
	Mild	1
	Moderate	2
	Severe	3
Air entry	Normal	0
	Decreased	1
	Severely decreased	2
Cyanosis	None	0
	With agitation	4
	At rest	5
Consciousness	Normal	0
	Altered	5
Add up the scores and grade as follows:		
0–3 mild croup		
4–6 moderate croup		
>6 severe croup		

d A Cochrane review 2004[7] suggested that dexamethasone 0.15 mg/kg should be first-line treatment, being most effective if used within 24 hours of onset of croup symptoms. One dose is often all that is necessary as the half-life is 54 hours!

e The vast majority of patients that present to the ED with croup will only require a single dose of dexamethasone and will be suitable for discharge home. However, in the deteriorating child with severe croup and respiratory distress, emergent action must be taken to preserve the airway:

- First, call for experienced help. Most EDs treating children have a paediatric 'stridor-call' which, like a cardiac arrest call, immediately summons experienced paediatric, anaesthetic and ENT help to the child with a threatened airway
- In the meantime, give **nebulized** adrenaline at 0.5 ml/kg (up to 5 ml) of 1:1000 adrenaline. Further doses of nebulized adrenaline can be given as beneficial effects are often temporary.

Case 8

a Clinical signs helpful in diagnosing diabetic ketoacidosis in children are:

- clinical dehydration (dry mucous membranes, sunken eyes, reduced skin turgor)
- ketotic breath
- reduced consciousness (as recoded by AVPU or GCS)
- hyperventilation (compensation for a metabolic acidosis).

b It is worth having a rough idea of the normal physiological values of children at different ages, for example:

Table 11.6

Age	Heart rate (min)	Systolic BP (mmHg)	Respiratory rate (min)
Infant <1 year	110–160	70–90	30–40
2–5 years	90–140	80–100	20–30
5–12 years	80–120	90–110	15–20
>12 year	60–90	100–120	12–16

c Signs of shock (e.g., hypotension) are treated with a bolus of 10 ml/kg of 0.9% saline, repeated up to twice over a 30 minute period to restore circulating volume. This is one circumstance when 10 mL rather than 20 mL/kg is used in resuscitation, predominantly to avoid the risk of cerebral oedema. Thus, this child would receive (age+4) × 2 × 10 mL = 200 mLs of 0.9% saline as a bolus.

d Cerebral oedema is a common and life-threatening complication of DKA in children, the risk of which is increased with too rapid fluid administration. So while adults with DKA are aggressively fluid resuscitated, in children with ketoacidosis IV fluids are given much more slowly. Typically, the calculated fluid requirement of the child is replaced over 48 hours, or even longer if any signs of cerebral swelling are present. Another difference is to deliberately delay starting the insulin infusion until **after** the first hour of IV fluids, again to reduce osmotic shift of water into the brain.

e Once adequate circulation has been attained and hypoglycaemia excluded, any neurological deterioration in a child with DKA (at any stage in treatment) can be assumed to be due to cerebral oedema. Maintain the airway and treat with osmotic agents:

- either hypertonic 2.7% saline 5 ml/kg IV
- or mannitol 0.5–1.0 g/kg IV over 20–30 mins.

In addition, reduce the rate of fluid administration by one half and transfer to a PICU.

The British Society for Paediatric Endocrinology and Diabetes have an excellent online resource for the management of DKA in children[8] which covers all the points raised in this question and expands them into a comprehensive guideline.

Case 9

a This patient is likely to have had a simple febrile convulsion. This is defined as a seizure that is associated with a fever, is isolated, generalized, tonic–clonic lasting less than 15 minutes, and does not recur within 24 hours or within the same febrile illness.

b Febrile convulsions usually occur between the ages of six months and six years of age with a peak incidence of 18 months. They may recur in around 30%. Family history of febrile convulsion exists in 25% of cases although only four per cent have a family history of 'epilepsy'. An important point to note is that any child with a diagnosis of epilepsy must be assumed to be having epileptic seizures whether there is a fever or not.

c Routine observations are required such as heart rate, CRT, oxygen saturations and respiratory rate. The two other essential bedside tests are blood glucose measurement and temperature.

d Unwell children with more serious infection (including suspicion of meningitis) complicated by seizure should, of course, be admitted but consideration should be given to referral and admission of the following with simple febrile convulsion:

- more than one convulsion in 24 hours
- on-going lethargy after an appropriate post-ictal period
- unrelenting high fever despite cooling measures in the ED (antipyretics and exposure)
- many hospitals admit children with their first febrile convulsion, or at least require paediatric team involvement before discharge
- parental concern
- poor social circumstances.

e In practice, most children with simple febrile convulsion can be safely discharged. In arranging discharge parental advice is important.[9] Ensure that:

- the family understand what a febrile convulsion is and be reassured that there will not be any lasting damage and that this does not mean the child is epileptic
- the precipitant infection should be identified to the parents and the

appropriate treatment explained
- advice must be given on treating fevers at home – maintain hydration, remove excess clothing, give anti-pyretics if the child is uncomfortable
- If the patient has a further seizure lasting greater than five minutes they must call 999 immediately.

Note, another common question topic is the management of status epilepticus in children (febrile or otherwise), for which useful guidance and a protocol can be found on the South Thames Retrieval Service (STRS) website.[10]

Case 10

a The combination of symptoms leads to mumps as the most likely unifying diagnosis with paramyxovirus the underlying infective organism. The introduction of a mumps vaccine in the 1950s and the subsequent combined MMR have reduced the incidence considerably. However, concerns surrounding the vaccine have produced a resurgence in cases in the last decade.

b It is important to be aware of the chronology of the UK immunization schedule.[11] Certain illnesses may need to be considered more closely if inadequate immunization has occurred due to the child's age, immigration status or through parental choice in declining immunization.

Table 11.7

Age	Immunization
2 months	Diptheria/tetanus/pertussus, polio, HiB, pneumococcal
3 months	DTP, polio, HiB, meningitis C
4 months	DTP, polio, HiB, meningitis C, pneumococcal
12 months	HiB, meningitis C
14 months	Mumps, measles, rubella, pneuonococcal
3–4 years	Diphtheria, tetanus, pertussis, polio Measles, mumps and rubella
Girls 12–13 years	HPV (human papillomavirus as a cause of cervical cancer)
13–18 years	Diphtheria, tetanus, polio

From this table, we can see that the boy in question should have received the mumps vaccination – in the UK as part of the MMR triple vaccine – at the age of 14 months and a second vaccination at three to four years.

c Acute scrotal/testicular pain and swelling must always be promptly addressed in the ED. The most likely diagnosis in this boy is mumps orchitis although it is important to consider the full differential diagnosis and investigation with ultrasound of the testes arranged to exclude testicular torsion.

- mumps orchitis
- testicular torsion
- other infective orchitis (bacterial /chlamydial)
- hydrocele.

Mumps orchitis affect up to 50% post-pubertal boys with mumps and may be unilateral (70%) or bilateral (30%). It is often associated with fever, chills, vomiting and abdominal pains. Testicular swelling occurs rapidly and may be up to four times its original size; in many, due to the severe scrotal oedema, the testes, themelves, are not palpable at all. Although the symptoms are dramatic, and some degree of testicular atrophy does occur, sterility is actually quite rare.

d The more common complications of mumps are:

- parotitis (most often the cause of presentation)
- orchitis (and oophoritis in females causing pelvic pain).

and the more rare:

- pancreatitis (remember the 'm' in 'get smashed'?)
- mumps meningitis (and meningo-encephalitis)
- spontaneous abortion
- myocarditis
- hearing loss.

e Treatment is entirely supportive, however, often anti-pyretics are required and possibly intravenous fluid rehydration if parotitis is limiting oral intake. Orchitis is also treated symptomatically with bed-rest, analgesia, scrotal supports and occasionally prophylactic antibiotics.

Case 11

a The differential diagnosis of non-traumatic hip pain in children is a frequently asked question in both RCPCH and CEM examinations. While the differential is wide, it can often be narrowed to a likely cause using the age of the child and clinical history.

Table 11.8

Age	Diagnosis to consider
All ages	Osteomyelitis Septic arthritis Synovitis (viral, bacterial, idiopathic) Trauma Non-accidental injury
0–4 years	Congenital dysplasia of the hip Non-accidental injury
4–10 years	Avascular necrosis of the femoral head (Perthe's disease) Epiphyseal injury Leukaemia Juvenile arthritis
10–16 years	Slipped upper femoral epiphysis (SUFE) Occult sports trauma/stress fracture

b The 'frog's legs' pelvic X-ray (Figure 11.1) shows posteromedial slippage of the femoral epiphysis at the right hip. The clinical history and radiological findings are, therefore, consistent with this boy having a slipped upper femoral epiphysis (SUFE). It is three times more common in boys with a peak age of 13 years of age, and is more common in the left hip although 40% have bilateral changes.

c SUFE is most commonly associated with obesity (most sufferers are above the 95th centile for weight) combined with skeletal immaturity. Endocrine abnormality (hypothyroidism, hypogonadism, hypopituitarism), previous radiation of the pelvis and previously missed septic arthritis of the joint are also recognized causes.

d The clinical examination of a hip with SUFE will vary depending upon the chronology of the presentation:

- acutely, the child may not be able to walk or may walk with an altered gait with external rotation of the hip and trunk shift. On examination, hip movements including internal rotation and abduction are often limited by pain
- chronic presentations show the patient may have mild to moderate leg shortening and associated atrophy of the thigh muscles.

e Titrated analgesia and bed-rest are the two key management steps to be initiated in the ED, along with referral to the orthopaedic team, for whom definitive treatment involves surgical closure of the epiphysis with screws.

Case 12

a The most likely underlying diagnosis here is non-accidental injury (NAI). The child is presenting late and the history inconsistent with the age of the child: babies under three months cannot roll over unaided. Thus, a high degree of suspicion of NAI is warranted and further investigation by the ED and paediatric teams is essential.

It is worth being familiar with the NICE guideline on when to suspect child maltreatment which divides the categories of abuse into physical, sexual, emotional and neglect. Examples of each are given in Box 11.3.

Box 11.3. Categories of child abuse[12]	
Category of abuse	**Examples**
Physical	Hitting, shaking, biting, burning, poisoning and suffocation
	Factitious illness by proxy (previously Munchausen's by proxy)
Sexual	Oral, vaginal and anal penetrative acts
	Involvement in pornography, sexual photography
	Sexualized behaviour
Emotional	Persistent emotional ill treatment
	Making the child feel worthless
	Bullying
	Unrealistic expectations

continued

Neglect	The persistent failure to meet a child's physical and psychological needs
	Not providing food or shelter
	Not enabling medical care
	Emotional neglect

b All healthcare staff dealing with children must always be vigilant to the possibility of NAI and all ED notes should now have a safeguarding checklist to be completed for all patients attending under the age of 16. In addition, certain risk factors put children at greater risk of NAI, and these can be divided into parental-factors, child-factors and environmental factors:

Table 11.9

Parental factors	Single, teenage, psychiatric illness, previous NAI, substance abuse, domestic violence, multiple young children and unwanted pregnancy
Child factors	Premature, low-birth weight, first-born, pre-verbal and pre-mobile infants. Excessive crying
Environmental factors	Areas of high unemployment, areas with high crime rates, and reduced access to social services

c Certain fracture patterns raise the suspicion of NAI. It is crucial to consider if the fractures in children are consistent with the history and mechanisms of trauma described by the accompanying adult(s). In addition, the following bony injuries are certainly suggestive of NAI:

- any fracture in the pre-mobile infant
- rib and spinal fractures (almost pathogmnemonic)
- skull fractures
- long bone fractures
- spiral fractures
- metaphyseal chip fractures (bucket-handle)
- multiple fractures of varying chronology.

d In all cases where NAI is suspected, it is paramount to escalate and involve the necessary specialists. These would include the ED consultant, the duty paediatric consultant, along with the named consultant for child protection, the duty social worker, the midwife or health visitor and the patient's GP. The child should not leave the hospital until reviewed by a senior decision-maker responsible for cases of NAI and not without an appropriate plan of action and follow-up in place.

Further Reading

1. Advanced Life Support Group. (2006) *Advanced Paediatric Life Support: The Practical Approach*, 4th edn. BMJ books and Blackwell Publishing.
2. Newberger X, *et al.* (2004) Diagnosis, Treatment, and Long-Term Management of Kawasaki Disease. *Circulation*; **110**:2747–71.
3. NICE Guideline – Feverish illness in children – Assessment and initial management in children younger than 5 years (2007). www.nice.org.uk/cg47

4. NICE Guideline CG102. (2010) Bacterial meningitis and meningococcal septicaemia. *www.nice.org.uk/Guidance/CG102*

5. BTS/SIGN British Guideline on the Management of Asthma (2009) www.britthoracic.org.uk/ClinicalInformation/Asthma/AsthmaGuidelines/tabid/83/Default.aspx

6. SIGN Bronchiolitis in Children – A National Clinical Guideline (Nov 2006) www.sign.ac.uk/pdf/sign91.pdf

7. Russell KF, Liang Y, O'Gorman K, *et al.* Cochrane review. Glucocorticoids for croup. Jan 2000 (Updated July 2010) www2.cochrane.org/reviews/en/ab001955.html

8. BPSE. Recommended DKA Guidelines (2009) Found at www.bsped.org.uk/professional/guidelines/docs/DKAGuideline.pdf

9. Febrile Convulsions – BMJ Patient Advice Leaflet. (2009) www.bestpractice.bmj.com/best-practice/pdf/patient-summaries/febrile-seizures-standard.pdf

10. Status Epilepticus Guidelines – South Thames Retrieval Service (STRS), London (2008) www.strs.nhs.uk/resources/pdf/guidelines/seizures.pdf

11. National Immunisation Schedules www.immunisation.nhs.uk/Immunisation_Schedule

12. NICE Guideline CG89. (2009) When to suspect child maltreatment. www.guidance.nice.org.uk/CG89

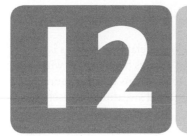

PSYCHIATRIC AND LEGAL EMERGENCIES

Mathew Hall

Introduction

Core topics

- the alcohol related admission
- assessing the self-harm patient
- acute psychosis
- rapid tranquilization of the acutely disturbed patient
- depression
- eating disorders
- consent and capacity
- compulsory detention and the Mental Health Act
- dementia
- Gillick competency
- do not resuscitate orders and living wills.

In this chapter are five SAQ style questions, covering a number of possible topics. While there is little data to interpret in psychiatric SAQs, we consider the following core knowledge highly useful both in the exam and day to day clinical practice.

- a solid understanding of symptoms, signs, and management of the main psychiatric illnesses (there are not many – schizophrenia, bipolar disorder, depression being most common)
- able to use correct terminology when describing symptoms of psychiatric illness (e.g., delusions, hallucinations, thought disorder, etc.)
- a risk assessment tool for use with self-harm patients (e.g., SAD persons score)
- the NICE guideline on Self-harm (2004)[2]
- components of the mental state examination (MSE)
- components of the mini-mental state examination (MMSE)
- criteria for capacity
- the Mental Health Act.

If psychiatry is not your strong suit then a good place to start is either the *Oxford Handbook of Emergency Medicine* (a little brief) or better, *The Oxford Clinical Handbook of Specialties* chapter on psychiatry.[1]

Case 1

A 54-year-old man with previous attendances for alcohol related problems is brought to the emergency department by his partner. He has been unwell with vomiting for the past few days and has been unable to drink his usual amount of alcohol. This evening, he has become confused and started sweating profusely. The following blood results have been obtained:

WCC	10.8×10^9/L
Hb	15.7 g/dL
MCV	105.3 fL
Na$^+$	137 mmol/L
K$^+$	3.9 mmol/L
AST	407 u/L
ALT	178 u/L
Bilirubin	43 μmol/L

a Explain the likely cause of the abnormalities in this patient's blood tests. [2]
b Give three features of acute delirium tremens (DT). [3]
c Outline the emergency department management of this patient. [4]
d What are the four questions of the CAGE questionnaire? [2]
[11]

Case 2

You receive a handover from the ambulance crew about a 38-year-old woman with a past history of depression who has taken an overdose of 24 of her own fluoxetine 20 mg tablets approximately 45 minutes previously, along with half a bottle of vodka. She is alert although appears distressed and tearful. Her alcometer reading is three times the legal maximum for driving. Otherwise, she appears asymptomatic.

a Give three steps in your medical management of this patient. [3]
b You are approached later in the shift by the nurse looking after the patient who says the patient is preparing to leave the department before completion of your treatment plan. Outline briefly how you would assess this patient's mental capacity to determine whether she can refuse treatment and self-discharge. [6]
c Give six features of a presentation with deliberate self-harm (DSH) which are widely recognized to increase the risk of completed suicide. [3]
d As well as a risk assessment, briefly name two further forms of assessment which should be undertaken as part of a comprehensive psychosocial assessment of the self-harm patient. [2]
[14]

Case 3

While on shift, you notice a commotion at the triage desk where three police officers are restraining a man in his twenties, whom they found behaving oddly after being arrested trying to gain access illegally to a television store. The man had said that he is hearing voices telling him to break into the store and smash all the televisions. He says that 'they' are hiding in the televisions and each time the picture changes this is evidence of 'their' presence. His speech jumps between seemingly random topics and makes little sense. The man is struggling violently and it is clear you need to intervene!

a What key features suggest the presence of psychosis in this patient? [3]
b Outline your approach to rapid tranquilization of the acutely disturbed patient. Give drugs with routes where included in your answer. [4]
c Give four causes of acute psychosis. [4]
d What features of the history and examination in a presentation of psychosis might make you suspicious of an organic (medical) rather than purely psychiatric cause? [2]

[13]

Case 4

An 17-year-old girl has been brought by her highly anxious parents. They say she has not been eating anything for months now and she is 'wasting away'. 'Just look at her doctor!'. The girl denies there is anything wrong and has refused to see her family doctor, though admits she is on a permanent diet. On examination, she is extremely thin and pale. The triage nurse has recorded her weight as 42 kg and her height as 1.73 cm on the casualty card.

a What is her body mass index (BMI)? [1]
b What are the four diagnostic criteria for anorexia nervosa? [2]
c Give four serious medical complications which indicate hospitalization for feeding may be required in patients with severe eating disorders. [4]
d After consultation with the psychiatric team, it is decided this patient needs emergency admission to hospital. However, she refuses to either see the psychiatrist or be admitted to hospital. The nurse in charge says you will have to 'section her'. Give two requirements for compulsory detention under current Mental Health Act legislation? [2]
e Which persons are required to make an application for a Section 2 under the Mental Health Act? [3]

[12]

Case 5

A 15-year-old girl attends your department early in the morning requesting emergency contraception. She had sexual intercourse the previous night with her boyfriend without any contraception. She is now afraid of becoming pregnant and even more afraid of her mother finding out she is sexually active.

a Briefly explain the legislation which allows prescription of emergency
contraception to a child below the age of 16 without parental knowledge.   [4]

b What other forms of medical treatment does this legislation apply to?   [1]

c Under what circumstances would it be appropriate to break confidentiality
of this minor?   [3]

d Give two medical contra-indications to the prescription of the emergency
contraception.   [2]

e You feel it is appropriate to prescribe emergency contraception to this
patient. What advice will you give with it?   [4]

    [14]

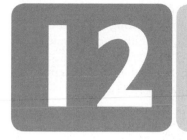

PSYCHIATRIC AND LEGAL EMERGENCIES – ANSWERS

Case 1

a Markedly raised mean corpuscular volume (MCV) with normal haemoglobin is consistent with chronic alcohol consumption. Also, the picture of a raised AST, raised ALT (AST rise greater than ALT rise) and raised bilirubin is typical of alcoholic liver disease.

b Around 5–10% of patients suffering alcohol withdrawal progress to delirium tremens or the DTs, an illness which carries a mortality of up to 30%, if untreated. It is, therefore, important to recognize delirium tremens as such patients require more aggressive management. The key features are:

- marked visual hallucinations
- confusion and disorientation
- autonomic hyperactivity (raised pulse, blood pressure and respiratory rate)
- uncontrollable course tremor.

Some patients may have seizures and or fever but these are not specific to the DTs.

c Important steps which should be taken in the early management of a patient with alcohol withdrawal and possibly delirium tremens include:

- place on a cardiac monitor; arrhythmia from acidosis and electrolyte disturbance is common
- think of hypoglycaemia and check the blood glucose level. If below 4.0 treat with glucagon 1 mg IM and/or an IV infusion of 250 ml 10% glucose. Hypoglycaemia is common with excess alcohol and may present similarly to acute withdrawal
- give vitamin B1 (thiamine) intravenously as pabrinex 2 high potency ampoules (total 250 mg thiamine) to treat thiamine deficiency and avert Wernicke's encephalopathy
- assess the degree of alcohol withdrawal, preferably using a validated scoring system, and prescribe a correspondingly appropriate regime of benzodiazepine treatment. The Clinical Institute Withdrawal Assessment (CIWA-Ar) scoring system[2] uses the following parameters to assess withdrawal: nausea and vomiting, tremors, anxiety, agitation, paroxysmal sweats, orientation, tactile disturbances, auditory hallucinations, visual disturbances and headache. Chlordiazepoxide 10–40 mg PO six hourly is most often used. Vomiting patients may need intravenous diazepam titrated in 5–10 mg doses until symptoms are controlled

- other supportive treatments include maintaining hydration with intravenous saline, treating electrolyte deficiency and stopping vomiting with anti-emetics (metaclopromide 10 mg IV) and a proton pump inhibitor (omeprazole 40 mg IV)
- look for co-existent illness, e.g., pneumonia, myocardial infarction, sepsis, pancreatitis etc. with blood tests, arterial gas analysis, ECG and chest X-ray. Treat what is found
- admit under the medical team. Critical care review if particularly unwell.

d The CAGE questionnaire is used to identify alcohol dependence and is particularly useful where patients are reluctant to give accurate details of their daily or weekly alcohol consumption (Box 12.1.)

Box 12.1 The CAGE questionnaire

Have you ever tried to **C**ut down your drinking?

Do you ever get **A**ngry when people talk to you about your drinking?

Do you ever feel **G**uilty about your drinking?

Do you ever take an '**E**ye opener' to get rid of a hangover in the morning?

Answering 'Yes' to 2 or more questions indicates likely alcohol dependence.

Case 2

a In general, the selective serotonin re-uptake inhibitors (SSRIs) of which fluoxetine is the most commonly prescribed are rarely harmful, even in large quantities. Amounts greater than 6 mg/kg are considered potentially harmful though in practice gram quantities are required to cause serious poisoning. This patient has ingested 480 mg of fluoxetine and appropriate steps in management would be:

- activated charcoal is indicated as the presentation is within 1 hour of ingestion, and as far as we have information, the patient is alert and not vomiting
- the National Poisons Information Service (NPIS) should be consulted online at Toxbase[3] and for fluoxetine overdose recommends routine blood tests, blood glucose level and an ECG
- Toxbase also recommends a minimum period of observation of 6 hours in asymptomatic patients. Thus, the patient should be admitted to a ward with regular nursing observations. Admission in this case also allows for 'sobering up' before further psychosocial assessment
- IV fluids might be given to encourage renal secretion of the drug, especially overnight when the patient is not drinking.

The National Poisons Information Service[3] do not recommend routine paracetamol and salicylate levels in patients who state they have not taken paracetamol or aspirin. Thus, while in many emergency departments it is commonplace to do so, this is probably an incorrect answer to this question.

b Mental capacity is assumed to be present in all adult patients and, therefore, to treat a patient against their wishes there must be evidence of incapacity. Incapacity implies an impairment of mental function or decision-making ability which renders the person unable to make an informed choice of whether to accept or refuse a particular treatment being offered. The criteria for capacity are set out in Box 12.2.

Box 12.2. Criteria for Capacity

The patient should be able to:
- Understand the need for treatment and exactly what the treatment entails
- Understand the main benefits and risks of treatment, as well as the consequences of not receiving treatment
- Be able to retain this information long enough to make a decision
- Weigh up the information and reach an effective decision

The decision should be free from coercion.

A patient judged to lack capacity and **who is likely to die or come to serious harm** in the absence of the proposed treatment, can be detained and receive emergency treatment against their wishes, under the common law doctrine of necessity, 'Common Law'. For the particular patient in the question, alcohol intoxication may be sufficient to impair her mental function and **temporarily** result in a lack of capacity, but on the other hand, she is unlikely to come to serious harm from the fluoxetine taken. The approach to capacity in the deliberate self harm (DSH) patient is discussed in detail in the NICE Guideline on Self-harm[4] and is well worth reading.

c The NICE Guideline on Self-harm[4] stress that it is NHS policy that everyone attending hospital with an episode of self-harm should receive a psychosocial assessment by trained personnel. An important part of the psychosocial assessment is an assessment of the risk of a future successful suicide attempt. There are a number of tools or scoring systems designed to facilitate risk assessment of suicide in the DSH patient, the SAD persons score being an example of one of the most widely used. However, they all rely on essentially the same set of factors relating to patient demographics, their mental state and features of the overdose attempt itself, which have been repeatedly shown to increase the risk of completed suicide. NICE summarize these as follows:

- age >55
- male sex
- unemployed
- socially isolated/without partner/living alone
- past psychiatric history (major depression, psychotic illness and/or in-patient treatment)
- previous attempts at suicide
- evidence of high intent (e.g., near fatal acts of self-harm such as drowning, hanging, jumping)
- painful, disabling or terminal physical illness

- expressions of hopelessness
- on-going high suicidal intent
- alcoholism.

d In addition, to a risk assessment, two further components of a complete psychosocial assessment are a mental state examination to look for psychiatric illness and a 'needs' assessment, which explores the patient's current life situation, along with the events which have brought them to this point of personal crisis. A needs assessment includes their social situation, personal relationships, current life difficulties and motivation for further self-harm, as well as uncovering problems with alcohol or drugs. From this information, a picture of the patient's vulnerabilities is gained and their needs clearly identified. A full psychosocial assessment, therefore, contributes to a management plan which addresses the future risk of serious self-harm, provides treatment of any psychiatric illness, and offers interventions to address patient needs and vulnerabilities; all designed to reduce further self-harming.

Case 3

a Correct terminology is required to answer this question. This patient believes that the picture changing on the television is evidence of the television being inhabited by other beings – this is a **delusion** (an unshakeable belief which is usually obviously false and, at the very least, is not in keeping with cultural norms). He is hearing voices telling him to do something – this is a **hallucination** (a sensory experience in the absence of corresponding stimulus). He also has a pattern of disordered speech and cannot carry through an intelligible train of thought – this is evidence of a **thought disorder**. Delusions, hallucinations and thought disorder are key features of psychosis; though remember psychosis is not a diagnosis in itself, but a clinical presentation.

b Before rapid tranquillization of an acutely disturbed patient, first check their blood glucose (sedation is not a treatment for hypoglycaemia!). Then, try and avoid it. Employ de-escalation techniques. Remove the patient to a quiet but safe area. Engage them openly in whatever they wish to talk about, whilst slowly reducing the level of restraint and presence of threatening stimuli. However, **do not put yourself or others at risk**. More often than not, this – and a bit of time – is all that is required to make a situation manageable. When required, give drugs proportionate to the situation. Mildly agitated patients can be given oral sedation in combination with 'talking down'. More disturbed un-cooperative patients may require parenteral sedatives; the intramuscular route is preferable, but where patient and staff are at risk from violent behaviour, as in this scenario, rapid intravenous tranquillization is the last resort.

In the exceptional circumstance when rapid intravenous tranquillization **is** required, do it properly. In very disturbed patients, and those with alcohol or drug dependence, large doses of sedatives can be required and their effects unpredictable. Key points are:

- the decision to use IV sedation should be made by senior staff. Full resuscitation equipment and facilities must be close to hand. All staff involved should be trained to immediate life support (ILS) level and, ideally, senior staff with airway management skills should be present and lead the team
- ensure adequate but not excessive restraint, to make drug delivery as safe as possible for you and the patient
- drugs recommended for use in rapid tranquillization of disturbed patients are lorazapam which can be given by any route or haloperidol, which is useful where psychotic features are also present. Other sedatives – diazepam, olanzapine and risperidone – are not recommended for this purpose
- as far as possible, titrate dose incrementally upward against response. Your goal is a calm patient, no longer posing a risk to themselves or others – not an unconscious or 'flat' patient. Allow time between doses to judge effect. Do not mix drugs
- closely observe tranquilized patients particularly for airway compromise and respiratory depression. Monitor blood pressure, pulse, respiratory rate, oxygen saturations and conscious level at frequent intervals
- Oh, and make sure you document your assessment of the patients capacity in the notes!

NICE has produced guidance entitled 'Violence. The short-term management of disturbed/violent behaviour in psychiatric in-patient settings and emergency departments' which covers all of the above points in more detail and contains an algorithm for rapid tranquilisation;[5]

c Acute psychosis can have both psychiatric and organic (non-psychological) causes:

Table 12.1

Psychiatric	Organic
Schizophrenia	Hypoglyceamia
Bipolar Disorder (mania)	Drug-induced (classically amphetamines and LSD 'magic mushrooms',
Severe depression	but also alcohol and cocaine)
Excessive psychosocial	CNS infection
stress	CNS trauma
	CNS tumour
	Electrolyte imbalances
	Post–partum
	Temporal lobe epilespsy
	Dementia
	AIDS

d The list of organic causes is longer than that of psychiatric causes (see Box 12.3.), although in practice, most psychotic patients presenting to ED have a background of psychotic illness (look for non-compliance with medication) or have a drug induced disturbance. It is important to identify the more unusual medical causes of psychosis as they require medical treatment rather than psychiatric care, at least at first. From the history and examination pointers to a medical cause include:

- no previous psychiatric history or **symptoms**
- evidence of a CNS illness (e.g., fever, meningeal signs, seizure, focal neurology)
- evidence of acute or chronic head injury
- evidence in the history or examination of chronic alcohol or recent illicit drug use
- reduced GCS or clouding of consciousness
- also remember, visual and tactile hallucinations are manifestations of organic pathology. The hallucinations of schizophrenia and mania are predominantly auditory or somatic.

Case 4

a Body mass index (BMI) is calculated using a person's weight and height (Box 12.3):

> **Box 12.3** Calculating body mass index (BMI)
>
> BMI (kg/m^2) = weight (kg)/height^2(m^2)
> Thus, this patient has a BMI of 42 kg/1.73^{2}m^2 = 42/3 = 14.0 kg/m^2
> Normal BMI is between 18.5 and 25.
>
> She is severely underweight.

b Anorexia nervosa is defined by the following four diagnostic criteria:

- refusal to eat resulting in unhealthy weight loss and BMI <17 (or <85% of expected weight for height, sex, age and population)
- intense fear of becoming fat, even though underweight
- delusional belief they are overweight, even when dramatically thin
- amenorrhea for longer than three consecutive menstrual cycles (for post-menarche females).

c Severe malnourishment has a dramatic effect on appearance with cachexia, hair loss, brittle nails and on mood with depression and para-suicide common. However, medical complications which need to be looked for and indicate the need for emergency treatment include:

- recurrent fainting
- hypokalaemia
- hypoglycaemia
- tachyarrythmia or long Q-T interval (low K^+/Mg^{2+} predispose)
- cardiovascular compromise (bradycardia and/or hypotension)
- extreme lethargy
- irregular menstrual periods.

d Only persons with a defined mental disorder may be detained using Mental Health Act (MHA) legislation.[6] The Mental Health Act (1983) was amended in 2007 and the new 2007 Act, defines mental disorder as any 'disorder or disability of the mind' but crucially – and this is where it differs from the 1983 act – excludes those with drug or alcohol dependence and those with learning disability. In addition, the act states that hospital detention **must** be required for the assessment and/or treatment of the patient's mental disorder. This implies: firstly, all means of treating the patient on a voluntary basis have been exhausted and only compulsory treatment remains; secondly, that compulsory treatment is in the best interests of the patient or required where the patient is a danger to themselves or others; and finally, that it is the mental disorder alone which is to be treated (although Section 2 does allow for the treatment of any physical disorder which has arisen as a direct result of the mental disorder).

e   Section 2 of the MHA is used where there is a need to admit for assessment. Three separate persons are required:

- an approved social worker (or a nearest relative) may make the application
- a doctor approved under guidance set out in the MHA, in practice a senior psychiatrist
- a doctor who is familiar with the patient in a professional capacity, i.e. their GP (where this is not possible the second doctor should also be 'approved' under the MHA).

Assembling the people and completing the paperwork for an application for compulsory detention takes time and, where there is a need for more urgent action, there is a Section 4 of the MHA which allows for up to 72 hours detention for emergency treatment and requires only an approved social worker (or nearest relative) and the recommendation of a single doctor. In practice, in the A&E department, it is Common Law under which detention and emergency treatment of both physical and psychiatric illness is given where deemed absolutely necessary.

Case 5

a   In 1985 an activist parent, Victoria Gillick, challenged the right of the doctor to prescribe the oral contraceptive to her daughter under the age of 16, without her knowledge or consent. The case (*Gillick vs W Norfolk and Wisbech AHA*) was referred to the House of Lords, which decided against Victoria Gillick and established the concept of Gillick competency, a concept summarized by Lord Scarman as 'the parental right yields to the child's right to make his own decisions when he reaches a sufficient understanding and intelligence to be capable of making up his own mind on the matter in question'. Thus, a minor who is judged sufficiently mature to understand the treatment proposed, can themselves give consent without parental knowledge or parental right to veto. The judgement as to the child's level of intelligence, understanding and maturity, i.e., whether they are Gillick competent, rests solely with the doctor concerned, and may be made either using the doctors prior knowledge of the patient, or through a formal assessment of capacity (see Box 12.2).

b In essence, the ruling in the Gillick case applies to all forms of medical treatment as it focuses on the issue of consent itself as a principle, and not on any particular action.

c Firstly, where a minor is judged not to be Gillick competent, the doctor is not required to maintain confidentiality and indeed may feel that parental involvement in any medical treatment **should** occur, regardless of the child's wishes. Furthermore, even if judged Gillick competent, the child's right to confidentiality can be overruled if it is judged in their best interests to do so. Such a situation may occur where the doctor suspects that the sex, for which the contraception is requested, is occurring as a result of coercion or abuse, or illegally with an adult. In such situations, involvement of the parents, social services, and possibly the police, may be necessary.

d The most common emergency contraceptive currently prescribed in the UK, is levonorgestrel (levonelle). It is most effective up to 72 hours after unprotected intercourse, and is taken as a single pill as soon as prescribed. Levonelle has few contraindications, the main ones being:

- pregnancy (always check urine pregnancy test before prescribing)
- hypersensitivity reaction to levornorgestrel
- severe migraine
- severe liver impairment
- it has no efficacy more than five days after unprotected intercourse.

e Advice to be given with emergency contraception should cover:

- if vomiting occurs soon after taking the pill, a second dose should be taken as soon as possible
- it is not 100% effective, therefore, the woman should take a pregnancy test if her next period is delayed more than five days
- emergency contraception does not provide on-going contraception. Thus, she should receive additional contraceptive advice to avoid a recurrence
- she should be advised about safe sex and given information on advice services for sexually active young people
- advice on sexually transmitted diseases, and referred to a genito-urinary medicine clinic, if this is a possibility.

Further Reading

1. Collier J, Longmore M, Turmezi T, *et al.* (2009) *Oxford Handbook of Clinical Specialties*, 8th edn. Oxford University Press. pp 312–409.
2. Sullivan JT, Swift R, Lewis DC. (1991) Benzodiazepine requirements during alcohol withdrawal syndrome: clinical implications of using a standardized withdrawal **scale**. *Journal of Clinical Psychopharmacology* **11**, 291–5.
3. UK National Poisons Information Service found at www.toxbase.org.
4. NICE Guideline CG16. Self-Harm: The short-term physical and psychological management and secondary prevention of self-harm in primary and secondary care (2004), www.nice.org.uk/Guidance/CG16

5. NICE Guideline CG25. Violence. The short-term management of disturbed/violent behaviour in psychiatric in-patient settings and emergency departments' (2005), www.nice.org.uk/Guidance/CG25
6. A useful succinct summary of compulsory detention using The Mental Health Act is found at www.patient.co.uk/showdoc/40000709/

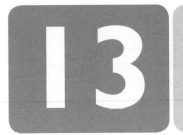

ENT AND MAXILLOFACIAL EMERGENCIES

Chet R Trivedy

Introduction

Core topics

ENT

- painful ear
- epistaxis
- nasal trauma
- sore throat
- foreign bodies
- facial nerve palsy
- salivary gland pathology.

Maxillofacial and dental

- anatomy and physiology of the facial structures (parotid duct, facial nerve, lacrimal duct)
- nasal fractures
- facial fractures (Le Fort classification, mandibular and zygomatic fractures)
- temperomandibular joint dislocation
- soft-tissue injuries (including tongue lacerations)
- normal dental development
- dental abscess
- avulsed permanent teeth
- post extraction complications.

It is also useful to be aware of the nomenclature and classification of the primary (children's) and adult dentition as this had come up on more than one occasion in CEM examinations.

A general primer for those interested in further reading on the topics covered in this chapter is '*Head, Neck and Dental Emergencies*', edited by Perry M. Oxford University Press. 2005.

Case 1

A three-year-old boy has a 1-day history of worsening pain in his right ear, accompanied by a purulent non-bloody discharge from the ear. He has a low-grade fever but is otherwise well. He has never suffered from earache before.

a What is the most likely diagnosis?   [1]
b List three organisms that may be linked with this condition.   [3]
c How would you treat this child in the ED?   [3]
d Give two specific indications for antibiotics in this child.   [2]
e List three possible complications that may arise from this condition. [3]

                                                                                                    [12]

Case 2

A 42-year-old man presents with a one-week day history of right-sided facial weakness. He is otherwise well and has no weakness of his limbs. All observations are within normal limits. He is concerned that he has had a stroke. The photograph below was taken whilst asking the patient to smile widely and close his eyes tightly (Figure 13.1).

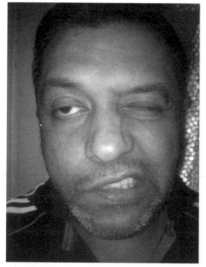

Figure 13.1

a Describe the clinical features shown in the photograph (Figure 13.1). [2]
b Assuming neurological examination of the limbs is normal, list three further clinical abnormalities you would examine for in this man to refine the diagnosis.   [3]
c Explain how you can distinguish between an upper (central) and lower (peripheral) motor neurone facial palsy.   [1]

d Following examination of this patient's cranial nerves, you conclude he has a lower motor neuron (LMN) facial palsy. Give a differential diagnosis of a lower motor neurone facial palsy. [3]

e How would you manage this patient with a LMN facial palsy (give doses and routes of any drugs used)? [3]

[12]

Case 3

A 65-year-old man presents with a nosebleed which began spontaneously and, despite simple measures to halt the flow of blood has now persisted for four hours. He is alert and otherwise well with a heart rate of 110 bpm regular and blood pressure 170/110 mmHg.

a List two local (to the nose) and two systemic contributory factors to the development of epistaxis. [4]

b Outline the arterial supply to Little's area of the nasal septum (Kiesselbach's plexus). [3]

c Describe three methods of controlling an anterior epistaxis. [3]

[10]

Case 4

A 25-year-old female patient presents to the Emergency Department (ED) with a 6-hour history of a sore throat, and difficulty in swallowing, as well as pain opening her mouth. Her observations at triage are heart rate 106 bpm, blood pressure 114/76 mmHg, respiratory rate 18 and temperature 38.4 °C. There is no airway obstruction.

a Give two bacteria and two viruses known to be common causes of acute tonsillitis. [4]

b What clinical signs on examination would indicate a peritonsillar abscess (give 3)? [3]

c Symptomatic treatments aside, outline the key steps in the management of a patient suspected of having a peritonsillar abscess. [4]

d What important structure may be damaged in the surgical treatment of a peritonsillar abscess? [1]

[12]

Case 5

A 40-year-old gentleman arrives in the ED after being assaulted and punched in the face. He is fully alert and the examining doctor notes extensive swelling and bruising over the left side of his face and eye. The patient's facial X-ray is shown below (Figure 13.2).

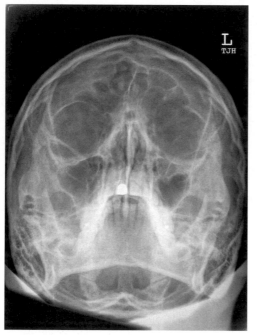

Figure 13.2

a List four clinical signs you would look for that suggest an underlying facial fracture. [4]
b Name a classification system used to describe fractures of the facial skeleton. [2]
c List the most appropriate types of plain X-ray views that would be of use in this scenario. [2]
d Describe the bony abnormality in the X-ray (Figure 13.2). [4]

[12]

Case 6

A 13-year-old boy presents to the emergency department after falling off his pushbike onto his face and losing his front teeth in the process (Figure 13.3). He has a GCS of 15 and has been cleared of any other significant injuries, and his front teeth are in a container of milk.

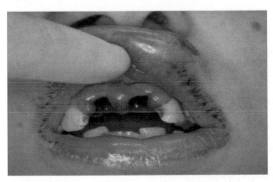

Figure 13.3

a Outline your immediate management of his dental injury (Figure 13.3). [4]
b List three prognostic factors that will affect successful replantation of his
   teeth. [1]
c Following treatment, what specific advice you would give this patient on
   discharge with regards to his dental injury. [1]
d List three contraindications for replanting teeth following avulsion. [3]
e Give a simple classification system for deciduous and permanent teeth. [4]
   [13]

Case 7

A 40-year-old male presents with a progressively enlarging swelling of the left side
of his face. He has limited mouth opening due to pain and complains of difficulty
in swallowing. He reports having toothache in a lower left molar tooth for some
time but had not yet seen a dentist. On examination, he is pyrexial at 38.6 °C and
has a marked tender swelling over his left cheek. Other observations are heart rate
110 bpm, oxygen saturation 98% on air, temperature 38.6 °C and blood glucose
18 mmo/L.

a List a differential diagnosis for diffuse non-traumatic unilateral facial
   swelling. [3]
b Which potential soft-tissue spaces of the face are at risk of infection from
   the lower **molar teeth**? [3]
c Outline the key steps in your management of this patient. [3]
d List the serious complications that may arise from this condition. [3]
   [12]

Case 8

A 30-year-old male is attacked with a machete sustaining a deep wound across the left side of his face. The laceration extends from the margin of the medial canthus of his right eye, crossing his cheek to the angle of the mandible, just below his ear. He is haemodynamically stable and his eye has escaped injury.

a List four structures that may have been damaged as a result of this injury. [4]
b Describe how you would assess for damage for three of the structures you describe. [3]
c Give three steps in the ED management of this patient. [3]
d Excluding aesthetics, list three important complications which might arise from this injury. [3]

[13]

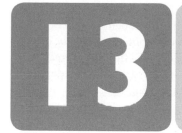

ENT AND MAXILLOFACIAL EMERGENCIES – ANSWERS

Case 1

a The most likely diagnosis is acute otitis media which has three hallmark features:

- acute onset
- middle ear inflammation (tympanic membrane erythema and pain which keeps the patient awake at night)
- signs of a middle ear effusion (bulging tympanic membrane or perforated tympanic membrane with discharge).

It is important to distinguish acute otitis media (AOM) from otitis media with effusion (OME or colloquially known as 'glue ear'); the latter being a chronic condition of middle ear fluid accumulation without signs of acute inflammation. Both are most common in early childhood and both may cause conductive hearing loss in the affected ear.

b Most AOM is associated with viral upper respiratory infection (Respiratory Syncitial Virus, Influenza, Parainfluenza, Enterovirus, Rhinovirus) and a smaller percentage being bacterial in origin (*Strep pneumonia, Haemophilus influenza, Moraxella catarrhalis, Group A streptococci, Staph. aureus*).

c Treatment of acute otitis media is generally supportive and antibiotics are usually not required. You should:[1]

- explain to the parents that the symptoms are self-limiting and in most cases (at least 80%) symptoms resolve in three to four days, without specific treatment
- advise regular analgesia e.g., paracetamol 20 mg/kg (max 1g) qds for discomfort
- any discharge should be swabbed for culture in case of persistent symptoms
- the child should be followed up by the GP to ensure the complaint is settling.

d For a child with uncomplicated otitis media antibiotics are generally not indicated. However antibiotics for a suspected bacterial AOM may be considered where:[2]

- the child is systemically unwell
- there is a history of recurrent infection
- symptoms worsen rather than improve after two to three days
- infection spreading beyond the middle ear is suspected (e.g., mastoiditis which requires admission under ENT and intravenous antibiotics)
- swabbing returns a positive result for bacterial infection.

e Complications of AOM are rare, as most cases go on to complete recovery. However, a small number of important sequelae are worth being aware of. Most tympanic membrane perforations heal within a month but, occasionally, can persist causing chronic hearing loss. Acute middle ear infection may spread to the adjacent mastoid air cells resulting in mastoiditis (evidenced by tenderness and erythema of the mastoid process) or further, a meningitis. Chronic middle ear infection also predisposes to cholesteatoma in adults.

Case 2

a The patient (Figure 13.1) clearly has a right-sided facial palsy and is unable to close their right eye. There is no evidence of a rash suggestive of a herpetic infection.

b Additional features to look for and which help with diagnosis are:

- eyebrow raising on the affected side to distinguish an upper and lower motor neurone palsy (see below for explanation)
- test for any impairment to the hearing or balance which is suggestive of a cause involving not just the facial nerve (e.g., acoustic neuroma)
- examine the external auditory meatus or palate for zoster lesions (crusty vesicles), which, in association with a facial palsy, indicates Ramsay–Hunt syndrome (herpes zoster oticus). Facial nerve dysfunction in this condition is due to re-activation of varicella zoster virus (VZV) in the geniculate ganglion of the facial nerve.

c Ask the patient to raise their eyebrows so that they wrinkle their forehead. Supplied by the temporal branch of the facial nerve, the occipto-frontalis muscle producing this action, has bilateral cortical representation and consequently, eyebrow raising and forehead wrinkling are **preserved** in focal central nervous system lesions affecting facial motor function. Conversely, the diagnostic sign of a lower (peripheral) motor neurone facial palsy is the **absence** of eyebrow raising and forehead wrinkling on the affected side. All other facial nerve motor functions are unilaterally cortically innervated and hence equally affected in both upper (central) and lower (peripheral) motor neurone facial weakness.

d Causes of isolated lower motor neurone facial nerve palsy include:

- idiopathic Bell's palsy (most common)
- trauma to the facial nerve (facial laceration or from fracture of the petrous temporal bone)
- invasive parotid tumour
- Lyme disease
- diabetes mellitus
- sarcoidosis (of the parotid)
- multiple sclerosis
- cerebellopontine angle tumour (acoustic neuroma).

e Drug treatment of an uncomplicated Bell's palsy is high-dose steroids such as prednisolone (1 mg/kg ; maximum 80 mg) for seven days. In addition, the inability to blink and close the eye puts the cornea at risk of injury, and patients with facial palsy of any cause should be given lubricant eye drops (e.g., viscotears prn) to use frequently and an eye patch to use at night. Follow-up in the ENT clinic should be organized. Recent studies suggest that in uncomplicated Bell's palsy antivirals do **not** offer any additional benefit when given in combination with steroids.[3,4] Also, reassure him he has not had a stroke but give a realistic assessment of prognosis; most recover fully in three months, 15% have some residual facial weakness and 5% do not recover at all.

Case 3

a Epistaxis is common, affecting up to 60% of the population at some time or another, and consequently accounts for an appreciable workload in the ED. The incidence is bimodal and clinically relevant epistaxis is most often seen in children below10 years and adults above age 50. Factors contributing towards epistaxis can be divided into local and systemic:

Local causes mostly predispose to anterior epistaxis (90% arise from Little's area) and include:

- trauma (nosepicking to nasal bone fracture)
- nasal polyps
- infection (URTI)
- allergy (allergic rhinitis)
- excessive drying of the nasal mucosa (increased respiration, central heating in winter)
- exposure to chemical irritants including the use of intranasal recreational drugs and alcohol!

Systemic factors contribute to both anterior and posterior epistaxis:
- anticoagulant use or clotting disorders
- platelet disorders
- uncontrolled hypertension (often overlooked).

b

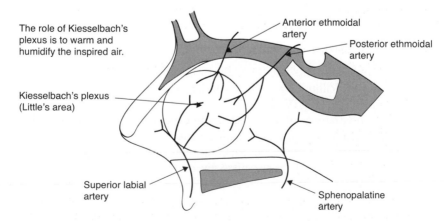

Figure 13.4

Little's area is the anteroinferior part of the nasal septum, where the three main arteries supplying the nasal septum anastamose in a vascular plexus called Kiesselbach's plexus. The three main arteries are the anterior ethmoidal artery (branch of the internal carotid), the sphenopalatine artery and the superior labial artery (both branches of the external carotid artery). The role of Kiesselbach's plexus is to warm and humidify the inspired air.

c Three methods of halting anterior epistaxis in order of execution:

- apply pressure to the fleshy part of the nose clamping the nares firmly together (for at least 15 minutes at a time)
- cautery of any causative vessels or bleeding points with a silver nitrate stick under direct vision
- anterior nasal tamponade with commercial packs, e.g. Mericel® nasal tampon or Rapid Rhino® pack (depending on local protocol).

Case 4

a Acute tonsillitis affects most children at some stage with most episodes of viral origin and linked to upper respiratory infections. Specific viruses include EBV (with or without full blown glandular fever), adenoviruses and HSV. Bacterial causes account for around 20% with Group A *β-haemolytic streptococci* most common probably followed by *Strep. pyogenes* and anaerobes.

b We might suspect the more serious complication of peritonsillar abscess (Quinsy) in this patient since she has painful mouth opening (trismus), which is not usually a symptom of tonsillitis alone. Additional clinical signs suggestive of peritonsillar abscess include:

- high fever/systemic toxicity
- complete dysphagia and drooling of saliva
- halitosis
- unilateral tonsillar swelling
- deviated uvula
- nasal sounding speech
- rarely airway obstruction.

c Key steps in managing a patient with peritonsillar abscess are:

- intravenous antibiotics to cover gram +ve streptococci and anaerobes e.g. Benzylpenicillin 1.2 g QDS (or clindamycin if penicillin allergic) and metronidzole 500 mg IV tds
- incision and drainage of the abscess by an experienced ENT surgeon is ideal. This can often be performed under local anaesthetic but where there is likely distress, trismus or airway concerns, a general anaesthetic is preferable
- dexamethasone 8 mg IV is also often given to minimise swelling and subsequent pain.

Untreated, a peritonsillar abscess can result in septicaemia as well as spread locally to the deeper tissue spaces in the neck causing parapharyngeal abscess, and from there to the mediastium, cavernous sinus, or even meninges.

d The parapharyngeal space lies just lateral to the tonsils and upper pharynx and importantly contains the internal carotid artery, as well as the internal jugular vein and a number of cranial nerves. Aspirations or incisions into the tonsils should be no more than 1 cm deep to avoid damage to vascular structures at a location where they cannot be compressed if haemorrhaging!

Case 5

a Clinical signs and symptoms that suggest an underlying fracture of the facial skeleton include:

- facial asymmetry
- bony tenderness on palpation of the facial skeleton
- a change in bite (malocclusion)
- diplopia
- opthalmoplegia
- limited or painful mouth opening
- paraesthesia in the infraorbital, mental or inferior alveolar distribution
- nasal complex deviation
- subconjunctival haemorrhage.

b The Le Fort classification of maxillary fractures was described in 1901 by Rene Le Fort following his experiments applying blunt forces to cadaveric skulls.[5] He described 3 patterns of injury which bear his name:

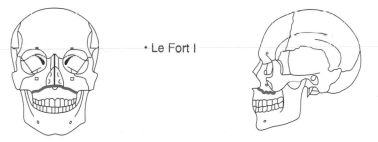

• Le Fort I

Horizontal fracture through the palate at a level above the roots of the teeth and extending back across the pterygoid plates. Clinically, separation of the palate results in an abnormal bite and bruising in the labial and buccal sulcus.

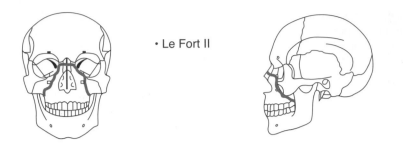

• Le Fort II

Pyramidal-shaped fracture involving the orbital floor and lacrimal bones extending from the nasal bridge and the frontal process of the maxilla inferiorly through the maxillary sinuses and across the pterygoids plates. Clinical features include swelling and distortion of the upper third of the face including bilateral periorbital ecchymosis (panda or raccoon eyes), infraorbital parasthaesia, epistaxis and subconjunctival haemorrhage.

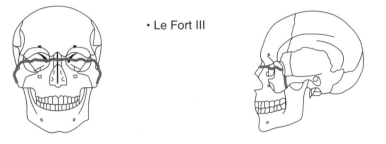

• Le Fort III

Transverse fracture causing craniofacial separation across the nasofrontal and nasomaxillary sutures. The fracture passes posteriorly through the orbit, ethmoid bones, vomer and pterygoids plates at the base of the sphenoid. The zygomatic arch and zygomaticofrontal suture are also disrupted. Clinical signs are similar as those of Le Fort II fracture but, in addition, CSF rhinorrhea and lengthening of facial height may occur.

Le Fort II and III fractures are also associated with the danger of airway compromise

c In this scenario, the most appropriate imaging is an occipitomental X-ray taken from two different angles which are usually at 15 and 30 degrees. These are the mainstay of facial views when there is an injury to the maxillary component of the facial skeleton. Mandibular views such as an orthopantamogram (OPG) or a posterior-anterior (PA) view of the mandible should only be requested if you are concerned about a mandibular injury. For a dental injury alone, an OPG would suffice. There are no indications for requesting a specialist temperomandibular joint (TMJ) view in the ED.

d The facial X-ray (Figure 13.2) shows a fracture of the left orbital floor with herniation of the orbital soft tissues into the maxillary antrum – 'tear drop' sign.

Case 6

a Manage a traumatic avulsion of incisor teeth as follows:[6]

- the priority is to replant the teeth back in their sockets. Successful re-plantation is time critical and intact avulsed teeth should be promptly replanted into the socket ideally, within 30 minutes of the injury. Prior to replanting avulsed teeth, the socket should also be examined and gently irrigated to remove any debris
- following replantation, the teeth ideally should be splinted in place. If no splinting material is available, the patient should be encouraged to bite on some gauze to keep the teeth in place and referred to a dental/maxillofacial specialist for splinting
- a soft diet should be advised until the teeth are secure
- refer for follow-up by their dental practitioner
- antibiotics are commonly given following this type of injury but there is no evidence base to support this.

b Prognostic indicators for successful re-plantation include:

- ensure you inspect the teeth and look for any damage. Minor trauma to the tooth is not a contraindication for re-plantation but if the tooth is fractured this may affect the prognosis
- time since avulsion. Teeth replanted within 30 minutes have the best prognosis
- the prognosis is poorer if the tooth is allowed to dry out, or if the root is handled. This may damage the periodontal ligament lining the root which is essential for reattachment
- poor oral hygiene, smoking and immunocompromised states may also reduce the prognosis.

c A soft diet should be advised to assist the healing phase of tooth reattachment to the alveolar socket. Excess movement of the teeth or axial loads on the tooth may impair the attachment of the periodontal ligament.

d Contraindications to tooth re-plantation may be absolute or relative. Deciduous (baby) teeth should never be replanted, due to risk of damage to the permanent teeth that follow. Teeth that have fractured roots or are otherwise badly damaged, should only be replanted following expert advice. Relative contraindications include replanting teeth in patients who have a poor dentition or who may have severe learning difficulties and may be unable to maintain good oral hygiene. Replanting teeth in patients where there is a risk of endocarditis may also be a relative contraindication.

e Deciduous teeth are classified as A–E and the adult teeth from 1–8. The key to classification is to start from the two front central incisor and count backwards. Children have 20 teeth, whereas adults have 32. One classification system involves identifying the quadrant the tooth is in, followed by the number or letter describing the tooth:

Upper right (UR)	Upper left (UL)	Lower right (LR)	Lower left (LL)

Hence, an upper first premolar on the right can be classified as UR4. Box 13.1 below lists the classification, as well as the eruption dates for adult and deciduous teeth. As this boy is 13, it is most likely that he has lost his adult front teeth. This is a time critical emergency where the teeth should be replanted ideally within 30–60 minutes of the injury to maximize the chances of survival. There should be minimal handling of the root and the tooth should be immobilized with a temporary splint.

Table 13.1: Classification of adult and deciduous teeth

Permanent maxillary teeth dates	Eruption dates	Deciduous maxillary teeth	Eruption dates
1. Central incisor	7–8 years	A. Central incisor	8–12 months
2. Lateral incisor	8–9 years	B. Lateral incisor	9–13 months
3. Canine	11–12 years	C. Canine	16–22 months
4. First premolar	10–11 years	D. First molar	13–19 months
5. Second premolar	10–12 years	E. Second molar	25–33 months
6. First molar	6–7 years		
7. Second molar	12–13 years		
8. Third molar	17–21 years		
Permanent mandibular teeth	Eruption dates	Deciduous mandibular teeth	Eruption dates
1. Central incisor	6–7 years	A. Central incisor	6–10 months
2. Lateral incisor	8–9 years	B. Lateral incisor	10–16 months
3. Canine	11–12 years	C. Canine	17–23 months
4. First premolar	10–11 years	D. First molar	14–18 months
5. Second premolar	10–12 years	E. Second molar	23–31 months
6. First molar	6–7 years		
7. Second molar	12–13 years		
8. Third molar	17–21 years		

Case 7

a The differential diagnosis of non-traumatic unilateral facial swelling commonly involves those causes arising from the parotid glands versus those arising from dental infection:

- parotid gland stones (sialolithiasis) with obstruction of the salivary duct. Suggested by pain and swelling prior to eating and drinking which subsides on hour or so after eating
- acute bacterial parotitis (most commonly follows salivary duct obstruction)
- mumps parotitis (20% have unilateral swelling)
- spreading dental infection/dental abscess

- Sjorgren's syndrome is a more unusual autoimmune cause (dry eyes, dry mouth, polyarthritis and Reynaud's)
- sarcoidosis.

b Infection initially localized to decayed teeth may progress to invade the peri-oral tissue, spread along fascial planes and settle in several potential spaces within the soft tissues of the face. Signs, symptoms and location of facial swelling relate to the precipitating teeth involved!

Table 13.2

Initial tooth infection	Infected soft tissue space	Signs and symptoms
Mandibular, canines and incisors	Submental space Sublingual space	Midline swelling under the chin Swelling floor of mouth with tongue elevation, dysphagia and change in speech
Mandibular molars	Submandibular space	Swelling submandibular triangle neck, often associated with trismus Ludwig's angina – serious invasive cellulitis of sublingual, submental and submandibular spaces. Tongue elevation and swelling, complete dysphagia with drooling and high risk of airway occlusion. Retropharyngeal and mediastinal spread is a further danger
Maxillary canines	Canine space/ maxillary sinus	Anterior cheek swelling and tenderness
Maxillary molars	Buccal space	Diffuse swelling of the cheek

Risk factors for complications from a simple dental infection include poor oral hygiene, recent dental extraction or root canal treatment and smoking or immunocompromise of any kind: diabetics, post-chemotherapy, HIV, chronic steroid use or medications such as methotrexate or azothioprine.

c This patient has an odontogenic sub-mandibular soft tissue infection/abscess and, in addition, is systemically unwell and has trismus, preventing mouth opening or swallowing. He requires:

- airway assessment by senior ED, ENT or anaesthetic personnel
- IV antibiotics to cover a wide range of possible aerobic and anaerobic organisms, e.g. amoxycillin 1 g TDS or co-amoxiclav 1.2 g TDS with metronidazole 500 mg TDS
- referral to maxillofacial surgeon for drainage of the abscess under general anaesthetic
- parenteral analgesia and antipyretic for symptomatic relief.

d Complications of spreading dental infection include:

- airway obstruction (seen with Ludwig's angina – a surgical emergency)
- retropharyngeal abscess (sore throat, anterior neck pain, dysphagia and airway compromise, swelling visible on lateral soft tissue X-ray of the neck)

- mediastinal spread (high mortality)
- systemic sepsis
- rarely, cavernous sinus (CS) thrombosis (infection spreads to the CS via the facial veins).

Case 8

a Trace the course of the laceration across an imaginary face and consider the anatomical structures underlying the skin at each point and which may, therefore, have been damaged. In this case, and in order from the medial canthus to the angle of the mandible, consider the:

1 lacrimal duct
2 orbicularis occuli muscles
3 infraorbital nerve
4 facial nerve as it passes through the parotid gland
5 superficial lobe of the parotid gland
6 parotid duct
7 transverse facial artery.

b Damage to these structures can be clinically assessed as follows:

Table 13.3

Structure	Test
Lacrimal duct	Any eyelid injury in the medial corner of the eye may involve the lacrimal duct. Probing of the lacrimal duct to test patency by an ophthalmologist is required
Orbicularis occuli	Test integrity of the blink reflex
Infraorbital nerve	Ask about parasthaesia and examine for anaesthesia over cheek and upper lip
Facial nerve (particularly the buccal, mandibular and cervical branches)	Test the muscles of facial expression (blow out your cheeks, grin widely, tense your neck)
Parotid gland and duct	Look for blood at the opening of the parotid duct. Retrograde sialogram for a specialist assessment of ductal injury
Transverse facial artery	The arterial supply of the face is highly anastomotic and while injury to the transverse facial artery need not be repaired, bleeding may be profuse

c The priority in managing this wound is managing haemostasis. Bleeding vessels should be identified and either tied or clamped with haemostats. Laceration of the facial artery can result in significant blood loss. Once haemostasis has been achieved, ED management involves appropriate analgesia, assessment of the extent of injury to underlying structures, gentle cleaning by irrigation of the wound with normal saline, and dressing of the wound, followed by immediate referral to maxillofacial surgeons for closure under general anaesthetic. Involve maxillofacial, plastics and ophthalmology specialists as required by clinical findings. Antibiotics are generally not indicated although ensuring up-to-date tetanus prophylaxis is.

d Tears to the parotid duct or the lacrimal duct may heal irregularly causing ductal stenosis which can impair the flow of tears and saliva. Damage to the eyelid may cause ectropion with consequent impairment of eyelid closing and corneal irritation.

Further Reading

1. Coker TR, Chan LS, Newberry SJ, *et al.* (2010) Diagnosis, microbial epidemiology, and antibiotic treatment of acute otitis media in children: a systematic review. *JAMA*; Nov 17; **304**:2161–9.
2. Rovers MM, Glasziou P, Appelman CL, *et al.* (2006) Antibiotics for acute otitis media: a meta-analysis with individual patient data. *Lancet*; **368**:1429–35.
3. Quant EC, Jeste SS, Muni RH, *et al.* (2009) The benefits of steroids versus steroids plus antivirals for treatment of Bell's palsy: a meta-analysis. *BMJ*; **339**:b3354.
4. Sullivan FM, *et al.* (2007) Early treatment with prednisolone or acyclovir in Bell's palsy. *N Engl J Med*; **357**:1598.
5. Tessier P. (1972) The classic reprint. Experimental study of fractures of the upper jaw. I and II. René Le Fort, MD. *Plast Reconstr Surg*; **50**(5):497–506.
6. Gregg TA, Boyd DH. (1998) Treatment of avulsed permanent teeth in children. UK National Guidelines in Paediatric Dentistry. Royal College of Surgeons, Faculty of Dental Surgery. *Int J Paediatr Dent*; **8**:75–81.

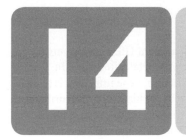

DERMATOLOGY AND RHEUMATOLOGY

Sam Thenabadu and Mathew Hall

Introduction

Core topics

- dermatological emergencies which may threaten life (erythroderma, pemphigus, Steven's Johnson syndrome and toxic epidermal necrolysis, staphylococcal scalded skin syndrome)
- urticaria and angio-oedema
- petechial and purpuric rashes
- erythema nodosum and erythema multiforme
- eczema (including eczema herpeticum)
- skin infection (erysipilas, cellulitis)
- impetigo
- herpes zoster
- varicella zoster, shingles and zoster opthalmicus
- childhood exanthems (see paediatric chapter)
- skin cancer, particularly malignant melanoma.

Being able to describe rashes using the correct terms is vital for answering dermatology SAQs. Although we give several examples in the questions in this chapter, it is beyond the scope of this book to teach how to diagnose rashes from their appearance. Obtain a concise dermatology text[1,2] and read the introduction with a view to learning both the key elements of the dermatological history and the correct terms in which to describe rashes and other common skin conditions.

- diagnosis and investigations of an acute monoarthritis
- diagnosis of polyarthritis
- septic arthritis
- crystal arthropathies (gout, pseudogout)
- rheumatoid disease (including complications of treatment)
- osteoarthritis
- ankylosing spondylitis.

Relevant knowledge for rheumatology SAQs, includes distinguishing radiological appearances of various joint diseases, the interpretation of joint aspiration results and do not forget the extra-articular manifestations of rheumatological disease – always a favourite of examiners!

Case 1

A 16-year-old boy is brought to the Emergency Department (ED) by his parents. For the previous four days, he has also been treated with cefalexin for a skin infection on both his legs but his parents are concerned that the infection is getting worse, as the boy is now complaining that the red areas on his shins are painful and tender. On questioning, the boy has had a bad sore throat and dry cough for the past week, although says this is now improving. He has a low-grade fever but all other observations are normal. Figure 14.1 shows the boy's lower legs.

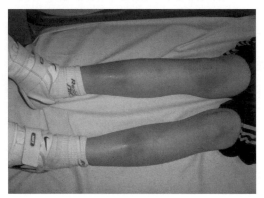

Figure 14.1 (see colour plate.)

a You do not think the rash is an infection. What is the correct diagnosis for this rash (Figure 14.1)? [2]

b Describe, in three stages, the natural progression of the lesions of this rash. [3]

c What is the likely cause of this rash in this boy given the history above? Give three further causes of such a rash in the general population. [4]

d What specific tests should be carried out on this boy to confirm the underlying cause of the rash? [2]

e What treatment would you prescribe for the rash and should the patient stop the antibiotics? [1]

[12]

Case 2

A mother brings her two-year-old son to the ED as she is concerned about a rash on his face that has been spreading over the last three days (Figure 14.2). The child is alert although miserable and trying to scratch at the facial lesions. His observations are temperature 37.2 °C, heart rate 120 bpm and respiratory rate 26/min. A photograph of the child's face is shown below (Figure 14.2).

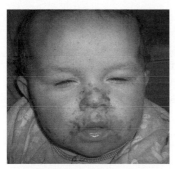

Figure 14.2 (see colour plate.)

What is the likely diagnosis based on the child's appearance in figure 14.2? [1]
b Give two organisms commonly responsible for this rash. [2]
c How is this condition classified so as to guide therapy? Include in your answer two clinical features of the infection that differ between the classes you describe. [4]
d How would you treat this child? [2]
e What advice should you give the family living in the same house? [3]

[12]

Case 3

A 13-year-old boy presents to the ED with a two-day history of a productive cough, myalgia and mild fevers. He has been tolerating oral fluids, and using regular anti-pyretics with good effect. Over the last day, however, he has developed a pronounced rash over his lower limbs with a few spots on his arms and torso. You are called to see him by the triage nurse who has correctly identified the rash as purpuric and is concerned. At triage, the boy appears well and initial observations are heart rate 95 bpm, blood pressure 110/75 mmHg, CRT less than 2 seconds, respiratory rate 20/min and temperature 37.3 °C.

a Define the following terms: petechiae, purpura and ecchymoses. [3]
b Name five distinct differential diagnoses for a petechial or purpuric rash. [5]
c Results of blood tests performed on this boy are given below:

WCC	11.9×10^9/L	INR	1.1
Hb	13.0 g/dL	APTT	1.2
Platelets	17×10^9/L		
Neutrophils	7.0×10^9/L		
Lymphocytes	4.0×10^9/L		

What is the likely cause of the rash in this patient? [1]
d Outline your approach to treatment of this young boy. [3]

[12]

Chapter 14 DERMATOLOGY AND RHEUMATOLOGY – Cases

Case 4

A 57-year-old woman presents to the ED with a four-hour history of spreading rash over her chest, back and upper limbs. She has a past medical history of asthma and a mild nut allergy. Apart from itching terribly, she feels fine and all her observations at triage are stable. A photograph of a section of the rash on her lower back is shown in Figure 14.3.

Figure 14.3 (see colour plate.)

a Describe the rash in Figure 14.3.   [2]
b Give three common causes of this type of rash.   [3]
c Give three drugs that can be used in the ED to treat this woman's rash.   [3]
d What is the pathophysiological difference between this condition and
   angio-oedema?   [2]
e Name two commonly prescribed drugs known to cause angio-oedema.   [2]
f What treatment options are available to treat a patient with hereditary
   angio-oedema who presents with potential airway compromise?   [2]
                                                                                        [14]

Case 5

A 65-year-old man presents following a worsening rash over the past few days. He is now completely covered with an itchy rash and is feeling unwell. The nurse takes his initial observations as heart rate 106 bpm, blood pressure 120/65 mmHg and temperature 35.0 °C. You are called to see him and note the rash in Figure 14.4.

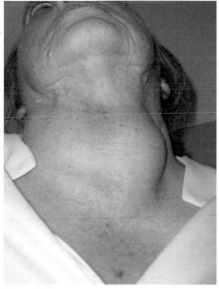

Figure 8.1

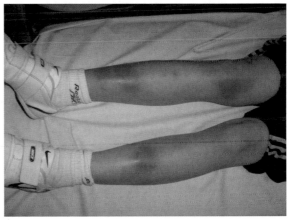

Figure 14.1

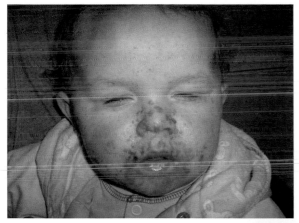

Figure 14.2

Figure 14.3
(photograph courtesy of Dr D Adler)

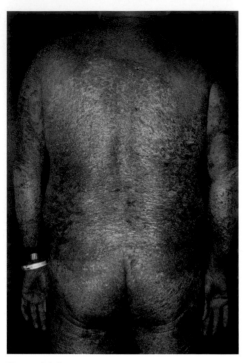

Figure 14.4
(photograph courtesy of Dr D Adler)

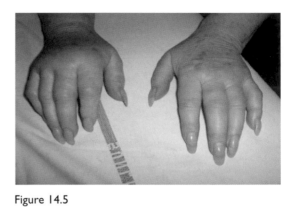

Figure 14.5

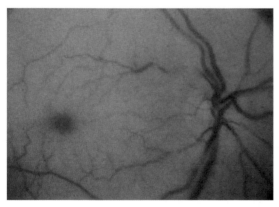

Figure 15.1

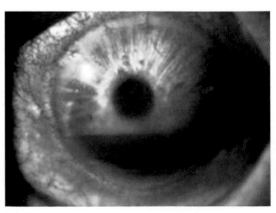

Figure 15.2

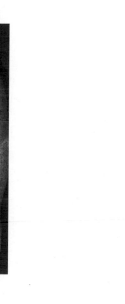

Figure 14.4 (see colour plate.)

a Describe the rash given in Figure 14.4 and what clinical condition does it represent? [4]
b Give four causes of this condition. [4]
c What serious complications may arise in this patient? [3]
d Describe three key steps in the ED management of this patient. [3]

[14]

Case 6

A three-year-old boy is brought by his mother to the paediatric ED with worsening eczema on his arms and legs. She had been to see her GP on numerous occasions about the problem but says, so far, the eczema is not improving with the creams prescribed for the child, and she wants a second opinion from the hospital. The child appears well and is playing happily as you examine him.

a Give four features of the typical rash of infantile atopic eczema. [4]
b Outline your stepwise approach to treating this child's eczema. [3]
c Give two serious complications of atopic eczema and how they should be managed? [4]
d What three further atopic conditions might this child be at greater risk of suffering? [3]

[14]

Case 7

A 45-year-old woman attending the local acute care centre, complains of swollen hands that have been getting steadily worse, 'especially over the knuckles', for the last three months. She describes the hands as being painful first thing in the morning but there is improvement after an hour or so. She has no significant past medical or family history of note. A photograph of her hands at presentation is shown below (Figure 14.5).

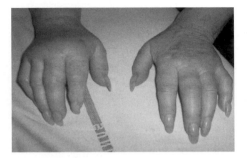

Figure 14.5 (see colour plate.)

a Describe the abnormalities in this patients hands (Figure 14.5). What diagnosis is likely? [2]

b Name two further abnormalities that may be found in the hands in patients with this condition. [2]

c Name four findings on plain X-ray associated with this disease. [4]

d Name two medications that the national guidelines recommend initiating in the first instance in this woman. [2]

e Patients with more severe arthritis are often placed on disease modifying anti-rheumatic drugs (DMARDs) by their rheumatologist. What serious side-effect may occur from DMARD therapy and give three symptoms which would raise suspicion that this side-effect may be present in a patient attending the ED who is taking DMARDs. [4]

[14]

Case 8

A 28-year-old Hungarian male presents to the ED with a one-week history of worsening lower back pain. He tells you, that when he lived in Budapest as a child, he was diagnosed with a 'back condition', but has not been followed up for the last ten years. He describes the pain as being a dull ache that wakes him at night, with associated stiffness, worse in the mornings. On examination, he has a tall and slender frame and is markedly stooped. He is tender on palpation of the hips and lumbar spine.

a What is the likely diagnosis and common genetic association? [2]
b Name the three clinical features required to diagnose this condition. [3]
c Name four extra articular features you will look for in this patient. [4]
d Give three X-ray findings you may see in this condition. [3]
e Name two pharmacological treatments you could initiate in the ED. [2]

[14]

Case 9

A 50-year-old man with alcohol dependence presents to the ED with a five-day history of worsening pain in his big toe, now so bad he can barely walk. He has multiple similar episodes of the same problem over the last five years but has never previously brought it to the attention of a doctor. On examination, he has a red, swollen and very tender first metatarsophalyngeal joint with a valgus deformity. An X-ray is performed (Figure 14.6) and you are asked to review the patient with a view to proposing treatment. He last attended your hospital one month ago suffering with peptic ulcer disease.

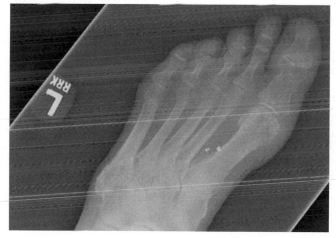

Figure 14.6

a Describe the abnormalities on the patient's foot X-ray (Figure 14.6) [2]
b What is your diagnosis? [1]
c Name four risk factors for the diagnosis you suspect in this patient. [4]
d What physical sign is associated with chronic recurrence of this condition? [1]
e How will you treat this particular man? Include in your answer both
medications and advice you would give. [3]

[11]

Case 10

A 42-year-old man presents to your ED with a two-day history of a red, hot, swollen right knee which he can no longer move without considerable pain. He denies any specific trauma but often scuffs his knee whilst working under cars in his job as a mechanic. He has no medical history of note and takes no regular medications.

a List an appropriate differential diagnosis for this patient (give four possible diagnoses).   [2]
b The patient's observations are heart rate 105 bpm, blood pressure 155/88 mmHg, respiratory rate 24/min and temperature 38.8 °C. You form a working diagnosis of septic arthritis. Briefly describe three routes through which bacteria may infect a joint.   [3]
c Give three common causative organisms in true septic arthritis.   [3]
d What diagnostic procedure is required and what four tests will you request from this?   [3]
e The diagnosis of septic arthritis is confirmed. Give your management of this patient in three key steps.   [3]

                                                                                   [14]

DERMATOLOGY AND RHEUMATOLOGY – ANSWERS

Case I

a The appearance in Figure 14.1 is classical of erythema nodosum (EN). EN is an immune-mediated inflammation (panniculitis) of the subcutaneous fat and presents initially, as shiny erythematous large nodules distributed over both shins (although it can occur on the arms or trunk), as in this picture. They are often painful and tender. EN occurs commonly in young females (female:male ratio of approximately 4:1) with ages 16–35 years most affected.

b The lesions of EN have a defined natural progression. They appear as shiny, red tender nodules 2–6 cm round with poorly defined borders. These nodules may coalesce into fluctuant areas similar to an abscess and with their colour changing to a blue–purple hue. Over a period of three to six weeks, the nodules regress into flatter macules and the colour fades to yellow then back to normal skin tone.

c Known associations include the following (there are many more):

- group A streptococcal infection
- bacterial infections of the GI tract (*Yersinia, Campylobacter,* and *Salmonella*)
- sarcoidosis
- inflammatory bowel disease (Crohn's disease and ulcerative colitis)
- drugs (sulfonylureas, gold and the OCP)
- Hodgkin's lymphoma
- tuberculosis.

In this patient with the preceding history of severe sore throat, a streptococcal throat infection – 'Strep throat' – is likely to be the cause of the erythema nodosum.

d In cases of suspected strep throat, a throat swab and an antistreptolysin-O (ASO) titre are relevant first-line investigations.

e EN is treated symptomatically with NSAIDs to reduce the inflammation and hence, alleviate the pain and tenderness of the lesions. Antibiotics do not help the skin rash but an oral cephalosporin is appropriate treatment for a streptococcal throat infection, both to shorten the throat infection and, to help avert the complications of group A streptococcus infection such as rheumatic fever and glomerulonephritis.

Case 2

a The rash in Figure 14.2 has the typical appearance of impetigo – red vesicles developing into honey crusted plaques around the mouth and nose – often pruritic. Impetigo is a very common superficial skin infection of pre-school children and young adults.

b The two common causative bacteria are *Staphylococcus aureus* and β-haemolytic streptococcus.

c Impetigo can be most usefully divided into bullous or non-bullous forms which have the following differing characteristics:

Table 14.1

Non-bullous impetigo	Bullous impetigo
70% of cases	30% of cases
Red vesicles and honey crusted plaques	Superficial bullae, often fragile and ruptured at time of presentation, with underlying erythematous dermis
Staphylococcus and streptococcus	Exotoxin secreting staphylococcus (the exotoxin attacks the dermal-epidermal junction proteins causing blistering)
Localized lymphadenopathy is common	Lymphadenopathy is rare
Systemic upset is rare	Systemic upset may be present (fever, GI symptoms)

Another system divides impetigo into primary or secondary, with secondary being superimposed on an underlying skin condition such as atopic dermatitis.

d Topical antibiotics such as fucidic acid are given for use on localized, small crops of lesions in systemically well children. Systemic antibiotics such as flucloxacillin can be considered in 'bullous' forms, more widespread disease or systemically unwell children. This child has widespread and worsening rash and so would benefit from both topical and systemic antibiotics treatment.

e Impetigo is highly contagious, through direct contact, so advice should be given to the patient and family about cleaning weeping areas of skin regularly, followed by thorough hand-washing, avoidance of sharing towels and bedsheets. If the rash responds poorly to treatment, or worsens, advise the parents to seek further medical help.

Case 3

a Haemorrhage into and just below the skin causes non-blanching rash correctly described by the following terms:

- petechiae – 1–2 mm purple or red spot caused by bleeding from surface capillaries
- purpura – 3–10 mm wide area of purple discolouration under the skin secondary to subcutaneous small vessel rupture
- echymoses – purpura measuring greater than 10 mm are termed echymoses, or in layman's terms, bruises.

b Think of the causes of a petechial or purpuric rash as being divided into those which cause the rash through low platelet numbers (thrombocytopaenia) and those which cause the rash through another mechanism.

Table 14.2

Thrombocytopaenic causes	Non-thrombocytopaenic causes
Idiopathic thrombocytopenia purpura	Meningococcal septicaemia
Disseminated Intravascular Coagulation	Vasculitis (e.g,. Henoch–Schonlein Purpura)
Leukaemia	Fragile vessels (senile purpura and steroid use)
Heparin-induced (HIT)	Bacterial endocarditis
	Trauma (direct pressure, tourniquets and coughing/vomiting in children)
	Simple viral illness
	Haemorrhagic fevers (typhus, dengue, ebola etc.)

c This young man has a very low platelet count with an otherwise normal full blood count and clotting studies, making idiopathic thrombocytopaenic purpura (ITP) the likely cause of his rash. ITP is due to an immunologically-mediated destruction of platelets which occurs as an acute mostly self-limiting form in children, but as a slower onset then chronic and recurrent form in adults. The immunological trigger for ITP is usually not known although in children, is thought most often to be an otherwise innocuous viral illness. As well as purpuric rash, bleeding may occur from the mucous membranes, gums and nose and there may be easy bruising; females may have menorrhagia.

d In managing ITP in a child, the following steps are important:

- make sure other diagnoses are excluded, particularly haematological malignancy
- assess bleeding risk. Platelet counts below 50×10^9/L are considered thrombocytopaenic, below 20×10^9/L, there is risk of spontaneous bleeding and below 10×10^9/L, there is risk of life-threatening intracerebral and gastrointestinal haemorrhage. Look for other risk factors for bleeding in the patients past medical history or medication list
- steroids (oral prednisolone) boost platelet numbers and are used for symptomatic bleeding and/or for platelet counts below 20×10^9/L
- IV immunoglobulin (IVIg) can be used to temporarily increase platelet numbers to halt severe bleeding
- platelet transfusions are not used (the immune process simply destroys the new platelets shortly after transfusion) except for life-threatening bleeding
- not all children with ITP need admission but all should be seen and assessed by the paediatrician prior to discharge.

Case 4

a Figure 14.3 shows an urticarial rash – raised pale red weals of various circular and irregular shapes covering a large area of skin. Although not evident from the picture, the weals are palpable and blanch with pressure.

b   Urticaria is a localized or generalized superficial oedema of the skin, caused
    by the release of potent inflammatory mediators such as histamine and
    bradykinin into the epidermis and mucous membranes, anywhere on the
    body. Urticaria may be acute (hours to six weeks) or chronic (greater than six
    weeks). In addition, the British Society of Dermatologists[3] divides the aetiology
    of urticaria into immunological (due to immune-mediated mast cell and
    basophil degranulation), non-immunological (release inflammatory mediators
    without immune triggers) or idiopathic (a large proportion of urticaria is cause
    unknown). However, the many actual causes of urticarial, do not all fall neatly
    into any of these classifications and the following may be of more practical use:

    ● ordinary urticaria – most common, idiopathic and usually lasts less than
      24 hours
    ● contact urticaria – nettle rash, latex allergy, animal dander
    ● allergic (type I hypersensitivity reaction) – nuts and food allergies, penicillin
      and other drugs, stings and other toxins
    ● physical urticaria – pressure, cold, vibration
    ● cholinergic urticaria – heat, exercise, emotional stress
    ● directly triggered release of histamine from mast cells – opiates
    ● histamine release without mast cell involvement – aspirin, NSAIDs
    ● vasculitic urticaria (often chronic) – SLE, autoimmune disease.

c   Urticaria may cause discomfort to distress but, alone, has no deleterious impact
    on health. Treatment proportionate to symptoms is with:

    ● H_1 antihistamines (2nd Generation) – cetirizine, loratadine, piriton
    ● H_2 antihistamines – cimetidine, ranitidine
    ● corticosteroids – for widespread/severe attacks, try short course prednisolone.

d   Angio-oedema arises from a similar pathological process as urticarial but, in
    contrast, causes inflammatory swelling deeper below the dermis of the skin
    (urticaria is above the dermis). As such, it is characterized by marked swelling
    of areas where the dermis is not tightly tethered, such as the lips, tongue, peri-
    orbitally and oropharynx and larynx. Angio-oedema is mostly self-limiting
    and benign, occurring with urticarial, in more than half affected patients. It is,
    however, treated with caution, as on occasion may cause difficult to treat life-
    threatening upper airway swelling. Angio-oedema is classified into idiopathic,
    immunological and hereditary.

e   Drugs commonly associated with angio-oedema include aspirin, ACE inhibitors,
    NSAIDs, statins, oestrogens and anti-psychotics. Note that symptoms of
    drug induced urticaria and angio-oedema (aspirin and NSAIDs-induced in
    particular) can suddenly arise, even after many years of drug use; being aware of
    this and withdrawing offending agents is often the key intervention to prevent
    recurrence.

f   Patients with hereditary angio-oedema lack circulating C1 esterase-inhibitor,
    a protease required to hold in check complement and inflammatory (kinin-
    kallikreinin) pathways, once triggered. Sufferers present from adolescence
    onward, with recurrent bouts of swelling of the skin, abdominal gut and of

the upper airway. Life-threatening laryngeal angio-oedema often occurs in this condition and, to add to the ED doctor's anxiety, is relatively resistant to conventional anti-allergy and anaphylaxis treatments. Thus, it is important to know that the emergency treatment of airway swelling in hereditary angio-oedema involves direct replacement of the missing enzyme by giving either IV C1-inhibitor concentrates (most EDs have access to this for emergencies) or 2–4 units of fresh frozen plasma, if concentrates are not available. Expert airway management may also be required.

Case 5

a This rash (Figure 14.4) is widespread and confluent (covering the vast majority of the body surface) as well as erythematous and exfoliative, as evidenced by large areas of silvery scales on underlying redness. Where greater than 90% of the skin is involved, the clinical condition is termed exfoliative dermatitis (or erythroderma) and is a dermatological emergency causing appreciable mortality.

b Exfoliative dermatitis has the following common causes:

- drug reaction (most common)
- psoriasis (erythrodermic psoriasis)
- haematological malignancy
- atopic dermatitis
- contact dermatitis
- 30% is idiopathic.

c Irrespective of cause, exfoliative dermatitis involves compromise of the integrity of the skin over virtually the entire body surface, which poses clinical issues, very similar to high percentage burns:

- fluid loss and the potential for dehydration and shock
- bacterial infection and sepsis
- body temperature dysregulation and hypothermia
- metabolic imbalances (hypoalbinaemia)
- high output cardiac failure due to cutaneous vasodilatation.

d Emergency department priorities in managing a patient with exfoliative dermatitis include:

- keep warm by taking measures to avoid hypothermia
- maintain hydration. Formulae for fluid replacement used in burns are not useful, as exfoliative dermatitis develops less acutely than a burn. Instead, chart fluid intake and output and aim to maintain urine output at greater than 30 mL/hr with IV normal saline as necessary (at least 3 L/day)
- dress 'wet' areas of skin with non-adherent dressings or wet gauze
- treat any evidence of bacterial infection with IV antibiotics to cover staphylococcus and streptococcus species (e.g., flucloxacillin 1 g IV qds and/or benzylpenicillin 1.2 g IV qds)

- moderate strength topical steroid creams are the mainstay of treatment e.g., betnovate (betamethasone 0.1%)
- antihistamines (e.g., chlorphenamine 4 mg p.o. qds) for pruritis
- admit the patient to hospital under the general medical team and refer immediately for review by a dermatologist.

Case 6

a The rash of atopic or infantile eczema is usually easy to recognize and has the following features:

- flexural distribution (anticubital fossa, popliteal fossa, buttocks, flexural aspect of the wrists, face and anterior neck)
- affected areas exhibit dry eythematous skin
- cracking of the skin and bleeding is often present
- itching
- excoriation from scratching.

b Eczema is a frequent cause of paediatric presentation to the ED. Despite rarely constituting an actual emergency, the variable efficacy of treatments initially prescribed in the community leads the carer to seek advice from the hospital. The treatment of atopic eczema is fairly straightforward, and escalates according to clinical severity, with the general principle that it should be managed with the least potent intervention which controls symptoms.

Avoid detergent soaps which remove natural skin oils and stop any other skin products in use

↓

Start with simple emollients applied to dry skin. Aqueous cream is a good start, moving up to greasier emollients such as diprobase, oilatum and epaderm, on severely dry skin

↓

Oral antihistamines (chlorphenamine 1 mg qds for a child aged three years) used to reduce itching, particularly at night, where the sedative effect of piriton is useful in children!

↓

Mild to moderate eczema, unresponsive to emollients, can be treated with weak topical corticosteroids such as hydrocortisone 1% cream or ointment applied twice daily to areas, until clinical improvement occurs

↓

More potent topical corticosteroids are used for severe atopic eczema and for acute flare-ups. They should really be used under specialist supervision and used on the limbs only (not the face) for short periods (one to two weeks max). By this stage, the child should be under the care of a dermatologist or eczema clinic

---

c The two main complications of eczema which can be sufficiently serious to require admission to hospital are, superinfection with bacteria, and infection with herpes simplex virus. Both may present as a flare-up of eczema and close examination should always be undertaken to ensure neither is present in patients of any age with worsening eczema.

Bacterial infection of eczematous skin is almost always staphylococcal and may give skin erosions, an impetigo-type picture or, most serious, a widespread cellulitis. Treatment of mild localized infection is with topical antibacterials (e.g, fucidic acid or mupuricin), although more widespread infection requires systemic antibiotics – oral or intravenous as clinically indicated.

Eczema herpeticum appears as a sudden outbreak of vesicles and pustules over active areas of eczema. The vesicles burst, crust over and form small ulcers very characteristic of this condition. Herpetic lesions may spread rapidly to involve large areas and, occasionally, become generalized and life-threatening. Topical steroids predispose to eczema herpeticum and must be stopped immediately. Further treatment is with anti-virals such as acyclovir or valcyclovir and again oral or intravenous, according to clinical situation.

d Infantile eczema is an atopic disease and children with one atopic illness are more at risk of the others which are hayfever, asthma, food and drug allergies as well as urticaria.

Case 7

a This patient has evolving rheumatoid arthritis (RA) with the photograph (Figure 14.5) showing 'sausage fingers' of early RA and bilaterally swollen metacarpo-phalangeal joints(MCPJs). The American College of Rheumatology sets out seven diagnostic clinical features of RA that are worth remembering (Box 14.1).

Box 14.1 American College of Rheumatology diagnostic features of rheumatoid arthritis:[4]

- symmetrical arthritis lasting at least 6 weeks
- swelling of the MCPJ, PIPJ or wrists for at least six weeks
- soft-tissue swelling of three or more areas for at least six weeks
- morning stiffness around joints improving after one hour and present for at least six weeks
- subcutaneous nodules
- positive test for Rheumatoid factor
- radiographic erosions +/- periarticular osteopaenia in the hands.

---

b Rheumatoid arthritis first manifests in the hands as digital swelling and swelling of the metacarpo-phalangeal joints (MCPJ) and proximal interphalangeal joints (PIPJ). Progresive synovitis at the MCPJs, causes the classic appearances of ulnar deviation and volar subluxation at these joints. Further structural abnormalities include swan neck deformity (PIPJ hyperextension and DIPJ flexion) and Boutonnière's deformity (PIP hyperflexion with DIP hyperextension) of the fingers distal to the knuckles. Rheumatoid nodules (firm lumps under the skin) may also be seen on the fingers.

c Radiological findings in rheumatoid arthritis include the following:

- soft-tissue swelling
- peri-articular osteoporosis
- joint space narrowing
- bony erosions/subluxations.

d The British Society for Rheumatology guidelines[5] suggest initiating paracetamol and NSAIDs in the ED to patients with newly diagnosed synovitis. Patients should also be directed back to their GP for referral to a specialist as per local guidelines.

e Disease-modifying anti-rheumatic drugs (DMARDs) such as methotrexate, sulfasalazine, gold, penicillamine, azothioprine, cyclosporine and leflunomide are all immunosuppressants used in treating moderate to severe rheumatoid disease under specialist guidance. In addition, monoclonal antibodies which inhibit TNF-alpha function such as etanercept and infliximab are also increasingly used having shown considerable benefits in severe RA.

It is important to be aware that all the DMARDS listed above, to a greater or lesser degree, can cause myelosuppression or bone marrow suppression. While it is obviously unnecessary to perform a full blood count on every patient taking DMARDs presenting the ED, it is important to recognize the features of myelosuppression so that any patient with this serious side-effect of their rheumatoid medication, is not missed. Clinical features which might raise suspicion of myelosuppression include:

- sore throat
- fever and other signs of infection
- unexpected bleeding or bruising
- purpura and rashes
- mouth ulcers
- cough or breathlessness.

Investigate with full blood count (low haemoglobin, neutropaenia and thrombocytopaenia) and, if present, stop the DMARD responsible, treat as per neutropaenic protocol and refer to the medical team on-call and haematologist.

Case 8

a This patient has ankylosing spondylitis (AS). This is a chronic seronegative spondyloarthropathy affecting the axial skeleton, and manifesting most commonly with sacroiliitis (inflammation of the sacroiliac joint) and spondylitis (inflammation of the vertebrae). Ninety-two per cent of patients with AS will be HLA B27 positive, compared to only 6% of the general population. It has a 5:1 male preponderance with onset classically between ages 15–25, with the highest prevalence amongst northern European populations.

b The British Society for Rheumatology outlines three clinical criteria for diagnosing ankolysing spondylitis:

- greater than three months lower back pain – improved by exercise; not relieved by rest
- reduced lumbar spine movement in flexion, extension and lateral flexion
- limitation of chest expansion.

The radiological finding of sacroiliitis with one or more of the above clinical features makes the diagnosis certain.

c Extra articular associations – the **'5 A's'** are:

- **a**nterior uveitis
- **a**pical fibrosis
- **a**ortitis
- **A**V conduction block
- **a**myloidosis.

d The diagnostic radiographic finding of sacroiliitis may not always be evident in early disease. A lumbar spine and pelvis X-ray must be ordered to look for early changes such as blurring in the lower part of the joint. Evolving changes are then bony erosions and/or sclerosis around the sacroiliac joints, and eventual fusion of the sacrum and ileum.

　　Spinal osteopaenia may be seen and changes such as 'squaring' of the vertebral bodies can occur with eventual ossification of the spinal ligaments and complete fusion of vertebrae, giving the classical 'bamboo spine' appearance.

e Treatment of AS in the ED should be with NSAIDs and oral steroids for acute exacerbations. These patients require rheumatology follow-up for consideration of steroid injections and anti-TNF alpha therapy in severe disease. Advise exercise – as much as tolerable and **not** rest for backpain. The physiotherapist may be able to help.

Case 9

a The X-ray (Figure 14.6) shows soft-tissue swelling around the MTPJ and punched out lesions (peri-articular erosions), at the MTPJ and IPJ of the big toe, both typical radiographic findings in gout. Loss of joint space and occasionally tophi are also seen in chronic disease.

b This patient has gout, a crystal arthropathy due to urate crystal accumulation in the joint. The metatarsophalangeal joint of the big toe is the most common site affected (>50% of acute presentations) while other common sites include the ankle, knee, midfoot, wrist and distal interphalangeal joints of the fingers. Investigations to support the diagnosis may come from a raised serum uric acid level but joint aspiration is the gold standard and will reveal monosodium urate crystals that are negatively birefringent on polarizing microscopy.

c Gout may be classified as primary or secondary. Primary gout occurs typically in middle-aged men who suffer recurrent attacks due to idiopathic hyperuricaemia. Secondary gout has an identifiable cause.

Table 14.3

Risk factors for primary gout	Identifiable causes in secondary gout
Male sex (9:1 male to female ratio)	Diuretic therapy (most common cause)
Alcohol (red wine!)	Polycytheamia
Red meat consumption	Chronic renal failure
Diabetes	Chronic alcohol excess
Obesity	Cytotoxic drug therapy
Hypertension	Osteoarthritis
	Joint trauma

d Recurrent episodes may lead to chronic tophi, irregular hard nodules found in the 1st MTPJ, ears, extensor surface of hands, fingers, elbow and the Achilles tendons. Chronic tophaceous gout is becoming less prevalent due to better management of the primary disease.

e Treat acute gout as follows:[6]

- affected joints should be rested
- a rapid acting oral NSAID at maximal doses (e.g., diclofenac 50 mg tds or indometacin 100 mg bd) is first-line treatment (consider need for gastric protection with proton pump inhibitor)
- where NSAIDs are contraindicated – hypersensitivity, peptic ulcer disease, asthma, and severe ischaemic heart disease – colchicine is next in line. Thus, the patient in this question who has active peptic ulcer disease should be treated with colchicine: give 1 mg STAT then 0.5 mg every six hours until pain relieved or either the side-effect of diarrhoea develops or the maximum dose of 6 mg for any one course is reached
- note that renal impairment is a contra-indication for both NSIADs and colchicine; try oral prednisolone
- allopurinol should be continued (but not started) during an acute attack.

Longer term management involves advising patients with gout to avoid alcohol, eat less red meat and lose weight. Reduce or stop diuretics, if appropriate and safe. Allopurinol should be started by their GP once the acute attack has subsided.[6]

Case 10

a The differential diagnosis of an acute non-traumatic monoarthropathy of the knee is as follows:

- septic arthritis (until proven otherwise)
- crystal arthropathy (gout, pseudogout)
- acute exacerbation of osteoarthritis
- bursitis/infected bursitis
- reactive arthritis (follows GI infection)
- psoriatic arthritis
- there are others (Reiter's disease, mono-articular rheumatoid disease etc.).

b Any acutely hot, swollen joint with restriction of movement is septic arthritis until proven not to be. In addition, the patient in the question has a fever and so septic arthritis becomes the working diagnosis. Joint sepsis is more common than we think occurring in 10–20/100 000 UK population and remains a serious problem not just because of the potential for irreversible joint destruction but also because of associated mortality of 10% (also irreversible!). There are five routes for joint infection:

Table 14.4

Route	Examples
Haematogenous spread	Bacteria seed into joint synovial fluid from the bloodstream (e.g., from a bacteraemia following a dental procedure or from IV drug abuse using unclean materials)
External puncture	Introduction of bacteria into the joint following penetrating trauma (e.g., infection of the 5th metacarpophalangeal joint after a bite wound to the overlying skin acquired during a punch to the face)
Iatrogenic	Following invasive procedures to the joint (e.g., arthroscopy, joint aspirations, therapeutic joint injections) also include post-operative prosthetic joint infection in this category
Spread from adjacent soft tissue infection	Spread from a bursitis, overlying cellulitis or abscess
Extension of osteomyelitis	Dissemination of organisms from infected bone to the joint medium

c The three most common causative organisms in septic arthritis are *Staphylococcus aureus*, *Haemophilus influenza* and streptococcal species. Think also of *Gonococcus* in young adults and consider gram –ve organism in the elderly, immunocompromised and those with prosthetic joints. Also, anaerobes (think *Clostridium*) in penetrating injury to a joint. Remember salmonella osteomyelitis occurs with sickle cell disease.

d This patient requires joint aspiration under an aseptic technique. The fluid should be sent urgently for:

- gram stain
- culture
- crystals
- cell count.

And the results interpreted as follows:

Table 14.5

	Normal fluid	Reactive fluid	Septic fluid
Colour	Colourless	Yellow	Yellow
Turbidity	Clear	Turbid	Purulent
Cell type	Mononuclear	Neutrophils	Neutrophils
Cell count	200–1000	3000–10 000	>10 000
Gram stain	None	None	Positive
Culture	Negative	Negative	Positive

e Three key steps in the ED management of a septic arthritis are:

- symptomatic treatment with analgesics, antipyretics and place the patient nil by mouth and on IV fluids
- start IV antibiotics immediately. IV flucloxacillin 1g qds and benzylpenicillin 1.2g qds in most cases, although add gentamycin where gram −ve infection is possible and metronidazole for penetrating injuries to the joint
- immediate referral to the orthopaedic team for joint wash-out in theatre.

Further Reading

1. Buxton PK. (2003) *ABC of Dermatology*, 4th edn. BMJ Publishing Group.
2. Collier OJ, Longmore M, Turmezi T, *et al.* (2009) *Oxford Handbook of Clinical Specialties*. 8th edn. Oxford University Press. pp 582–611.
3. Grattan CEH, Humphreys FY. (Dec 2007) British Association of Dermatologists. Guidelines for evaluation and management of urticaria in adults and children. *Br J Dermatology*, **157**, pp 1116–23. Also found on the British Association of Dermatologists website www.bad.org.uk
4. American College of Rheumatologists. (2010) The 2010 ACR–EULAR classification criteria for rheumatoid arthritis. www.rheumatology.org/practice/clinical/classification/ra/_2010.asp
5. British Society for Rheumatology. (2006) British Society for Rheumatology and British Health Professionals in Rheumatology Guideline for the Management of Rheumatoid Arthritis. www.rheumatology.org.uk/includes/documents/cm_docs/2009/m/management_of_rheumatoid_arthritis_first_2_years.pdf
6. British Society for Rheumatology. (2007) British Society for Rheumatology and British Health Professionals in Rheumatology Guideline for the Management of Gout. www.rheumatology.org.uk/includes/documents/cm_docs/2009/m/management_of_gout.pdf

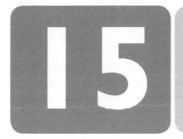

OPHTHALMIC EMERGENCIES

Mathew Hall

Introduction

Core topics

- the red eye
- the painful eye
- sudden loss of vision
- eye infection
- acute glaucoma
- iritis/episcleritis
- chemical eye injury
- ocular trauma (blunt, penetrating and foreign bodies)
- orbital and peri-orbital cellulitis
- retinopathy (hypertensive and diabetic)
- diplopia.

It is vital to know the serious and not so serious causes of red eye and how to identify and manage each one (Box 15.1). In addition, know the differential diagnosis for sudden visual loss and revise the management of all ocular trauma from a simple foreign body to penetrating injuries, globe rupture and chemical eye injury, as all have appeared as SAQs.[1] Also, be able to express visual acuity as measured using a typical Emergency Department (ED) Snellen chart – remember 6/9 means that, at best, the subject could read the line marked nine at six metres from the chart.[2]

Box 15.1

Serious and uncommon (requiring specialist management)	Not so serious but common (ED care in the first instance)
Acute angle closure glaucoma (AACG)	Conjunctivitis (allergic, bacterial and viral)
Iritis (anterior uveitis)	Subconjunctival haemorrhage
Scleritis and episcleritis	Simple foreign body
Corneal ulceration (especially in contact lens wearer)	Corneal abrasions
Orbital cellulitis and endopthalmitis (intraocular infection)	
Chemical eye injury	

Case 1

A 70-year old Afro-Caribbean woman complains of a 'boring' pain behind her left eye, associated with blurring of vision the same eye. The pain woke her in the middle of the night and is getting progressively worse. You suspect she has acute angle closure glaucoma.

a Give four signs of acute angle closure glaucoma for which you would examine in this woman. [4]

b Briefly outline the patho-physiology behind this condition. [2]

c Give three treatments (with drug names and routes) that are used to lower intraocular pressure in an emergency. [4]

d What is the definitive management of acute angle closure glaucoma? [1]

e Name two drugs which may precipitate acute glaucoma in susceptible individuals. [2]

[13]

Case 2

The emergency nurse practitioner asks for your opinion on a 32-year-old man with bilateral red eyes. He gives no history of trauma or foreign body but reports discomfort in both eyes and some sensitivity to light.

a List three signs or symptoms which you would look for and which suggest a sinister cause of acute 'red eye'. [3]

b Briefly describe how scleritis or episcleritis differs in appearance from conjunctivitis. [2]

c You suspect this man has conjunctivitis. Give three questions you would ask him to identify a specific cause or pathogen. [3]

d How would you treat, and what advice would you give, this man with presumed conjunctivitis? [4]

[12]

Case 3

A 66-year-old woman comes to the ED straight from the local theatre. While watching the play, she suddenly noticed she had lost sight in the right eye. She has no other symptoms and the vision in her left eye is unaffected. It is now 45 minutes since the onset of blindness. Below is a picture of her right retina visualized with fundoscopy (Figure 15.1).

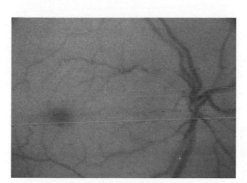

Figure 15.1 (see colour plate.)

a List a differential diagnosis for sudden loss of vision in one eye. [4]
b Describe the abnormalities in the picture (Figure 15.1) and give your
diagnosis for this woman's sudden loss of vision. [3]
c Give two predisposing conditions for the diagnosis you have made. [2]
d Describe two interventions which you might try in the ED to save this
woman's sight. [2]

[11]

Case 4

A 46-year-old insulin-dependent diabetic man is referred by the out-of-hours
GP service for suspected orbital cellulitis. He is feverish and in considerable pain
in his left eye. Triage observations indicate a pulse of 90 bpm and blood pressure
140/90 mmHg.

a Give four clinical signs that distinguish orbital cellulitis from peri-orbital
cellulitis. [4]
b Describe three modes of transmission of infection into the orbit. [3]
c Name the two most common organisms responsible for orbital cellulitis. [2]
d Outline the key steps in your management plan for this patient with orbital
cellulitis. [3]

[12]

Case 5

A 38-year-old man has been struck in the right eye by a fast moving squash ball. Since then, he has had severe pain and reduced vision in the left eye which is weeping profusely. An FY2 doctor has examined the eye and calls you to review her findings (Figure 15.2).

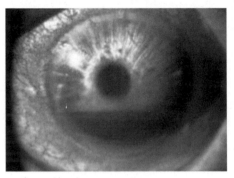

Figure 15.2 (see colour plate.)

a Give six components of the comprehensive eye examination you would
 perform. [6]
b Describe the abnormality in the picture. [1]
c What steps will you take in managing this patient? [3]
d While you are examining the patient, he tells you that he saw flashing lights
 at the moment when the ball struck his eye. What additional complication
 does this indicate? [2]
[12]

Case 6

A six-year-old child is brought to the ED screaming. The history is that half an hour earlier the child was playing with a sachet of concentrated washing liquid. The sachet burst and the contents sprayed into the child's eyes. The child has a red weeping left eye which he will not allow anyone near.

a Give two chemicals or classes of chemical, which are particularly harmful
 to the eye. [2]
b Describe your immediate management of this child. [4]
c What examination will you perform once immediate management is
 complete? [2]
d Give two clinical signs which suggest severe eye injury. [2]
e What is the definitive management of this patient? [2]
[12]

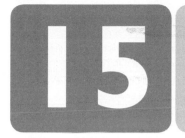

OPHTHALMIC EMERGENCIES – ANSWERS

Case 1

a Acute angle closure glaucoma (AACG) is an ophthalmological emergency caused by rapid rise of intraocular pressure. Classic presentation is as a unilateral red eye associated with pain, vomiting, and impaired vision. The onset is swift, over a few hours is typical, and there may be a recent history of similar attacks which spontaneously abated. Often, there is a preceding history of seeing haloes around lights, particularly at night. Clinical signs to look for include:

- corneal and scleral injection (red eye)
- semi-dilated pupil
- the pupil may be unresponsive to light
- reduced intraocular movements
- hazy oedematous cornea (visible with or without the slit lamp)
- decreased visual acuity (finger counting only)
- tender, hard globe to palpation
- a shallow anterior chamber may be noted on slit lamp examination.

Fundoscopy may indeed show optic disc cupping although may not be possible through a cloudy cornea. Also remember that mydriatics will exacerbate angle closure and are strictly contra-indicated. Overall, therefore, fundoscopy is often unhelpful in AACG.

b In predisposed individuals, the iris may closely appose the lens inhibiting the flow of vitreous fluid from posterior to anterior chamber. Consequently, the lens bulges forward under the increasing backpressure and blocks the trabecular meshwork and canal of Schlemm which drains vitreous fluid from the anterior chamber. Vitreous fluid production continues but its drainage is now completely blocked and the intraocular pressure rises quickly causing the ciliary body, lens and cornea to become ischaemic and the eye blind.

c Urgent treatment is required with drugs to lower intraocular pressure. The following can be used:

Table 15.1

Drug	Action
Acetazolamide 500 mg PO/IV	Carbonic anhydrase inhibitor which reduces the production of aqueous fluid in the eye
Pilocarpine (2% or 4%) eye drops. Give hourly until definitive treatment	Constricting the pupil pulls it away from the iris and reduces obstruction of the drainage system
β-adrenergic eye drops (Timolol 0.5% or levobunolol 0.5%)	Reduces aqueous humour production
Apraclonidine (0.5% or 1%) eye drops	Alpha-adrenergic agent which reduces intraocular pressure in both acute and chronic glaucoma
Mannitol	Powerful osmotic diuretic used to reduce intraocular pressure pre-operatively (one for the ophthalmologist to advise on!)

d Patients with AACG are referred immediately to an ophthalmic surgeon for definitive treatment – peripheral iridectomy either by surgery or laser.

e Drugs which may precipitate AACG in patients at risk (i.e., the long-sighted, those with shallow anterior chambers and narrow angles, and those with a previous history of AACG) include mydriatic eye drops, anticholinergic agents and antidepressants. In addition, rapid correction of hyperglycaemia may cause osmotic movement of water into the eye with accompanying sudden increase in pressure.

Case 2

a The acute non-traumatic red eye is a frequent and easy to mismanage ED presentation. First, ask yourself are there any features of a sinister cause such as:

● significant pain
● reduced or loss of vision
● pupil abnormalities
● corneal abnormalities

In addition, a unilateral red eye should always be viewed with more suspicion than bilateral. The above features are associated with the following serious causes of red eye:

Table 15.2

Serious cause of red eye	Pain	Visual acuity	Pupil abnormality	Corneal abnormality
Acute angle closure glaucoma	+++	Reduced	Semi-dilated and unresponsive to light	Cloudy
Iritis (anterior uveitis)	++	Reduced	Constricted	Normal
Corneal ulceration	+++	Normal or reduced (depending on location ulcer)	Normal	Ulceration visible with fluorescein staining

continued

| Scleritis | ++ | Normal or reduced | Normal | Normal |
| Orbital cellulitis | ++++ | Normal early/reduced later | Pain on eye movements. Ophthalmoplegia | Chemosed |

b The episclera lies just below the conjunctiva whilst the sclera forms the protective outer coat all around the eye. Both may become inflamed, either idiopathically, or in association with systemic autoimmune disease, to give a unilateral or sometimes bilateral red eye. Episcleritis is usually self-limiting whereas scleritis is more serious carrying the danger of globe perforation. When suspected, both should be referred to the ophthalmologist. They are distinguishable from conjunctivitis by: more localized or focal nature of the visible inflammation; larger size of inflamed vessels; more painful; and globe tenderness.

c Uncomplicated conjunctivitis presents with none of the above sinister features. Instead, one or both eyes are uniformly inflamed, feel gritty and there may be clear or purulent discharge. Vision, pupils and cornea are all normal. Questions to ask to ascertain the cause or pathogen responsible in a young man should include:

- are your eyes sticky or crusty in the morning? Is the discharge purulent? Sticky mucopurulent discharge indicates bacterial conjunctivitis with the most common organisms being Staphylococcal and Streptococcal commensals, *Haemophilus influenza* and *Corynebacterium* sp
- do you wear contact lenses? An important question. Contact lens use predisposes to pseudomonal infection, which may rapidly progress to corneal ulceration, abscess and irreversible blindness. Examine the eye of contact lens wearers with fluorescein and refer immediately those with suspected corneal ulceration
- do you have any genital discharge or lesions? *Chlamydia* and gonorrhoea both cause a florid conjunctivitis associated with the venereal symptoms and require systemic, as well as topical treatment; *Chlamydia* with tetracycline for 4 weeks and gonorrhoea with a penicillin
- are your eyes very itchy? Allergic conjunctivitis is common, affects both eyes and may have concomitant history of allergen contact. Along with conjunctival injection, there is corneal oedema and even swollen papillae on the underside of the eyelids. Treatment is with sodium cromoglycate eye drops and allergen avoidance.

d Uncomplicated conjunctivitis is treated with chloramphenicol eye drops two to four hourly and ointment at night. Gentamycin eye drops and ointment are an alternative. Swab any discharge and send for culture. Importantly, conjunctivitis is contagious and viral conjunctivitis highly so. Thus, advise strict hygiene with hand-washing after touching eyes and different towels and face products for each member of the family. Tell them not to worry if a unilateral conjunctivitis becomes bilateral, and to apply the same treatment to both eyes, if this occurs. They must return to the ED if pain develops or vision becomes impaired: corneal ulceration and abscess are uncommon complications but do occur.

Case 3

a The differential diagnosis of sudden unilateral loss of vision may be helpfully divided into painless and painful causes:

Table 15.3

Painless	Painful
Central retinal vein occlusion (and branch retinal vein occlusion) Central retinal artery occlusion Amaurosis fugax (temporary loss of vision) Vitreous haemorrhage (diabetics with severe retinopathy) Retinal detachment (idiopathic, trauma and diabetic retinopathy)	Acute angle closure glaucoma Traumatic globe rupture Rarely visual loss may accompany migraine

b The photograph (Figure 15.1) shows a pale retina with absence of normal vessels and presence of the pathognomonic 'cherry red spot'. This is the fundoscopic appearance of central retinal artery occlusion (CRAO). Devoid of its arterial supply, the retina appears pale with the only colouration at the macular, the thinnest part of the retina where the underlying, and unaffected, choroidal circulation is visible as an area of redness, the 'cherry red spot'. Blindness results from retinal ischaemia.

c Like any other occlusive arterial disease, CRAO may be due to thrombus, emboli, vasculitis or hyperviscosity. Anatomically, the retinal artery is a branch of the ophthalmic artery which branches from the internal carotid artery. Thus, carotid artery atherosclerotic disease may provide a source of emboli aimed at the retinal circulation whilst temporal arteritis (giant cell arteritis) does not just affect the temporal arteries but causes granulomatous inflammation with occlusion of similar sized vessels such as the ophthalmic and retinal arteries. It is important to recognize these two predisposing conditions as treatment with anti-platelet agents and endarterectomy for carotid disease, or with steroids for giant cell arteritis, is required to reduce the risk of blindness in the other eye.

d Clear evidence is lacking in support of any particular treatment regime for CRAO but most authorities advise at least trying the following if presentation is within one to two hours of symptom onset. Ocular massage may be attempted to break up the occluding embolus by repeatedly pushing firmly on the eyeball for 15 seconds and then quickly releasing the pressure. Alternatively, medical therapy involves lowering intraocular pressure to improve perfusion with acetozolamide 500 mg PO/IV and β-adrenergic agents such as timolol eye drops. Urgent ophthalmology review is also required.

Case 4

a The orbital septum is a protective fascial sheet extending from the periosteum of the orbital rim to the tarsal plates and separates peri-orbital soft tissue from contents of the eye socket. Peri-orbital (pre-septal) cellulitis describes bacterial infection of the skin around the eye, anterior to the orbital septum, whilst orbital cellulitis is post-septal and involves the eye itself. Thus, signs specific to orbital cellulitis include:

- ocular tenderness is an early sign, then
- conjunctival chemosis (oedema)
- ophthalmoplegia
- proptosis
- decreased visual acuity (including complete blindness of the affected eye)
- fever is usually present.

Marked swelling of the eyelids occurs with both peri-orbital and orbital cellulitis and it is not until the eyelids are prised open and the eye itself examined for the features above that the two are distinguished.

b Infection may enter the orbital cavity from a number of sources:

- most common, particularly in children, is the extension of infection from adjacent paranasal sinuses. Particularly, ethmoid sinus suppuration invades the orbit through perforations in the thin bony wall separating the two cavities. The patient may have a history of preceding sinusitis with nasal discharge
- other sources of local spread are dental abscesses, primary globe infections or through orbital wall fractures
- inoculation from penetrating eye injury or intra-ocular foreign body
- as a post-operative complication of eye surgery
- haematogenous spread is rare but can always occur.

High risk groups are the very young, diabetics and those with immuno-compromise.

c Given that the sinuses are the most common source of orbital infection, the most common infecting organisms are those of the upper respiratory tract – *Haemophilus influenza type B, Staphylococcus aureus* and *Streptococcus sp.* Gram –ve organisms can be found particularly if spread is from an oral source. The immunocompromised are at risk of fungal infection.

d Treatment must be prompt and aggressive to save the eye:

- culture blood and any nasal discharge
- start broad spectrum IV antibiotics covering upper respiratory gram +ve and gram –ve flora (co-amoxiclav or third generation cephalosporin) straight away in the ED
- analgesia titrated to pain (IV morphine if severe) and other supportive measures, as required
- immediate referral for admission by an ophthalmologist/ophthalmic surgeon. Orbital abscess drainage may be required
- also involve an ENT specialist for evaluation and treatment of a causative sinusitis
- investigate with CT imaging of the orbit and sinuses.

For completeness, loss of sight in the affected eye is the most common complication of orbital cellulitis (roughly 10%) although spread of unchecked disease may also cause frontal brain abscesses, meningitis and cavernous sinus thrombosis.

Case 5

a A comprehensive examination of the injured eye includes the steps below. Note, however, that where globe rupture is suspected, any pressure on the eyeball is avoided and topical eye drops (including fluorescein, cycloplegics and local anaesthetic drops) are contraindicated.

- **general inspection**. Severe injury may be obvious with enopthalmus (recession of the globe within the orbit) and/or prolapse of tissue outwards from a ruptured globe
- **visual acuity**. Both eyes should be tested separately using a Snellen chart. If vision is too poor to read the first line of the chart, record whether the patient is able to see fingers placed in the line of vision, then whether or not there is any light perception in the affected eye
- **eye movements**. Ophthalmoplegia is a sign of serious eye injury. Diplopia after blunt trauma prompts consideration of orbital floor fracture with prolapsed orbital contents
- **pupil shape, size, and reaction to light**. The pupil may be irregular if lacerated, or dilated and unreactive in serious globe trauma causing paralysis of the iris muscles
- **examine for one (or more) foreign bodies**. Evert the eyelids, examine the cornea with a slit lamp and view the anterior chamber for intraocular FBs
- **seidel test**. This looks for fluid leakage from the anterior chamber as a positive sign of globe rupture. Gently place a fluorescein dye strip onto the cornea at the site of injury and examine with a cobalt blue light. Streaming of darkened fluorescein down away from the site indicates fluid leakage as does dilution of the fluorescein colour at the tip of the strip. Very useful
- **examine for a corneal abrasion**. Once globe rupture is excluded, instil fluorescein drops and examine the cornea under a cobalt blue light. Abrasions show as green areas over the cornea invariant with blinking
- **fundoscopy**. Look for retinal detachment and vitreous haemorrhage as signs of posterior segment injury
- **do not forget to look for eyelid injuries or damage to the lacrimal ducts**. Lacerations of the eyelid margins and lacrimal duct injuries require specialist repair
- **examine the peri-orbital soft tissues and bones**. Important with blunt trauma, and facial X-rays may be required.

b Figure 15.2 shows a hyphaema or collection of blood in the anterior chamber, often forming a fluid level of dependent blood. Hyphaema arise from significant blunt or penetrating trauma to the globe, rupturing the blood vessels of the iris.

c   Management of a hyphaema involves:

- analgesia (e.g., ibuprofen 400 mg PO)
- use an eye shield (not a soft patch) to protect from any further external pressure
- all traumatic globe injuries with hyphaema need specialist assessment, so refer to the ophthalmologist immediately. Small hyphaema are treated conservatively and clear spontaneously, while larger hyphaema, particularly where the anterior chamber is completely filled with blood – the 'eight ball' hyphaema – may require surgical drainage
- the complication of most concern is raised ocular pressure; some treat with steroids to reduce this risk.

d   Flashing lights at the moment of impact raise the possibility of retinal detachment. Test for visual field defects and examine the fundi carefully. Refer to the ophthalmologist all patients with symptoms of retinal detachment (flashing lights, multiple floaters, field defects) even if you cannot detect an abnormality with fundoscopy.

Case 6

a   Chemical eye burns are common occupational injuries but also arise from household cleaning products; the classic is the young child splashed with a burst sachet of concentrated washing detergent (strongly alkaline). Most damaging to the eye are strong alkali (pH >10) and strong acids (particularly hydrofluoric acid).

b   All eyes subject to chemical injury should be irrigated to neutral pH (7.0–7.5). Instil local anaesthetic eye drops and irrigate directly with 1–2 litres of 0.9% saline or sterile water. Recheck the pH of the eye with litmus paper and continue irrigation until it reads neutral.

c   Once irrigated, try to examine the eye under direct vision and using a slit lamp. Instil fluorescein drops and look for a corneal epithelial defect (shows bright green with cobalt blue light). Test visual acuity.

d   Unsurprisingly, signs of severe chemical eye injury are reduced visual acuity or loss of vision and a whitened or opaque cornea, indicating irreversible corneal ischaemia 'white eye'.

e   All, except the most benign, chemical eye injuries should be seen by the ophthalmologist – refer with urgency related to degree of apparent injury. Chloramphenicol eye drops should also be given as prophylaxis against infection.

Further Reading

1. Khaw PT and Pilkington AR. (1999) *ABC of Eyes,* 3rd edn. BMJ Publishing Group.
2. Collier JAB, Longmore JM, Turmezei T, *et al.* (2009) Oxford Handbook of Clinical Specialties, 8th edn. Oxford University Press, pp 410–65.

16 OBSTETRIC AND GYNAECOLOGICAL EMERGENCIES

Sam Thenabadu

Introduction

Core topics

- ectopic (tubal) pregnancy
- antepartum haemorrhage
- hyperemesis gravidarum
- pre-eclampsia, eclampsia and the HELLP syndrome
- miscarriage (cervical shock)
- use of anti-D immunoglobulin to prevent rhesus haemolytic disease
- trauma in the pregnant woman
- intermenstrual bleeding
- vaginal discharge and sexually transmitted diseases
- pelvic inflammatory disease
- pelvic pain in the non-pregnant woman (ovarian cysts, ovarian torsion, endometriosis)
- presentations of gynaecological cancer.

The Royal College of Obstetrics and Gynaecology (RCOG) publish online and regularly update a series of guidelines on the management of obstetric and gynaecological problems known as the Green Top guidelines. They are readily found at the RCOG website www.rcog.org.uk. Another excellent source of revision is the *Oxford Handbook of Clinical Specialties* (8th edn) chapters on Obstetrics and Gynaecology.

Case I

A 36-year-old female, who is 30 weeks pregnant, presents to the Emergency Department (ED) with vaginal bleeding for the previous six hours. She has had no abdominal pains. It is her second pregnancy and she knows her blood group is AB negative. Her observations are heart rate 110 bpm, blood pressure 100/55 mmHg and respiratory rate 24/min.

a What are the two common causes of vaginal bleeding in later pregnancy? [2]
b Give four clinical features which would help distinguish between the two
   causes you give in answer to **a.** above. [4]
c What examination must be avoided and why? [2]
d Give four management steps in the ED. [4]
e Name four indications for giving anti-D immunoglobulin in the ED. [2]
   [14]

Case 2

A 28-year-old woman who is 32 weeks pregnant presents to the ED with a six-hour history of frontal headache and blurred vision. She has not attended any of her antenatal appointments since the booking scan at 11 weeks, where a single intrauterine pregnancy was seen.

a What three features are required for the diagnosis of pre-eclampsia? [3]
b Which pregnancies are at risk of pre-eclampsia? Give four maternal risk
   factors as your answer. [2]
c You suspect pre-eclampsia in this patient. Give three further clinical signs
   which might indicate the mother has severe pre-eclampsia and is in danger
   of eclampsia and seizures. [3]
d Before you have appreciated the full seriousness of the situation, the woman
   suffers a tonic-clonic seizure in the ED. What pharmacological treatment is
   required now (gives dose and route)? [3]
e The full blood count for this patient show a normal white cell count and
   haemoglobin level but a platelet count of 45×10^9/L. What important
   diagnosis, related to pre-eclampsia, does this result indicate is present and
   what, apart from thrombocytopenia, are the other clinical features of this
   diagnosis (give two)? [3]
   [14]

Case 3

A 22-year-old primipara, who is 10 weeks pregnant, presents to the ED with severe vomiting. She had suffered from early morning vomiting since six weeks into the pregnancy but over the past five days the vomiting has become continuous and she now feels weak and lightheaded on standing. Her initial observations are heart rate 105 bpm, blood pressure 105/65 mmHg and temperature 37.2 °C.

a Apart from continuous nausea and vomiting, give three features which help diagnose hyperemesis gravidarum. [3]
b Name two urinary investigations which should be performed in the ED for this patient. [2]
c The FY2 doctor who has initially assessed this patient asks for advice on what blood tests to perform. What blood tests would be of value in this situation giving your reasons (give two blood investigations)? [2]
d Give three pharmacological treatments of use in severe hyperemesis gravidarum. [3]
e Give two conditions associated with hyperemesis gravidarum which can be looked for on ultrasound examination. [2]

[12]

Case 4

A 31-year-old African lady presents with a 1-day history of worsening PV bleeding and mild lower abdominal cramps. Her LMP was approximately eight weeks ago and she says she had a positive home pregnancy test two weeks previously. She has had three previous miscarriages and one pregnancy which went to term. Her observations at triage are heart rate 90 bpm, blood pressure 130/75 mmHg and temperature 37.2 °C.

a What bedside investigation should be performed first? [1]
b What are the four possible categories of miscarriage? Give a short definition for each. [4]
c Give three risk factors associated with miscarriage. [3]
d The patient develops increased bleeding and passes some pale tissue and clots. She becomes light-headed and her repeat observations demonstrate a pulse of 45 bpm and a BP of 85/60 mmHg. What is likely to have occurred and how should this be managed in the ED? [4]
e Give two medications that can be used to slow bleeding due to miscarriage. [2]

[14]

Case 5

A 34-year-old woman is brought to the ED by her husband with worsening left pelvic pain since the morning. She is bent over with pain in the lower abdomen and needs helping onto the couch. She reports being pregnant with her last menstrual period seven weeks previously and a positive home pregnancy test one week ago. She has had no vaginal bleeding. She looks pale and her initial observations are heart rate 112 bpm, blood pressure 98/46 mmHg and temperature 36.7 °C.

a What is the differential diagnosis for this woman? [2]
b Give four risk factors for the most likely diagnosis in this woman. [4]
c Describe your management of this woman in the ED (give four key steps). [4]
d If this woman had presented earlier and before becoming haemodynamically unstable what two investigations might be performed to diagnose her condition? [2]

[12]

Case 6

A 25-year-old woman presents to the ED with a 10-day history of worsening lower abdominal pain and vaginal discharge. She describes the pain as a dull ache and states that it is only minimally relieved by NSAIDs. She is currently sexually active. You are concerned she may have pelvic inflammatory disease. Her observations are: heart rate 105 bpm, blood pressure 115/75 mmHg and temperature 38.2 °C

a Name four of the common features that the Royal College of Obstetrics & Gynaecology (RCOG) suggest makes a diagnosis of PID likely? [4]
b Name two common sexually transmitted organisms that can lead to PID? [2]
c Give four investigations relevant to the diagnosis of PID. [2]
d Name one outpatient drug regime for treating PID? [2]
e Name four possible sequelae of PID? [4]

[14]

Case 7

A 27-year- old pregnant woman is blue-lighted to the ED having been a front seat passenger in a car which collided, at speed, with a stationary vehicle approximately 30 minutes previously. She was wearing her seatbelt but the car had no airbags. She is 35 weeks pregnant. On arrival in the ED, she is conscious, three-point immobilized and is complaining of worsening lower abdominal pains while also drawing your attention to a deformed left wrist. Initial observations are heart rate 120 bpm, blood pressure 100/80 mmHg, respiratory rate 28/min and oxygen saturations 95% on room air.

a Name four specialties whose assistance you would call for from the outset? [4]
b Give four initial management steps you will undertake. [4]
c What is the ideal position to nurse a pregnant patient, why is this and how will you achieve it? [3]
d Name the four most urgent radiological investigations that should be performed? [2]
e It is now evident the patient is bleeding profusely from her vagina and is becoming increasingly hypotensive. What management is now required? [1]

[14]

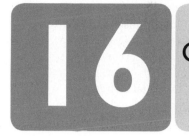

OBSTETRIC AND GYNAECOLOGICAL EMERGENCIES – ANSWERS

Case 1

a Bleeding per vaginum (PV) after 20 weeks gestation is termed antepartum haemorrhage and occurs in 3–5% of all pregnancies. The two major causes of antepartum haemorrhage are:

- **placenta Praevia** occurs when placenta occupies the lower segment of the uterus and may even cover the cervical os. As pregnancy progresses and the uterus expands, the placenta may stretch, rupturing vessels and causing bleeding both into the uterus and PV
- **placental Abruption** is separation of part of the normally situated placenta from the uterine wall, resulting mainly in bleeding into the uterus although some blood escapes into the vagina.

b Both placenta praevia and placenta abruption can present with PV blood loss and hypovolaemic shock, although other clinical features can help distinguish between the two as follows:

Table 16.1

Placenta Praevia	Placental Abruption
Painless	Constant pelvic pain
Non-tender uterus	Tense tender uterus on examination
No signs of foetal distress	Foetal distress (absent/slow foetal heart rate)
Clinical shock in proportion to visible PV blood loss	Clinical shock out of proportion to PV blood loss (bleeding is intrauterine)

c Digital vaginal examination must not be conducted in antepartum haemorrhage as if placenta praevia is present because this may promote further bleeding; it also adds little to immediate management. The obstetrician may wish to perform a speculum examination but this should not be done as part of the ED care of the patient.

d Management of antepartum haemorrhage depends on its cause, and the amount of bleeding. **All** patients, even those with small bleeds, should be admitted under the obstetric team. Heavily bleeding or shocked patients require resuscitation and urgent obstetric involvement. For the patient in this question (who is tachycardic and hypotensive) do the following:

- oxygen 15 L/min via reservoir bag
- insert two large bore cannulae and initiate intravenous fluid resuscitation

- cross-match six units of blood and transfuse, as required. Patients presenting in hypovolaemic shock may need O negative blood while awaiting cross-matched blood
- call immediately for senior obstetric help
- send blood for FBC, clotting and renal function
- institute cardiotocography (CTG) to monitor for foetal distress
- the obstetrician will decide on further tests, ultrasound and speculum examinations, or whether emergency C-section is the priority.

e A Rh–ve mother exposed to the blood of a Rh+ve foetus can rapidly develop antibodies (anti-D IgG), against the Rh antigen. While the pregnancy in situ is unaffected by this, further pregnancies with a RH+ve foetus could see the maternal anti-D antibodies cross the placenta and attack foetal RBCs, causing either anaemia at birth or, more seriously, foetal death. This is known as rhesus haemolytic disease.[1]

To avert rhesus haemolytic disease anti-D immunoglobulin is given after 12 weeks of pregnancy to a rhesus negative mother exposed to foeto-maternal haemorrhage such as: threatened miscarriage, ruptured ectopic pregnancy, chorionic villus sampling, amniocentesis, placenta praevia, placenta abruption or labour itself (the most common cause of mixing of foetal and maternal blood!).

Case 2

a Pre-eclampsia is a multisystem disorder of later pregnancy which is diagnosed by the presence of two of the following three features:

- blood pressure >140/90 mmHg
- proteinuria
- oedema

b Maternal risk factors for pre-eclampsia include: primipara or first pregnancy with new partner, BMI >35, age >40, Afro-Caribbean ethnicity, multiple pregnancy, family history of pre-eclampsia, pre-existing hypertension, diabetes or renal disease.

c Symptomatic severe pre-eclampsia is ominous, as the progression from symptoms to eclamptic seizure or death from stroke, hepatic or renal failure can be swift (<24 hours). Symptoms and signs include:[2]

- severe headache
- visual disturbances
- upper abdominal pain and vomiting
- tenderness over the liver
- elevated liver enzymes
- altered mental status/irritability
- hyperreflexia and/or clonus
- papilloedema
- signs of foetal distress
- thrombocytopaenia (platelets $<50 \times 10^9$/L)

d A large randomized control trial of magnesium sulphate versus diazepam[3] in eclamptic seizures demonstrated that magnesium sulphate was superior to benzodiazepine in preventing further seizures, and is now considered the treatment of choice. Thus, to a patient with eclamptic seizure give magnesium sulphate 4 g slow IV followed by an infusion of 1 g/hour for a minimum of 24 hours as initial treatment. A further 2 g magnesium sulphate can be given if the patient continues to fit.

Urgent delivery of the baby is required as definitive treatment, although be aware that eclampsia can also occur in the early post-partum period.

e The HELLP syndrome occurs in about 3% of patients with pre-eclampsia and is marked by the additional presence of clotting cascade activation, intravascular haemolysis and liver dysfunction. The letters HELLP stand for **H**aemolysis, **E**levated **L**iver enzymes and **L**ow **P**latelets. Recognition of HELLP is important, as it is an indication for urgent delivery of the foetus, to prevent progression to acute liver decompensation, coagulopathy (DIC), renal failure and eclamptic seizures.

Case 3

a Some degree of nausea and vomiting (morning sickness) occurs in the majority of pregnancies but, intractable vomiting resulting in fluid, electrolyte or nutritional disturbance, complicates around one in three hundred pregnancies and is termed hyperemesis gravidarum. Hyperemesis gravidarum has the following features:

- persistent nausea and vomiting
- dehydration
- ketonuria
- electrolyte imbalances (hyponatraemia, hypokalaemia)
- weight loss >5% of pre-pregnancy weight
- nutritional deficiency (particularly thiamine deficiency)

b In a woman with suspected hyperemesis, you would want to look for urinary ketones indicative of metabolic upset, as well as confirm they are pregnant with a urine pregnancy test. A urine sample should also be tested for leucocytes and nitrites, and an MSU sent for culture, in case urinary tract infection is contributing towards the vomiting.

c Blood investigations would include FBC to look for a raised haematocrit often seen with dehydration, electrolytes to look for hyponatraemia and hypokalaemia, as well as urea and creatinine to look for evidence of pre-renal renal failure, secondary to dehydration. Check the blood glucose as hypoglycaemia is more common in pregnancy.

d Pharmacological approaches to hyperemesis include:

- fluid and electrolyte replacement. Give normal saline according to clinical signs. Dextrose solutions should be used with caution, due to the risk of precipitating Wernicke's encephalopathy, if the woman has become thiamine deficient

- give potassium supplementation, if hypokalaemic
- antihistamines are effective in alleviating vomiting and promethazine 25 mg IV is recommended as first-line treatment due to good data indicating it is safe in early pregnancy
- prochlorperazine or metaclopromide are also used with good effect as antiemetics during pregnancy although absolute data on safety is lacking
- give thiamine 100 mg QDS to treat likely deficiency (IV thiamine, if required and serious danger of Wernicke's encephalopathy)
- other multivitamins orally when tolerated.

e   Hyperemesis gravidarum is associated with multiple pregnancies (twins, triplets etc.) and trophoblastic pregnancy (hydatiform mole) both of which are detected with ultrasound imaging. Other risk factors for hyperemesis include previous hyperemesis, a family history of hyperemesis, age <30, maternal obesity, non-smokers and a female foetus.

Case 4

a   First, establish if the patient is pregnant with a urine pregnancy test. At the same time, perform a dipstick test for infection. If the pregnancy test is negative but the LMP is significantly delayed, blood can be sent to the lab for β-HCG levels.

b   Miscarriage is generally divided into the following categories:[4]

Table 16.2

Type	Definition
Threatened miscarriage	Mild symptoms of bleeding rarely with pain. Cervical Os is closed.
Incomplete miscarriage	Heavy bleeding with clots and pain. Cervical Os is open but conception sac or placenta remains.
Complete miscarriage	Some bleeding may continue but all products of conception are passed. The cervical os is closed.
Missed miscarriage	The foetus has died but has been retained. No foetal heart activity will be visualized.

c   Risk factors for miscarriage include:

- age >30
- increased parity
- poorly controlled diabetes
- connective tissue diseases (e.g., SLE and the anti-phospholipid syndrome)
- excess alcohol or illicit drug use.

Exercise and sexual intercourse do not increase the risk of miscarriage.

d   In incomplete miscarriage, the product of conception may become lodged in the cervical canal causing profound vagal stimulation and can precipitate bradycardia, hypotension and potential syncope – a condition known as **cervical shock**. Management of cervical shock involves IV fluid resuscitation, immediate speculum examination with the use of sponge forceps to remove any products that may have become lodged in the cervical canal.

e Heavy bleeding during or after miscarriage can be treated with ergometrine 500 mcg IM (vasoconstricts uterine vessels and contracts uterine smooth muscle) or tranexamic acid 1 g PO (antifibrinolytic).

Case 5

a The differential diagnosis in a woman in early pregnancy, who has lower abdominal pain and haemodynamic instability, is an ectopic pregnancy until proven otherwise. Ectopics occur in around 1 in 100 pregnancies and cause around 4 maternal deaths a year. The diagnosis should be considered in all women of childbearing age with abdominal pain, PV bleeding or shock – do the pregnancy test no matter how sure they are that they are not pregnant! Other pitfalls include considering other diagnoses first (it is the ectopic that will kill the quickest), thinking it is too early in pregnancy to have symptoms from an ectopic (they may present even before a period is missed), and rejecting the diagnosis because of the absence of PV bleeding (blood loss from the vagina need not be present even with ruptured ectopics and heavy internal bleeding).

Once an ectopic pregnancy has been ruled out, the differential widens to include all other causes of an acute abdomen in a young woman.

b Risk factors for ectopic pregnancy are well known:

- in vitro-fertilization
- pelvic inflammatory disease or salpingitis
- previous ectopic
- surgery to the fallopian tubes
- endometriosis
- intrauterine contraceptive device.

c All women with any suggestion of ectopic pregnancy should be referred to the gynaecology team for evaluation. Shocked patients with suspected ectopic pregnancy need the operating theatre straight away.[5] In this woman:

- manage in the resuscitation area
- call the senior gynaecologist immediately to the bedside
- cross-match 6 units of blood and give as needed (O neg if peri-arrest)
- set up two IV lines and infuse colloid. Do not aim for normal blood pressure, aim to keep the patient conscious long enough to reach theatre
- initiate preparation for theatre: call the anaesthetist and ask the junior gynaecologist to inform theatres
- do not waste time with unnecessary tests and consults!

d Stable patients with suspected ectopic should be made safe in the ED (IV cannula and blood sent for group and save) then managed by the gynaecology team. They will perform pelvic ultrasound to look for the location of the foetus and, if in doubt, measure serial β-HCG levels in the blood. In normal pregnancy, the serum β-HCG increases 50% every 48 hours or so; slower rise is suspicious of ectopic pregnancy. Medical therapy with methotrexate is often used in stable women with minimal symptoms and low levels of serum β-HCG.[5]

Case 6

a The Royal College of Obstetrics and Gynaecology (RCOG) green top guidelines state seven features that may suggest pelvic inflammatory disease (PID):[6]

- bilateral lower abdominal tenderness
- abnormal vaginal or cervical discharge
- fever >38 °C
- abnormal vaginal bleeding
- deep dyspareunia (pain on sexual intercourse)
- cervical motion or adnexal tenderness on bimanual examination.

b *Chlamydia trachomatis* and *Neisseria gonorrhoeae* are most commonly implicated in PID although genital mycoplasma and endogenous vaginal flora can also be responsible.

c Young women presenting with abdominal pain should, first and foremost, have a urinary pregnancy test performed to exclude ectopic pregnancy. Urine should also be checked for leucocytes and nitrites as signs of urinary tract infection. Blood tests would include inflammatory markers – FBC, CRP. High vaginal and endocervical swabs should be performed either by the gynaecologist-on-call or an ED doctor with experience of performing such swabs (in inexperienced hands they are low-yield and uncomfortable).

Aside from investigations, patients with PID need symptomatic management with analgesia and antipyretics, and may need to be admitted by the gynaecologist if systemically unwell or septic, vomiting and so unable to take oral medications or where pain is poorly controlled. Follow-up for discharged patients should be made with the gynaecologist for the results of swabs and further care.

d The RCOG guidelines[6] give two potential outpatient regimes although local policies will be adjusted to regional sensitivities and resistances.

- ofloxacin 400 mg bd + metronidazole 400 mg bd orally for 14 days
- intramuscular ceftriaxone 250 mg (single dose) followed by oral doxycycline 100 mg bd + metronidazole 400 mg bd for 14 days.

e The complications of PID include infertility, ectopic pregnancy, chronic pelvic pain, tubal abscess formation, peri-hepatitis (Fitz-Hugh-Curtis syndrome), Reiter's syndrome and pre-term delivery.

Case 7

a A trauma-call should be put out for this patient that should bring the anaesthetist, surgeon, orthopaedic specialists but, for a near-term pregnant woman, we also need a senior obstetrician and the neonatal resuscitation team (paediatricians) present.

b The primary survey remains grossly the same as in the non-pregnant patient, with the mother remaining the priority.

- give oxygen at 15 L via reservoir bag
- secure cervical spine immobilization
- obtain two large IV cannulae and take blood for FBC, clotting, cross-match and rhesus status
- set up an IVI (normal saline) at a rate indicated by clinical assessment
- monitoring is required for the mother and the foetus (the obstetrician can set up cardiotocography)
- a nasogastric tube is required to reduce the risk of regurgitation (greater in pregnancy again due to the upward pressure of the uterus on the stomach)
- analgesia titrated to pain (morphine if required).

c In the supine position, the heavily gravid uterus compresses the vena cava to reduce cardiac preload and exacerbate hypotension. Thus, manually displace the uterus to the left to relieve pressure on the IVC. Once the entire spine has been cleared of injury, a Cardiff wedge can be used to the same end.

d This patient needs a full trauma series of X-rays – cervical spine, chest X-ray and pelvis X-ray – as the risk of missing significant injuries still outweighs any possible sequelae for the foetus (although radiation is most harmful in the first trimester). An ultrasound and/or focused assessment by sonography in trauma (FAST) scan may also be performed in the ED to look for intra-abdominal blood (rule in methodology) and/or to monitor the foetal heartbeat.

e This patient has placental abruption caused by blunt trauma to the abdomen and is in hypovolaemic shock. A crash caesarean section is now required to deliver the foetus while still viable, and to clamp the placental vessels to avert maternal death from massive haemorrhage. Remember to give anti-D immunoglobulin if the mother is Rh–ve.

Further Reading

1. Use of Anti-D Immunoglobulin for Rh Prophylaxis (Green-top 22). RCOG (May 2002) Found at· www.rcog.org.uk/womens-health/clinical-guidance/use-anti-d-immunoglobulin-rh-prophylaxis-green-top-22

2. The Management of Severe Pre-Eclampsia/Eclampsia (Green-top 10A). RCOG (2006) Found at: www.rcog.org.uk/womens-health/clinical-guidance/management-severe-pre-eclampsiaeclampsia-green-top-10a

3. Which anticonvulsant for women with eclampsia? Evidence from the Collaborative Eclampsia Trial. (1995) *Lancet*; **345**(8963): 1455–62.

4. Management of early pregnancy loss (Green-top 26) RCOG (March 2006). Found at: www.rcog.org.uk/files/rcog-corp/uploadedfiles/GT25ManagementofEarlyPregnancyLoss2006.pdf

5. Management of tubal pregnancy (green top-21). RCOG (2004) Found at www.rcog.org.uk/womens-health/clinical-guidance/management-tubal-pregnancy-21-may-2004

6. Management of Acute Pelvic Inflammatory Disease (Green-top 32) RCOG March 2006. (Revised 2009) Found at: www.rcog.org.uk/womens-health/clinical-guidance/management-acute-pelvic-inflammatory-disease-32

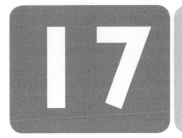

PAIN AND ANAESTHETICS

Mathew Hall

Introduction

Core topics

- assessment and treatment of pain in adults and children
- appropriate use of analgesics in different conditions
- use of local anaesthetics
- haematoma block
- intravenous regional anaesthesia (Bier's block)
- femoral nerve block
- airway management
- safe procedural sedation
- rapid sequence induction
- general anaesthetics: risks and contraindications
- emergency department care of the critically ill patient
- transfer of the critically ill/injured patient between hospitals.

Managing pain is an important element of Emergency Department (ED) practice and one which the CEM is striving to improve through clear guidance and regular audit. Pain is probably a feature of the majority of ED presentations and so questions on managing pain can crop up in SAQs on virtually any topic – and they do! Thus, we would recommend committing to memory the CEM guidelines on the management of pain in both adults and children, and we have referenced these at the end of this chapter.[1,5] In addition know about:

- pain scores and corresponding analgesic ladders
- pharmacology, contraindications and side effects of commonly used analgesics, sedatives and anaesthetic agents
- safe maximal doses of local anaesthetics
- landmarks and procedures for nerve blocks, central venous access and surgical cricothyroidotomy.

Case 1

A 74-year-old woman presents having fallen outside her home. She is complaining of a painful right wrist but is otherwise unhurt. She gives a good history of mechanical fall. She has only hypertension in the background and has no allergies. Below is the X-ray of her injured wrist (Figure 17.1).

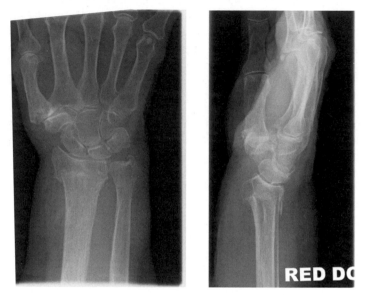

Figure 17.1

a Accurately describe the fracture in the X-ray (Figure 17.1).   [2]
b In your hospital, it is protocol to manipulate wrist fractures under regional
   anaesthesia. Describe in six steps how you would perform a Bier's block
   (including which local anaesthetic you would use).   [6]
c Give two properties of the local anaesthetic you use in answer to **b.** above
   that makes it particularly well-suited for regional anaesthesia.   [2]
d What is the safe maximal dose in adults and children of the local anaesthetic
   you have used in answer to **b.** above?   [2]
e Give two drugs you could use to treat severe, life-threatening local
   anaesthetic toxicity.   [2]
                                                                                                   [14]

Case 2

A four-year-old boy has pulled a cup of boiling water from the kitchen worktop onto his anterior torso. A large area of his chest and anterior of both arms have blistered but the face and neck are spared. His mother immediately doused him in cold water and brought him to the ED straight away. He weighs 18 kg and is screaming in distress.

a Describe a pain scoring system you might use to assess this child's pain. [5]
b Your assessment indicates the child is in severe pain (pain score 8). How would you manage his pain (give routes and doses of any drugs used)? [3]
c Once the child is more settled, you calculate the percentage burn using a paediatric burns chart. What is the approximate percentage burn in a child of this age, above which IV fluid is required as part of their burns care? [1]
d The child returns to your department some days later for a change of dressing on his burns. What non-pharmacological method of pain management, if available, could be used to facilitate the dressing change? [1]
[10]

Case 3

A 57-year-old man with no significant past medical history presents with a deformed left elbow, after an awkward fall, whilst ice-skating with his grandson. He has no other injuries but is in severe pain, despite liberally using the ambulance crew's entonox. You are asked to assess him at triage. His elbow X-ray is shown in Figure 17.2.

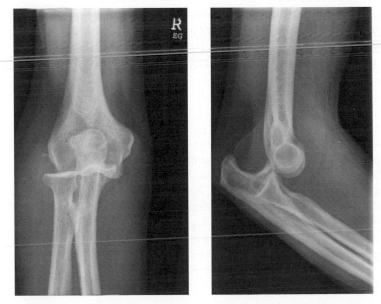

Figure 17.2

a Give two **non-bony** structures which are most often damaged as a result of the injury depicted in the X-ray (Figure 17.2) and, for both, give one clinical test of integrity. [4]

b How would you initially manage this man's pain? [1]

c It will be necessary to sedate this patient in order to treat this injury. In preparation for safe procedural sedation, give three important questions you would ask the patient. [3]

d Describe your **use of drugs** to achieve safe sedation in this patient (state doses and routes for any drugs used). [3]

e Just in case of respiratory compromise during sedation, you have a bag and mask close to hand. List four anatomical features evident on general inspection which make bag and mask ventilation difficult in a patient. [2]

[13]

Case 4

The ambulance service calls ahead to say there is a 57-year-old woman being brought to your hospital with severe difficulty in breathing. On arrival, she is cyanosed and struggling for breath with an audible stridor. She is at risk of imminent respiratory arrest.

a Give four causes of stridor you would think of in a woman of this age? [2]

b On rapid assessment, she is toxic with a temperature of 38.9 °C, drooling saliva and has a markedly swollen anterior neck along with protruding tongue. What is the likely diagnosis? [1]

c Securing the airway is the priority for this patient. Give three approaches that might be considered to achieve this. [3]

d It becomes clear that a surgical airway is required to avert impending respiratory arrest. Draw an annotated diagram indicating the landmarks for locating the site of incision for an emergency cricothyroidotomy. [4]

e What are the early complications of emergency cricothyroidotomy? [2]

[12]

Case 5

A 57-year-old man, known to drink heavily, is brought into resus after falling down a flight of twelve stairs, striking his head on the concrete floor at the bottom. He is quite unresponsive although he can groan, open his eyes and flex his arms in response to pain. You manage to perform a primary survey where his airway, breathing and circulation are all stable and, although he has an obvious haematoma over his right forehead, there do not appear to be any torso or limb injuries. The nurse has attached a monitor and placed him on oxygen.

a What is the patient's GCS?   [1]
b List three steps in managing this patient before obtaining a CT scan of the
   head.   [3]
c The patient requires transfer to a neurosurgical centre 30 minutes from your
   hospital. Describe how you will arrange safe transfer, including what
   equipment is required, who needs to go with the patient and how you will
   ensure good communication with the receiving centre.   [6]
                                                                                  [10]

Case 6

A 79-year-old man with a history of chronic obstructive pulmonary disease
(COPD), and very poor exercise tolerance, is brought in by blue-light ambulance
very short of breath. He is an ex-smoker of 80 pack years and carries both a blue
and green inhaler which he uses when his breathing is bad. He has had previous
admissions where he required treatment with non-invasive ventilation. He is alert
but in respiratory distress with a respiration rate of 34/min and oxygen saturations
of 77% on air.

a Outline your initial approach of this patient's oxygen therapy.   [2]
b You make a working diagnosis of exacerbation of COPD and initiate medical
   therapy with bronchodilators and IV steroid. What are the indications for
   non-invasive ventilation (NIV) in patients with exacerbations of COPD?   [3]
c Briefly describe the physiological mechanism whereby NIV helps patients
   with respiratory failure.   [2]
d What 'mode' of NIV is best suited to this patient and what initial settings for
   inspiratory and expiratory pressure, (IPAP and EPAP) would you use?   [3]
e Name two conditions other than COPD which can be treated with NIV.   [2]
                                                                                  [12]

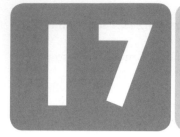

PAIN AND ANAESTHETICS – ANSWERS

Case 1

a The X-ray (Figure 17.1) shows an impacted, dorsally angulated fracture of the distal radius.

b Intravenous regional anaesthesia or Bier's block is a simple technique for anaesthesia of a distal limb, first described by August Bier in 1808. It is used for procedures of less than 40 minutes on either the lower arm or leg, and is well-suited for fracture manipulation as it also provides a good degree of muscle relaxation. When correctly performed, it is safe and only contraindicated where there is hypersensitivity to local anaesthetic, or where a short period of hypoxia may cause harm to the limb; for example, injuries with already ischaemic or devitalized tissue and in patients with Reynaud's disorder or sickle cell disease. It requires two trained personnel (one a doctor) to perform and the key steps for a Bier's block of the upper arm are as follows:

- prepare for the procedure by taking the patient's blood pressure and inserting a small cannula into a vein on the back of the hand of the arm to be anaesthetized
- exsanguinate the limb by elevating for a minute with pressure over the brachial artery
- apply a blood pressure cuff to the arm and inflate to 50 mmHg above the patient's systolic blood pressure. An assistant must be solely responsible for watching the cuff pressure and maintaining it at 50 mmHg above systolic. Sometimes a double cuff is used where the outer cuff is first inflated, the anaesthetic applied and then the inner cuff inflated over an already anaesthetized area and the outer cuff deflated, so as to reduce the discomfort felt by the patient from the tourniquet
- inject 40 mL 0.5% prilocaine into the cannula on the back of the hand and flush with saline
- complete anaesthesia is obtained within three to five minutes and the procedure performed
- the cuff must stay inflated for at least 20 minutes from injection of local anaesthetic to allow the anaesthetic to distribute into fat. Warn the patient they may experience mild peri-oral tingling and tinnitus, and then deflate the cuff. Sensation rapidly returns to the limb.

c Prilocaine is used for Bier's block because it is the least cardio-toxic of the local anaesthetic agents and has a short half-life (30–60 minutes) matching the requirements of the procedure.

d The following table gives the safe maximal doses of local anaesthetics in common use and is well worth committing to memory.

Table 17.1

	Lidocaine	Bupivicaine	Prilocaine
Max safe adult dose	200 mg (20 mL of 1% solution)	150 mg (30 mL of 0.5% solution)	400 mg (40 mL of 1% solution)
Max dose with epinephrine	500 mg (50 mL of 1% solution)	Same as without epinephrine	Rarely used
Max safe dose in children (and adults <70 kg)	3 mg/kg	2 mg/kg	6 mg/kg
Speed of onset of analgesia	2–5 minutes	20 minutes	2–5 minutes
Duration of action	30–60 minutes (longer if given with epinephrine)	4–6 hours	30–60 minutes
Main uses	Local infiltration anaesthesia	Nerve blocks (longest duration action)	Bier's block (lowest cardiotoxicity)

e Early features of local anaesthetic (LA) toxicity are peri-oral tingling, slurred speech and tinnitus which may progress with severe toxicity to convulsion, coma, cardiac arrhythmia, shock and cardiac arrest. Life-threatening LA toxicity is treated with intralipid, an IV lipid emulsion which neutralizes circulating local anaesthetic. Other drugs of use would be oxygen, benzodiazapines for seizures, IV normal saline for shock, amiodarone and atropine for tachy or brady-arrythmias respectively.

Case 2

a The CEM stress that the recognition and alleviation of pain in children is an emergency department priority and annually carries out an national audit on this subject. The College guidelines[1] recommend the use of an established pain-scoring system to assess pain in children, and as a guide to selecting appropriate analgesia. There are a number of different pain scoring systems in use which generally involve grading pain from none (score 0) to severe or worst ever (score 10) and rely on an either observational assessment or self-reporting of pain by the child.[2] Interestingly, few are actually validated for the emergency department environment. A simple observational pain score is described in the CEM gridlines and summarized below:

Table 17.2

Pain level	Self-report	Behaviour	Score
No pain	Smiling face	Normal activities/playing happily	0
Mild	Neutral face	A few problems but can interact normally	1–3
Moderate	Unhappy face not moving affected part, complaining of pain	Consolable crying	3–6
Severe	Crying face	Complaining of lots of pain/ Inconsolable crying	7–10

b Severe pain should be managed aggressively but safely and the CEM recommend[1] either:

- intranasal diamorphine 0.1 mg/kg in 0.2 mL volume sterile water (1.8 mg in this child)
- **and/or** intravenous morphine 0.1–0.2 mg/kg (therefore 1.8–3.6 mg in this child)
- **and** children with severe pain should also receive oral analgesia such as ibuprofen 10 mg/kg (max 400 mg) and paracetamol 20 mg/kg (max 1g)
- non-pharmacological pain relief such as splinting broken limbs or applying cool burns dressings as in this case should be done as soon as possible
- the child should be reassessed after 20 minutes and further pain relief given as required.

c IV fluids are required in the treatment of children with burns greater than 10% body surface area. This figure is lower than in adults – where 15% is generally taken as the cut-off for a 'resuscitation burn' – because children have a relatively greater body surface area compared to volume, and so, will lose a greater percentage of body fluid for the same size burn. Children with greater than 10% surface area burns require transfer to a specialist burns unit with critical care facilities.

Calculating burn area in children is done with a paediatric burn chart or, where one is not available, using the child's hand to represent 1% of their body surface area. The 'rule of 9s', commonly used in estimating adult burns, is not accurate in younger children and should not be used below age 14.

Although not asked in this question, for completeness Box 17.1 sets out how to calculate the amount of fluid to be given to a child with greater than 10% body surface area burn.

> **Box 17.1** Calculating IV fluid requirements for children with greater than 10% surface area burns.[3]
>
> Additional fluid required **per day** (mL) = percentage burn(%) × weight (kg) × 4
> Importantly for the ED care of such patients, half of this daily amount should be given in the first eight hours **from the time of the burn**.

d Play specialists are skilled professionals who can facilitate minor procedures on children such as uncomfortable dressing changes. They may also participate in the management of children's pain, anxiety and distress surrounding more serious problems.

Case 3

a The X-ray (Figure 17.2) demonstrates a posterior dislocation of the elbow. The most common neurovascular structures injured as a result of elbow dislocation are the ulnar nerve, the median nerve and the brachial artery. The likelihood of neurovascular damage increases with anterior and open elbow dislocations. For brevity, we will give a single test for each of these structures, but a more detailed account of anatomy and functional testing of particularly the peripheral nerves can be found in a good orthopaedic text.[4]

Table 17.3

Structure	Anatomy	Example test
Ulnar nerve	Innervates adductor pollicis in the hand (among others)	Froment's test which involves the patient holding a sheet of paper between the thumbs and lateral border of the index fingers, while the examiner attempts to withdraw it. Paralysis of adductor pollicis causes weakness of grasp in the affected thumb, and the thumb flexes involuntarily at the interphalangeal joint
Median nerve	Innervates abductor pollicis brevis in the hand (amongst others)	Ask the patient to place his hand flat on the table palm upwards, then to raise his thumb to touch the examiners finger held above it. If the patient is able to do this, test strength in abductor pollicis brevis by attempting to push the thumb back to its original position, while the patient resists and compare to the unaffected side
Brachial artery	Divides into both the radial and ulnar arteries in the cubital fossa of the elbow	Brachial artery compression may be evidenced by weak or absent radial and ulnar artery pulses at the wrist, and by pallor or mottling of the distal limb with prolonged capillary refill time

b Severe pain in adults is managed with opiates, for example 0.1–0.2 mg/kg morphine sulphate IV or IM.[5] Exceptions include colicky pain where rectal diclofenac and smooth muscle relaxants are as effective and can be used prior to opiates.

c The goal of procedural sedation is to give a short period of reduced anxiety and amnesia to allow an otherwise painful and distressing procedure to be carried out. Verbal responsiveness and airway reflexes must be preserved, otherwise it is a general anaesthetic! Full assessment of the patient is required beforehand to establish suitability. Important questions to ask are:

- co-morbidities and general fitness (patients with serious co-morbid disease – cardiac, chest, renal – or with significant disability are not suitable for sedation in the ED)
- ask about smoking and the possibility of COPD
- previous bad reactions or problems with a general anaesthetic

- any previous airway problems (e.g. sleep apnoea)
- when did they last eat/drink?

d At the time of writing, IV midazolam remains the most widespread agent used for procedural sedation in the UK. Although propofol and ketamine are gaining traction for use by more senior ED personnel, there is still considerable anxiety surrounding their use by non-anaesthetists. Thus, in answering exam questions, stick to safe ground.

- give oxygen via facemask before and during the sedation
- CEM recommends starting with 2 mg midazolam IV and then titrating upwards 1 mg/minute until suitable sedation is achieved – i.e., the patient ceases voluntary interaction but responds to verbal prompts. Maximum adult doses of 7.5 mg midazolam, less in the elderly.

Perform the procedure as quickly as possible and institute post-procedure care, with regular observation from a member of the nursing staff dedicated to the patient, until they are once again fully alert. In general, reversal of sedation with flumazanil is not recommended unless in an emergency.

On their website, the CEM have a guideline for sedation of adults in the ED[6] on which this question was based. In addition, the Royal College of Anaesthetists have also published a guideline document on safe sedation practice.[7]

e Anatomical features which make bag-mask ventilation difficult are summarized by the mnemonic 'OBESE': Obesity, Beards, Elderly, Snorers, Edentulous.

For completeness, predictors of a difficult **airway** include the above, as well as limited mouth-opening, limited neck movement, small chin, large incisors, large tongue and Mallampati score three to four.

Case 4

a Stridor, a harsh high-pitched sound on inspiration, expiration or both, indicates partial obstruction of the upper airway and, when acute, warns a medical emergency is present. The most likely causes of acute stridor in adults are:

- foreign body inhalation
- anaphylaxis
- infection (acute laryngitis, epiglottitis, retropharyngeal abscess, Ludwig's angina)
- laryngospasm and laryngeal oedema, most commonly from inhalation injury
- sudden expansion of a tumour either intrinsic to the airway (laryngeal tumour) or extrinsic (thyroid mass, lung carcinoma).

b Ludwig's angina, or submandibular abscess, presents with fever associated with pain and firm swelling of the floor of the mouth, causing the tongue to rise and protrude. As the disease progresses, oesophageal compression causes drooling of saliva, and airway compression causes stridor. Respiratory arrest is a fatal complication.

c Securing the airway in Ludwig's angina poses a considerable anaesthetic challenge. Oral intubation should be considered but is often difficult or impossible due to the intraoral swelling and fibreoptic nasotracheal intubation can be used as an alternative method of securing the airway. Where swelling has progressed to make intubation impossible, a surgical airway is required with emergency cricothyroidotomy or, if there is sufficient time, formal tracheostomy.

d The incision for a surgical cricothyroidotomy is made through the cricothyroid membrane, a palpable depression between the thyroid and cricoid cartilages. Your annotated diagram should look something like this figure:

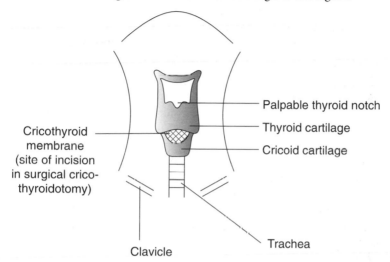

Figure 17.3

e Complications which may occur immediately or shortly after performing an emergency cricothyroidotomy are:

- haemorrhage/haematoma
- aspiration of blood
- vocal cord paralysis
- oesophageal perforation leading to mediastinitis
- tracheal perforation leading to mediastinal emphysema
- failure of procedure and subsequent death from failure to establish an airway.

Case 5

a The Glasgow coma score (GCS) is reproduced in Box 17.2.

Box 17.2 The Glasgow Coma Score (GCS)	
Best eye response	*Score*
Spontaneous eye opening	4
Eye opening to verbal command	3
Eye opening to pain	2
No eye opening	1
Best verbal response	
Oriented	5
Confused	4
Inappropriate words	3
Incomprehensible sounds	2
No verbal response	1
Best motor response	
Obeys commands	6
Localizes pain	5
Withdraws from pain	4
Flexion to pain	3
Extension to pain	2
No motor response	1
Add the best scores under each heading, eye opening, verbal response and motor response. A score of 13 or higher correlates with a mild brain injury, 9–12 is a moderate injury and 8 or less a severe brain injury.	

This patient opens his eyes to pain (scoring 2), makes only incomprehensible sounds (scores 2) and can flex to pain (scores 3) giving a total GCS of 7/15, and a diagnosis of severe brain injury.

b Three important steps to perform before considering CT brain are:

- immobilize the cervical spine (it is at risk and cannot be 'cleared' clinically in this patient)
- secure the airway (the patients' GCS is below eight putting the airway in danger)
- check the blood glucose (in any patient with altered mental status).

c Safe transfer of the intubated, ventilated and potentially deteriorating head injured patient between hospitals requires careful planning. Think about:

Table 17.4

Equipment	Personnel	Communication
Full portable monitoring equipment Capnograph Oxygen cylinders All necessary drugs, particularly anaesthetic and resuscitation drugs, and fluids Infusion pumps (and backup batteries) Resuscitation bag carrying full resuscitation and airway management equipment	An experienced anaesthetist must accompany the patient Trained critical care or emergency department nurse Ideally a paramedic ambulance crew	Initial phone referral including taking name and details of the neurosurgeon accepting the patient A copy of the patients notes, observations chart and CT scan should accompany the patient Phone the receiving hospital when the patient leaves the department with an estimated time of arrival

Case 6

a   This patient with severe COPD and who has previously been treated with non-invasive ventilation is clearly at risk of hypercapnoeic respiratory failure. The BTS guideline for emergency oxygen use in adult patients[8] advises the following:

- COPD patients should still receive higher flow rates of oxygen when critically ill, and/or severely hypoxic and controlled oxygen therapy instituted, as soon as possible guided by blood gases
- as soon as possible, place COPD patients at risk of hypercapnia on controlled oxygen therapy using either a 24% Venturi mask at 2–4 L/min or 28% Venturi mask 4 L/min and aiming for target saturations of 88–92%
- take urgent blood gases to guide further oxygen therapy. If the pH is normal or high but pCO_2 raised, then maintain the patient on controlled oxygen aiming for saturations 88–92% and recheck the blood gas in 30–60 minutes.

b   Non-invasive ventilation (NIV) is indicated in exacerbations of COPD, unresponsive to immediate medical therapy, and with respiratory acidosis, i.e.:

- low pH (<7.35)
- high pCO_2 (>6.5 kPa)

The BTS guideline on COPD[9, 10] recommend starting NIV within 60 minutes, preferably 30 minutes, of hospital arrival, in patients with persisting respiratory acidosis despite maximal medical treatment including controlled oxygen therapy. It is important to initiate NIV early rather than waiting for the patient to deteriorate, as its efficacy decreases with worsening acidosis below pH 7.25.

   Although not specifically asked in this question, we should also be aware of those situations where NIV is either contraindicated or should be used with caution:

- where life-threatening hypoxia is present
- obtunded or unconscious patients
- patients unable to protect their airway

- patient's non-compliance
- significant facial trauma
- where excessive secretions, blood or vomitus is present
- where invasive ventilation is more appropriate, i.e., pH <7.25 and patient co-morbidity does not preclude treatment on an intensive therapy unit
- NIV can lower blood pressure and so should be used with caution in haemodynamically unstable patients.

c The physiological benefits of NIV are to increase tidal volume thereby increasing alveolar minute ventilation which stimulates CO_2 loss in the lung. Importantly, NIV also reduces the work of breathing and so helps avoid either formal intubation or deterioration in exhausted COPD patients.

d There are two main types of NIV; continuous positive airways pressure ventilation (CPAP) where the inspiratory (IPAP) and expiratory pressures (EPAP) are identical and bi-level positive airways pressure ventilation (BiPAP) where the inspiratory and expiratory pressures differ.

CPAP is used mainly for type I respiratory failure where CO_2 retention is not so much a concern (such as in acute pulmonary oedema) whilst type II respiratory failure in COPD is best treated with BiPAP. Furthermore, NIV machines delivering BiPAP may be set to spontaneous mode meaning that the machine augments the spontaneous breaths of the alert patient, or timed mode where they deliver a set number of breaths per minute. In the emergency department, most exacerbations of COPD will be treated with BiPAP in spontaneous mode.

In setting up BiPAP on a patient, it is necessary to specify the inspiratory positive airway pressure (IPAP) and the expiratory positive airway pressure (EPAP). Typical starting pressures are: IPAP 10 cmH$_2$O and EPAP 5 cm H$_2$O.[10] IPAP should be incrementally increased until a good therapeutic response is gained or a maximum of around 20 cm H$_2$O achieved. Oxygen may also be entrained if required to achieve target saturations of 88–92%.

e NIV is also used as an acute treatment in cardiogenic pulmonary oedema, as well as in the treatment of respiratory failure, due to neuromuscular disease or chest wall deformities. CPAP is, of course, also a treatment of obstructive sleep apnoea.

Further Reading

1. CEM Clinical Effectiveness Committee guideline on the management of pain in children. (2004) Can currently be found at www.collemergencymed.ac.uk/CEM/default.asp then go to Clinical Effectiveness Committee (CEC) and then CEC Guidelines on the left hand menu.
2. Shavit I, Kofman M, Leder M, *et al.* (2008) Observational pain assessment versus self-report in paediatric triage. *Emergency Medicine Journal*; **25**:552–5.
3. *Advanced Paediatric Life Support*. 4th edn. (2005) The Advanced life support Group. Blackwell Publishing.
4. McRae R. *Pocketbook of Orthopaedics and Fractures*. (1989) Churchill Livingstone.

5. CEM Clinical Effectiveness Committee guideline on the management of pain in adults. (2004) Can currently be found at www.collemergencymed.ac.uk/CEM/default.asp then go to Clinical Effectiveness Committee (CEC) and then CEC Guidelines on the left hand menu.

6. Ikkede. U. Sedation guideline and pro-forma for adults in A&E. (2008) Found on the College of Emergency Medicine website at www.collemergencymed.ac.uk/asp/resources.asp?c=2

7. Implementing and ensuring Safe Sedation Practice for healthcare procedures in adults. Report of the intercollegiate Working Party chaired by the Royal College of Anaesthetists. (2001) Found at www.rcoa.ac.uk/docs/safesedationpractice.pdf.

8. British Thoracic Society (BTS) Emergency Oxygen Guideline Development Group. BTS guideline for emergency oxygen use in adult patients. (2008) *Thorax;* **63**: Suppl VI. Also online at www.brit-thoracic.org.uk.

9. NICE Guideline CG12. Chronic obstructive pulmonary disease (2004), www.nice.org.uk/Guidance/CG162. In addition, the section of the guideline relating to the management of exacerbations of COPD is published online at www.thorax.bmj.com/cgi/reprint/59/suppl_1/i131

10. Non-invasive ventilation in chronic obstructive pulmonary disease: management of type 2 respiratory failure. Concise guidance to good practice. British Thoracic Society and Royal College of Physicians (2008) Found online at www.rcplondon.ac.uk/pubs/brochure.aspx?e=258

SURGICAL EMERGENCIES

Jane Richmond

Introduction

Core topics

- the acute abdomen
- lower GI bleeding
- perforated bowel
- acute bowel obstruction
- acute appendicitis
- pancreatitis
- diverticulitis
- ischaemic bowel
- urinary retention
- testicular torsion
- epidydimo-orchitis
- scrotal gangrene
- ruptured abdominal aortic aneurysm
- the ischaemic limb
- surgical problems in children – pyloric stenosis, intersussception, volvulus.

A large variety of data may be included in stems for surgical questions. Blood tests may include white cell count and CRP for signs of infection/inflammation, liver function tests (know the different pictures of pre-, intra- and post-hepatic jaundice) and raised amylase in pancreatitis. Metabolic acidosis on an arterial blood gas points to sepsis or bowel ischaemia. Be able to interpret the urine dipstick testing and never forget the urine pregnancy test in women of childbearing age with abdominal pathology!

Be able to interpret the abdominal X-ray.[1] Also know the **indications** for abdominal X-ray (suspected obstruction, clinical peritonitis, ingested or per rectum radio-opaque foreign body, suspected renal calculus)[2] and avoid investigating with plain films, where either surgical intervention, ultrasound or CT imaging is more appropriate.

Oh, and be sure to carry in your mind a list of the differential diagnosis of abdominal pain in each quadrant (epigastric, RUQ, LUQ, RIF, LIF, suprapubic, flanks)!

Case 1

A 45-year-old man presents to the Emergency Department (ED) with a one-day history of epigastric pain, radiating through to his back and, accompanied by profuse vomiting. He is known to binge-drink, and admits to drinking a bottle of vodka every day for the past five days. He is also a heavy smoker. On examination, he has a very tender epigastrium with localized guarding.

His observations are: heart rate 128 bpm, blood pressure 100/60 mmHg, oxygen saturations 94% on air and temperature 36.8 °C.

a Other than acute pancreatitis give four further potential diagnoses to consider? [2]
b List four causes of acute pancreatitis. [4]
c The Glasgow scoring system can be used to risk-stratify patients with acute pancreatitis. Name four parameters in this scoring strategy with their respective values? [4]
d This patient's amylase is 1765 u/dL confirming your suspected diagnosis of pancreatitis. Give four important treatments to be initiated in the emergency department. [2]
[12]

Case 2

You are asked to see a 14-year-old boy with acute right testicular pain. It came on a couple of hours ago whilst playing rugby but the patient cannot remember any specific injury to his scrotum. He is in severe pain, and has been vomiting over the last half hour. He has no past medical history of note.

a Give a differential diagnosis of acute testicular pain and indicate which you would consider most likely in this patient. [4]
b Briefly describe the pathophysiology behind the likely diagnosis you give in answer to part **a.** above. [2]
c Assuming your working diagnosis is correct, what clinical features would you expect to find on examination of this patient's scrotum? [3]
d Give a three-point management plan for this patient in the ED. [3]
[12]

Case 3

You meet an emergency ambulance bringing a 72-year-old with both abdominal and lower back pain. He is pale and sweaty on arrival and has an easily felt pulsatile abdominal mass. His initial pulse is 110 bpm, blood pressure 90/69 mmHg, respiratory rate 28/min. One of your senior colleagues is able to perform a bedside ultrasound looking for an abdominal aortic aneurysm (AAA).

a Give two steps in your immediate management of this patient on arrival in
   the ED.   [2]
b What is the normal diameter of the abdominal aorta and at what diameter
   is the abdominal aorta considered to be aneurysmal?   [2]
c Name three ways of differentiating between the aorta and inferior vena cava
   (IVC) on ultrasound imaging.   [3]
d Describe your approach to managing this patient's fluid resuscitation.   [3]
e Give two options for surgical management of leaking AAA by a vascular
   specialist.   [2]
                                                                           [12]

Case 4

A 85-year-old nursing home resident is brought to the ED with a three-day
history of vomiting and abdominal distension. The carers at the home say she
has not opened her bowels for at least five days. Despite these factors she is only
complaining of minimal abdominal pain. Triage observations indicate she is
haemodynamically stable but with a mild fever of 37.4 °C. Her abdominal X-ray is
shown below (Figure 18.1):

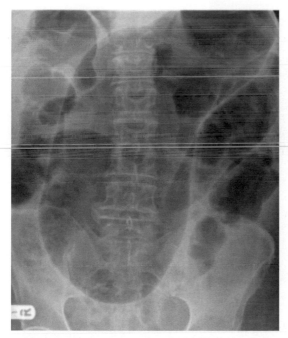

Figure 18.1

a Describe the abnormality on the abdominal X-ray of this patient (Figure 18.1). [3]
b What are the upper limits of normal for the diameter of large bowel? [1]
c List four causes of large bowel obstruction. [4]
d In the patient above, give a management plan with at least four points to be carried out in the ED. [4]
e What definitive treatment options exist for this condition? [2]
[14]

Case 5

A 38-year-old woman arrives in the ED after 48 hours of central abdominal pain and bilious vomiting on attempting any oral intake. She now feels weak and unable to bear the steadily worsening pain. She has a past surgical history of hysterectomy for uncontrollable menorrhagia five years ago. She is afebrile and has a heart rate 106 bpm with blood pressure of 126/80 mmHg. An abdominal X-ray is taken and shown below (Figure 18.2).

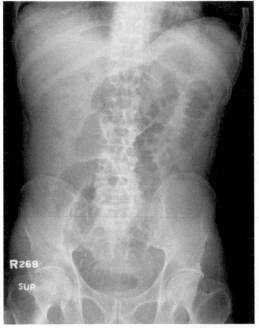

Figure 18.2

a Give four indications for requesting an abdominal X-ray in the ED. [4]
b Describe three abnormalities of the bowel shown in the X-ray of this patient (Fgure 18.2) and what diagnosis is indicated? [3]
c List four causes of this condition in adults. [2]
d Briefly outline what you understand by the term 'ileus'. [2]
e What is the most common cause of this condition in children? [1]
[12]

Case 6

You are asked to review a four-week-old male child with several episodes of projectile vomiting. He was an uncomplicated term delivery although, since birth, has gained little weight despite always wanting to feed. His mother has changed from breast milk to bottle milk but has seen no improvement. The baby is alert but appears dehydrated. A capillary blood gas is taken:

pH	7.56
pCO_2	4.5 kPa
pO_2	13.1 kPa
HCO_3^-	29.0 mEq/L
BE	+7

a Describe the abnormality on the capillary blood gas given above. [2]
b What is the likely diagnosis for the baby in this question and briefly explain the pathophysiology of this condition? [3]
c What clinical features may be found on examination of a baby presenting acutely with this condition? [4]
d Name two radiological investigations that can be used to diagnose this condition. [2]
e What is the definitive treatment for this condition? [1]
[12]

Case 7

A 72-year-old Asian male presents to the ED, having become unwell over the last six hours, with excruciating but poorly localized abdominal pain. His past medical history includes a 'heart attack' three months ago and type II diabetes. His abdominal examination reveals minimal abdominal tenderness with no guarding or rebound and no palpable aneurysm, despite his description of 10/10 pain severity. His pulse is 110 bpm irregular and blood pressure 95/55 mmHg with temperature 36.9 °C. The results of his blood tests are shown below:

WCC	21.0×10^9/L	Na^+	141 mmol/L
Neutrophils	19.0×10^9/L	K^+	5.4 mmol/L
Hb	10.9 g/dl	Urea	8.0 mmol/L
Glucose	4.3 mmol/L	Cl^-	88 mEq/L

ABG (on air):

pH	7.01
pO_2	12.0 kPa
pCO_2	2.3 kPa
Base excess	−14.2
HCO_3^-	−7.0 mEq/L
Lactate	11.7 mmol/L

a Interpret the abnormalities in this patients arterial blood gas (ABG) above. [3]
b What is the likely diagnosis and explain the pathophysiology of this
   condition? [3]
c Is the anion gap likely to be raised in this patient? Include your reason. [2]
d Give your initial management steps in the ED. [4]
e Name the investigation of choice and what is the definitive surgical
   treatment in this condition? [2]
   [14]

Case 8

A 65-year-old male, heavy smoker, is triaged to minors with acute pain in his left
lower leg. He is known to have peripheral vascular disease (PVD) and, for some
months, his walking has been limited by claudication pain. As of a couple of hours
previously, he cannot walk at all.

a What clinical features suggest that a patient's peripheral vascular disease
   (PVD) is progressing to critical ischaemia where they may be at risk of
   gangrene? [3]
b Name two bedside tests you can perform to assess the degree of arterial
   insufficiency in a patient with peripheral vascular disease. [2]
c List the six classic signs/symptoms of an acutely ischaemic limb? [3]
d Give four different causes of acute limb ischaemia. [2]
e What immediate action is called for in the ED, and name one surgical
   intervention used in the definitive management of an acute ischaemic limb? [3]
   [13]

Case 9

A 17-year-old female presents to the ED with two days of worsening right-sided
abdominal pain. She is nauseated but has not vomited. She has no past medical
history of note and currently denies any urinary symptoms and states her last
menstrual period was ten days ago and normal. Her triage record indicates initial
observations of temperature 37.8 °C, heart rate 102 bpm and blood pressure
105/75 mmHg. On examination, you elicit tenderness and guarding in the right
iliac fossa.

a Give four possible differential diagnoses in this patient? [4]
b What investigations would you perform in the ED for this patient (give four)? [2]
c Name three immediate management interventions. [3]
d Name six parts of the 'Alvarado scoring system' that are used to risk-stratify
   the most likely diagnosis in this patient? [3]
   [12]

Case 10

You next see a 74-year-old woman who has had some left mild, lower quadrant pains for five days and today, some fresh rectal bleeding. She tells you she had a similar episode one year ago which was diagnosed as diverticulitis, and she was treated by the GP with tablets. She is pyrexial at 37.8 °C, with heart rate 110 bpm and blood pressure 115/75mmHg. On examination, she is tender but not guarding in the left lower quadrant and with dark blood present on PR examination.

a Other than diverticulitis give four causes of lower GI bleeding.   [2]
b Briefly explain the difference between diverticulosis and diverticulitis.   [2]
c Other than pain and PR bleeding, list four symptoms of diverticulitis that
   you would ask about.   [2]
d Give four treatments you would give this patient in the ED?   [4]
e On questioning specifically about urinary symptoms, she confesses to recently
   passing frothy foul-smelling urine. What might be the explanation for this? [2]
                                                                              [12]

Case 11

A 44-year-old overweight Caucasian woman complains of three days of vomiting, sweats and abdominal pain. On examination, she is febrile with a fever of 38.8 °C although alert and haemodynamically stable. She is also noted to be jaundiced and tender to palpation in the right hypochondrium. The results of blood tests requested in the ED are shown below:

WCC	18.2×10^9/L
Hb	12.3 g/dL
Platelets	645 × 10^9/L
Neutrophils	16.2×10^9/L
AST	87 u/L
ALP	640 u/L
Bilirubin	132 µmol/L
Amylase	180 u/dL

a Interpret the blood results above for this patient.   [3]
b What is your working diagnosis based on the information given?   [1]
c Give two common causes and two causative organisms for the diagnosis
   you give in answer to in part **b**. above.   [4]
d Outline your management of this patient in the ED.   [4]
                                                                            [12]

SURGICAL EMERGENCIES – ANSWERS

Case 1

a This patient has the signs and symptoms of acute pancreatitis. Due to inflammation then autodigestion of the pancreas by its own exocrine hormones,[3] pancreatitis is responsible for 3% of all acute abdominal pain admitted to hospital in the UK. However, the wider differential diagnosis of upper abdominal pain should always be considered and in this patient – a smoker with heavy alcohol use – includes:

- perforated peptic ulcer
- basal pneumonia
- acute cholecystitis
- leaking/ruptured AAA
- small bowel obstruction
- an inferior myocardial infarction.

b The two most common causes of pancreatitis are gallstones and alcohol, accounting for up to 80% of cases. It is paramount to consider these two diagnoses first and foremost and take detailed histories to identify related risk factors. An easy way to remember the other causes is by the much loved mnemonic **GET SMASHED**: **G**allstones, **E**thanol, **T**rauma (blunt), **S**teroids, **M**umps, **A**utoimmune, **S**corpion bites(!), **H**yperlipidaemia/calcaemia, **E**RCP, **D**rugs (azathioprine, thiazides, valproate).

c Several scoring systems exist to risk stratify patients with likely pancreatitis with the aim of identifying the level of dependency the patient will require. Ranson's criteria, Apache II score and Glasgow scoring systems are the most commonly used.[4] The Glasgow scoring system is an easy to use score for the Emergency Department (ED) and can be recalled by using yet another mnemonic! **PANCREAS**.

Table 18.1

Parameter	Value
PaO$_2$	<8 kPa
Age	>55 years
Neutrophils	>15x10^9/L
Calcium	< 2 mmol/L
Raised urea	> 16 mmol/L
Elevated LDH	>600 U/L
Albumin	<32 g/L
Sugar (glucose)	>10 mmol/L (fasting)

Presence of three or more of these parameters both on admission and on subsequent tests within 48 hours indicates severe disease and the likely need for HDU/ITU care.

d Patients with acute pancreatitis can be significantly unwell requiring urgent resuscitation in the ED.[5] The following are the priorities:

- oxygen to give saturations 94–98%
- fluid resuscitation – start with normal saline 1 L IV stat and reassess aiming for adequate urine output (>0.5 mL/kg urine)
- analgesia. Use morphine IV, in 2.5 mg aliquots and titrate to pain with anti-emetic cover (metaclopromide 10 mg IV)
- nasogastric tube to avoid aspirations
- catheterize for accurate monitoring of urine output
- broad spectrum antibiotics e.g., cefuroxime IV 1.5 g, and metronidazole IV 500 mg if severe episode or signs of septic shock (the evidenced-based jury is still out on the efficacy of routine antibiotics in all cases of pancreatitis)
- prompt referral to the surgical team on call.

Case 2

a Acute testicular pain is an important time critical presentation to the ED.[6] The most important diagnosis to consider is testicular torsion because of the need for urgent surgical detorsion within four to six hours to salvage the affected testicle. Thus, testicular torsion is always the working diagnosis until proven otherwise for the presentation of acute testicular pain. Other diagnoses which present similarly include:

- orchitis and epididymo-orchitis
- torsion of the hydatid of Morgagni
- trauma
- incarcerated inguinal hernia
- mumps
- rarely hydrocele.

b The normal testicle is firmly fixed in the scrotum by the tunica vaginalis which attaches to the posterior scrotal wall and prevents any rotation of the testicle. Anatomically defective attachment of the tunica vaginalis allows the testis and epididymis to hang within the scrotal sac, and spontaneously twist about its axis, with occlusion of the testicular blood supply and resultant testicular necrosis. Torsion is most common in adolescence with peak incidence at 13 years although neonates are also vulnerable.

c The classic features of acute testicular torsion are those of a swollen, tender testis that is retracted and often lying horizontally. There is usually reddening of the scrotal skin and absence of the cremasteric reflex (more reliable in children than adults) may also be seen.

d A three-point plan for management of torsion in the ED might be:

- the pain of torsion is severe and distressing. Give morphine – for a 14-year-old, either oral (oromorph 10–15 mg PO) or intravenous (morphine sulphate 0.1–0.2 mg/kg) until comfortable
- place the patient nil by mouth and start IV fluids in preparation for surgery
- this is a urological emergency and thus **immediate** surgical referral is necessary with a view to prompt exploration. If the testis is viable, then it is surgically fixed (orchidopexy); often this is performed bilaterally as there is an increased incidence of torsion in the other testes. Testicular colour Doppler is a test which can be requested to confirm torsion, but this is primarily a clinical diagnosis, and unnecessary investigation should never delay surgical exploration.

Case 3

a The clinical scenario suggests this patient has a leaking or ruptured abdominal aortic aneurysm (AAA). Immediate management priorities in the ED are:

- establishing intravenous access (two large bore intravenous cannulae)
- sending blood for cross-match 10 units red cells
- pain relief, most likely with IV morphine 2.5–10 mg titrated to response
- establishing the diagnosis of ruptured AAA as quickly as possible; either on purely clinical grounds or using bedside ultrasound in the hands of ultrasound trained ED personnel
- referral to a vascular surgical team as soon as possible.

b Bedside ultrasound in the ED performed by an ultrasound trained ED physician is an excellent method, to quickly assess the diameter of the abdominal aorta. Normal is generally less than 2 cm on entering the abdomen and 1.5 cm prior to its bifurcation. The abdominal aorta is considered to be aneurysmal if the diameter is greater than 4 cm and considered to be 'ectatic' (dilated) if measuring between 2–4 cm. The risk of rupture rises appreciably once above 5 cm in diameter.[6]

c Ultrasonographic differences in the appearance of the aorta and vena cava include:

Table 18.2

Aorta	Vena cava
Non-compressible	Easily compressible
Thicker walled	Thinner walled
Pulsatile	Non-pulsatile
To the patient's left	To the patient's right
No variation with respiration	Variation with respiration

d Evidence from other conditions involving life-threatening bleeding, such as major GI haemorrhage and penetrating trauma, has indicated that **limiting** IV resuscitation pre-operatively – with the aim of reducing pressure driven blood loss and avoiding coagulopathy from large volume IV fluid administration – is beneficial and improves outcome. Although direct trial evidence for this in ruptured AAA is lacking, the practice of tolerating relative hypotension and holding off fluid resuscitation unless absolutely necessary, has been widely adopted for the ED management of these patients.[7] Thus, in managing the IV fluid resuscitation of this patient with a ruptured AAA:

- tolerate a relative hypotension of around 90 mmHg systolic blood pressure (permissive hypotension) without action
- give fluid resuscitation only where the blood pressure falls dangerously low (<60–80 mmHg – local protocols vary) or where there is evidence of organ hypoperfusion (e.g., deteriorating conscious level)
- resuscitate with blood, as far as possible, as it is blood they are losing
- aggressively correct any coagulopathy guided by clotting results.

e The two definitive surgical management options for ruptured AAA are:

- open surgical repair of the aneurysm. This involves midline laparotomy, clamping of the abdominal aorta as it exits the diaphragm, and then replacement of the damaged section with a synthetic vessel-like graft (e.g., Dacron®). Mortality of open surgical repair of ruptured AAA is 40–50%
- alternatively, endovascular stenting of the aneurysm can be attempted, usually where the patient is deemed not fit for the open procedure, because of age and co-morbidity. This option, however, is unsuitable for many patients due to anatomical considerations such as infra-renal extension of the aneurysm.

Case 4

a The X-ray (Figure 18.1) shows a single grossly-dilated large bowel loop extending up to the xiphisternum, with the classic 'kidney or coffee bean sign'; note also, that the gross dilatation has caused loss of the usual large bowel haustra. The X-ray appearance and, indeed, the history are consistent with a diagnosis of sigmoid volvulus.

Sigmoid volvulus (abnormal twisting of the intestine resulting in intestinal obstruction) is the most common type of volvulus and accounts for up to 8% of intestinal obstruction. It is most common in the elderly population[8] with chronic constipation, leading to a relative atonic segment of sigmoid colon. The faecally and gas-loaded segment twists on its mesenteric pedicle causing a closed loop obstruction. Progressive distension can then cause venous infarction and subsequent faecal peritonitis. On the abdominal X-ray, the classic appearance of volvulus is of a single hugely distended loop of bowel folded over on itself to give a 'bean' shape with the apex of the bean pointing away from the source of the volvulus, either sigmoid or caecal.

b Normal diameter of large bowel is 3–5 cm, with the caecum sometimes larger having a maximal diameter of 8 cm. Distension of the colon of more than 9 cm can signal impending perforation.

c The common causes of large bowel obstruction are:

- colonic tumour (most common in the developed world)
- volvulus
- diverticular disease
- inflammatory bowel disease
- faecal impaction
- extra-luminal tumours (e.g., gyneacological).

d ED management is symptomatic and supportive followed by surgical referral:

- nil by mouth
- nasogastric tube
- obtain IV access and rehydrate with normal saline (amount is guided by patient's haemodynamic status, cardiac and renal function)
- IV analgesia (use IV morphine 2.5–10 mg titrated until comfortable)
- refer to the surgical team.

e Surgical treatment of volvulus is by urgent decompression using sigmoidoscopy with a rectal decompression tube to release the flatus and build-up of liquid faeces, and this tube is left in situ for 24–48 hours. Over 60% of patients, however, will have a recurrence with conservative management alone. Definite treatment thus involves surgery with either sigmoid colectomy or fixation of the bowel to the abdominal wall to prevent rotation on the mesenteric axis.

Case 5

a An abdominal X-ray involves radiation exposure 30–50 times that of a chest X-ray and should therefore be requested only when likely to influence management. Consequently, the trend in ED practice is very much against unnecessary abdominal radiography, and recent studies have proposed a limited set of indications for such a request.[2] These are:

- suspected bowel obstruction (most common indication)
- suspected perforation (in conjunction with erect chest X-ray)

- peritonitis (though CT is better if readily available)
- acute severe colitis (looking for megacolon)
- suspected renal calculi (90% renal calculi are supposedly radio-opaque)
- suspected ingested foreign body (specifically sharp objects, button batteries and drugs bodypackers) and per rectum foreign bodies. Most ingested innocuous foreign bodies, classically coins swallowed by young children, need only a chest X-ray to demonstrate passage beyond the lower oesophageal sphincter and therefore likely passage unimpeded through the entire bowel.

b The diagnosis is small bowel obstruction. The normal radiological appearance of small bowel is that of a series of centrally located blobs of dark gas on a pretty amorphous grey background of fluid filled intestine. However, as seen in the X-ray shown (Figure 18.2), **obstructed** small bowel appears:[1]

- dilated (normal small bowel is less than 3 cm in diameter, obstructed bowel larger)
- prominent (visible whole loops of small bowel are suspicious; multiple loops are certainly abnormal)
- centrally located (to distinguish from peripherally located large bowel)
- with visible valvulae conniventes (these concentric rings of fibrous tissue extending across the whole diameter of small bowel are usually only evident as a result of small bowel dilatation).

c In the UK, common causes of mechanical small bowel obstruction include:

- post-operative adhesions (by far the most common)
- strangulated hernias
- Crohn's disease (strictures)
- neoplasm (lymphoma, extra-luminal tumours of gastric and pancreatic origin)
- gallstone ileus
- ingested foreign bodies (e.g., bezoars)
- radiation enteritis.

d Ileus describes a non-mechanical obstruction to the passage of food and fluid due to the cessation of the normal peristaltic action of the bowel. Most often, ileus is a post-operative complication after manual handling of the bowel during abdominal surgery. Other causes include electrolyte disturbance (classically hypokalaemia), drugs (opiates and L-dopa), intra-abdominal inflammation (pancreatitis, peritonitis) and more rarely bowel infarction.

e In young children, the most common cause of small bowel obstruction is intussusception. Intussusception describes the invagination or telescoping of one part of the bowel into a more distal part of the bowel; most commonly the terminal ileum into the proximal colon. Children between three months and six years are most at risk, although adults are not immune. The classic X-ray appearance of intussusception is of a sausage-shaped section of horizontal bowel in the left upper quadrant. The classic presentation is of a vomiting child with legs drawn up due to pain and with or without the redcurrant jelly stool.

Diagnosis, under the guidance of a paediatric surgeon, is via contrast-enema. Treatment, in the first instance, is with air insufflation per rectum.

Case 6

a The capillary blood gas demonstrates a raised pH with normal pCO_2 and excess base (elevated HCO_3^- and base excess). This is a metabolic alkalosis.

b The most likely diagnosis is hypertrophic pyloric stenosis. The underlying pathology is a hypertrophy and hyperplasia of the smooth muscle of the antrum and pylorus-blocking passage of feeds out of the stomach. This usually manifests between the first four-to-eight weeks of life, with failure to thrive and projectile non-bilious vomiting. First-born male infants are most at risk, and there may also be a positive family history.

Classically, the blood gas in pyloric stenosis shows a metabolic alkalosis due to the loss of hydrochloric acid (HCL) from constant vomiting (we examine the causes of metabolic alkalosis in more detail in Chapter 8, Question 8). Additional electrolyte abnormalities often seen are hypochloraemia, as a result of chloride ion loss in vomitus, and hypokalaemia from the intracellular shift of potassium to try and electrically balance the extracellular shift of H^+ ions which go to replace the lost acid.

c Textbooks describe clinical signs such as visible peristalsis and state that on palpation of the abdomen an 'olive'-shaped mass may be felt in the epigastrium, during a test feed. This is actually the thickened pylorus that can be felt. More reliably, affected children will be clinically dehydrated with signs of dry mucous membranes, sunken fontanelle, delayed CRT, lethargy and dry nappies, depending on the extent of dehydration.

d The two main imaging modalities used for diagnosis are:

- ultrasound to show the hypertrophied pylorus. It is highly sensitive and specific when used by an experienced operator, and is both easy to perform and non-invasive
- barium swallow will show the narrowing of the distal antrum and pylorus of the stomach. This is called the 'string-sign'. It also has the advantage of highlighting alternative diagnoses such as gastric reflux.

e The definitive treatment after fluid and electrolyte correction and confirmation of diagnosis is a Ramstedt's pyloromyotomy. This can now be carried out laparoscopically.

Case 7

a The ABG demonstrates a severe metabolic acidosis (low pH with reduced HCO_3^- and base excess) with respiratory compensation (low pCO_2). In addition, the lactate is raised (normal 0–2 mmol/L) indicating tissue hypoperfusion.

b The most likely diagnosis in this patient with significant ischaemic and thrombotic risk factors, severe pain but relatively normal abdominal examination and a metabolic (lactic) acidosis is clearly mesenteric ischaemia. Mesenteric ischaemia is caused by compromised blood flow to a region of the gut from blockage of one of the three major gastrointestinal arteries that arise from the aorta (the celiac axis, the superior mesenteric artery and the inferior mesenteric artery). The precipitants are:

● arterial embolism e.g., AF, embolus from mural thrombus post left ventricular infarction
● arterial thrombosis in patients who have pre-existing atherosclerosis of the mesenteric arteries
● non-occlusive causes e.g., hypotension secondary to sepsis, venous thrombosis.

c Lactate is an anion and, thus, when present in excess (as indicated from this patient's ABG) is a cause of a raised anion gap.

We could be more thorough – and in patients with a metabolic acidosis, it is good practice to be so – and calculate the anion gap directly. The anion gap is calculated by the equation $(Na+K) - (HCO_3+Cl)$[9] and is useful to identify the specific cause of an acidosis.

In this patient: $(141+5.4) - (7+88) = 51.4$. Normal is 14–18 so this is a raised anion gap. The causes can be remembered by the mnemonics **MUDPILES** and **PUSHAR**:

Table 18.3

Raised Anion Gap Acidosis	Normal Anion Gap Acidosis
Methanol	**P**ancreatic fistulae
Uraemia	**U**reto gastric conduit
DKA	**S**aline administration/spironolactone
Paraldehyde	**H**yperparathyroidism
Isoniazid/Iron	**A**cetazolamide/ammonium chloride
Lactate	**R**enal tubular acidosis
Ethanol/Ethylene Glycol	
Salicylate	

d The mortality from mesenteric ischaemia remains very high often due to the difficulty (and hence delay) in making the diagnosis. A high index of suspicion is thus needed especially when the degree of pain is out of context from the clinical examination. Prompt management in the ED involves:

● oxygen 15 L via reservoir bag
● IV fluid resuscitation with normal saline
● analgesia – IV morphine 2.5–10 mg titrated to pain
● IV antibiotics –e.g., metronidazole IV 500 mg, ceftriaxone IV 1.5 g
● prompt surgical referral.

e The gold standard investigation for mesenteric ischaemia is angiography.[10] This has the added advantage of being potentially therapeutic e.g. intra-arterial thrombolysis. Urgent laparotomy and resection of the length of necrosed bowel is indicated in patients with diagnostic angiography, or in those patients whom the diagnosis is suspected but prompt angiography unavailable.

Case 8

a Features of critical ischaemia of a limb in a patient with peripheral vascular disease include:

- rest pain – burning pain in the foot particularly at night and relieved by placing the limb into dependant position (dangling the feet over the edge of the bed)
- absent foot pulses
- sensory loss
- mottling/cyanotic colour of the skin
- ulceration
- gangrene, usually of the toes.

b Two bedside tests of arterial insufficiency to the leg are Buerger's test and the ankle-brachial pressure index (ABPI).[11]

Buerger's test is performed in two stages. Lie the patient flat then elevate the legs to an angle of 45 degrees and hold for two minutes. Pallor of the feet indicates arterial insufficiency (i.e., the arterial pressure in the limb cannot overcome gravity). The lower the angle at which pallor is observed, the greater the degree of arterial insufficiency – pallor observed at 45 degrees indicates severe insufficiency; at 25 degrees or less critical ischaemia. Then sit the patient up and ask them to hang their legs over the side of the bed with knees flexed at 90 degrees. Blood and colour returns to the ischaemic leg under gravity. The ischaemic limb first goes blue as deoxygenated blood passes through the ischaemic tissue, then red due to reactive hyperaemia from post hypoxic vasodilatation.

The ankle-brachial pressure index (ABPI) is the ratio of the highest systolic arterial pressure taken at the ankle over that taken at the brachial artery. At both locations, the systolic pressure is measured using a Doppler probe to monitor the arterial pulsation as a blood pressure cuff is deflated from above arterial pressure. The sphygmomanometer reading at the moment the Doppler once again picks up the pulse is taken as the highest systolic arterial pressure. An ABPI of around 1 is normal, 0.5–0.8 indicates moderate arterial disease whilst below 0.5 is critical ischaemia.

c The worry in this gentleman is that he now has acute limb ischaemia. The acutely ischaemic limb is classically (and in practice) identified by the **6 'P's** –

- **p**ain
- **p**arasthaesia
- **p**ulselessness
- **p**allor
- **p**aralysis
- and **p**erishingly cold!

d Arterial emboli and thrombosis *in situ* on an already atherosclerotic artery account for the majority of acute ischaemic limbs. The heart is the most common source of emboli – AF, prosthetic heart valves, vegetations on normal or prosthetic valves, post-MI mural thrombus and rheumatic fever all being predisposing factors. Emboli may also arise from aneurysms – aortic, femoral or popliteal. Thrombosis can develop at locations of established atheromatous disease and all the same risk factors as for ischaemic heart disease apply. Thinking more broadly, trauma, arterial dissection and compartment syndrome are all causes of acute limb ischaemia.

e When faced with an acute ischaemic limb in the ED the priority is to move quickly! Immediate management includes pain relief and anticoagulation with unfractionated heparin, as well as transfer of the patient's care to a vascular surgeon, as soon as possible. Searching for the cause is important but not as important as saving the limb.

The vascular surgeon can use on-table angiography to decide definitive treatment, either:

- embolectomy
- intra-arterial thrombolysis
- angioplasty
- or bypass graft surgery.

Case 9

a From the clinical history given, this patient is most likely to have appendicitis. However the differential diagnoses for right iliac fossa (RIF) pain are plentiful although of particular importance is the exclusion of pregnancy – and therefore the potential for ruptured ectopic – in any woman of child bearing age with abdominal pains.

Table 18.4

System	Differential diagnosis of RIF pain
Surgical	Acute appendicitis Strangulated hernia (inguinal and femoral) Diverticulitis Caecal carcinoma
Gynaecological	Ectopic pregnancy Ovarian torsion Ovarian cyst Pelvic inflammatory disease
Urological	Urinary tract infection Renal calculi
Gastroenterological	Gastroenteritis Constipation Crohn's disease/abscess
Others	Psoas abscess Gallbladder mucocele Mesenteric adenitis

b ED investigations of a female with abdominal pain should include:

● urinary pregnancy test
● urine dip stick for infection
● WCC and CRP for signs of infection/inflammation
● U&E, LFTs, and amylase in all patients with clinically significant abdominal pain
● serum β-hcg, if there is doubt about the result of urinary pregnancy tests.

NB. Abdominal radiographs are not part of the routine workup of suspected appendicitis and should not be requested in the ED for this reason. If the surgeon-on-call wants an abdominal X-ray, let them request it themselves!

c Investigations aside, ED management priorities are pain relief (likely IV morphine if pain is severe), and preparation of the patient for surgery: place them nil by mouth (NBM) and start IV fluid rehydration. Antibiotics are not recommended as a routine part of management in suspected appendicitis.

d The Alvarado scoring system can be used to risk stratify patients with the potential diagnosis of appendicitis.[12] A score out of ten is constructed from three signs, three symptoms and two laboratory tests: below four indicates appendicitis is unlikely while above seven considered 'probable'. This scoring system is thought to be most reliable at the ends of the range. An easy mnemonic to remember the components is **MANTRELS**.

Table 18.5

Feature	Score
Migratory right iliac fossa pain	1
Anorexia	1
Nausea or vomiting	1
Tenderness in the RIF	2
Rebound tenderness	1
Elevated temperature	1
Leukocytosis	2
Shift of white cells – Neutrophilia	1

Case 10

a Causes of **significant** lower GI blood loss in adults are:

● diverticulitis (most common)
● angiodysplasia (sudden and painless)
● colitis of infective, inflammatory or ischaemic origin all cause blood PR mixed in with stool and accompanied by abdominal pain
● ano-rectal causes such as anal fissure of haemorrhoids produce fresh red bleeding not mixed with stool and localised anal pain
● colorectal carcinoma may give fresh bleeding or slow GI blood loss resulting in anaemia

- brisk upper GI source of bleeding (e.g., bleeding peptic ulcer) with rapid transit of blood through the GI tract may mimic a lower GI bleed with large amounts of 'plum-red' coloured blood passed PR.

b Diverticula are pathological out-pouchings or small herniations of the gut wall, involving both mucosa and smooth muscle. They can be present at any point through the GI tract but are most commonly seen in the sigmoid and descending colon. The presence of diverticula without any symptoms is commonly known as diverticulosis. Patients whose diverticula progress to cause symptoms have diverticular disease, a problem of developed countries (low-fibre diet) with the sigmoid colon the affected site in 95% of patients.

In contrast, diverticulitis is a disease characterized by inflammation of large bowel diverticula causing localized signs to the area of active disease and systemic diverticula may also rupture and bleed causing complications of bowel perforation and GI haemorrhage.

c Signs and symptoms in diverticulitis can be quite non-specific but the following are also often present:

Table 18.6

Symptoms	Signs
Altered bowel habits	Low-grade pyrexia
Tenesmus	Localized tenderness
Bloating and flatulence	Local peritonitis (general peritonitis if perforated
Abdominal pain (most commonly left lower	diverticulum)
quadrant)	Abdominal distention
Fever	Left lower quadrant mass (diverticular abscess)
PR bleeding	Tachycardia and postural hypotension with blood
Nausea and vomiting	loss
Anorexia	

d This patient has pain, sickness and is passing blood PR. Your management in the ED must include:

- large bore IV access
- IV fluid rehydration with normal saline
- send blood for FBC, clotting, CRP and ESR (inflammatory markers all raised in active diverticulitis)
- group and save blood for further potential haemorrhage
- analgesia (IV morphine sulphate 2.5–10 mg titrated to pain and anti-emetic (metaclopromide IV 10 mg) for sickness
- antibiotics should be given to cover both gram positive and gram negative organisms. Local policies will vary but a third generation cephalosporin (cefuroxime IV 1.5 g) and metronidazole IV 500 mg would be a failsafe option
- refer early to the surgical team (as many as 20% of severely affected patients may need bowel resection).

e The presence of frothy urine (pneumaturia) should always be asked about as it is an ominous sign that a colovesicular fistula has occurred. An expanding fistula allows faecal material to pass through into the bladder and faecaluria is seen.

Another potential complication of diverticulitis is a colovaginal fistula and the presence of stool being passed through the vagina is pathognomonic, however, there may be earlier clues such as the presence of recurrent vaginal infections with purulent discharge.

Case 11

a The blood results given indicate the presence of infection (high WCC with neutrophilia) and of obstructive jaundice (raised bilirubin with raised ALP but normal AST). The amylase is only slightly above the normal range making acute pancreatitis unlikely.

b The working diagnosis in this case has to be acute or ascending cholangitis. Charcot's triad, first quoted in 1877, is the combination of 'fever, jaundice and right upper quadrant pain' as diagnostic of acute cholangitis. Still today up to 70% of patients with cholangitis will exhibit all three of Charcot's features. Unchecked disease leads to life threatening sepsis.

c Acute cholangitis arises due to initial mechanical compromise of the biliary tract allowing ascending infection by bowel organisms. Causes therefore include:

- gallstones causing biliary obstruction
- secondary to instrumentation of the biliary tract during Endoscopic Retrograde Cholangiopancreatography (ERCP)
- obstruction from other causes – pancreatic carcinoma, cholangiocarcinoma and bile duct strictures
- in travellers from abroad, parasitic infections such as river fluke and roundworms should be considered.

While the most common organisms which then infect the biliary tract are *Klebsiella*, *E. Coli*, *Enterobacter*, *Enterococci* and *Streptococci*, and it is common for cultures to grow more than one organism.

d Management of acute cholangitis in the ED should be along the following lines:

- pain relief (intravenous morphine 2.5–10 mg most likely required)
- IV access and fluid resuscitation/rehydration as guided by clinical status
- blood cultures
- start empirical antibiotics to cover both gram negative bowel organisms and anaerobes (intravenous ampicillin, gentamycin and metranidozole would be a typical regimen)
- referral to the surgical team for further investigation and management
- ultrasound of the biliary tract for diagnosis.

Further Reading

1. Begg JD. (1999) *Abdominal X-rays made easy*. Churchill Livingstone.
2. Smith J, Hall EJ. (2009) The use of plain abdominal X-rays in the emergency department. *Emerg. Med J*; **26**; 160–3.
3. Frossard J, Steer M, Pastor C .(2008) Acute pancreatitis. **12**; 371(9607):143–52.

4. UK Guidelines for the management of Pancreatitis (2005) www.bsg.org.uk/pdf_word_docs/pancreatic.pdf
5. Acute scrotum in children. Guidelines on paediatric urology. (2008) European Association of Urology.
6. Cosford P, Leng G. (2007) Screening for abdominal aortic aneurysm. Cochrane Database Systematic Review. Apr 18; (2):CD002945.
7. Lecky F. Best Bets: Fluid resuscitation in acute abdominal aortic aneurysm. (2003) www.bestbets.org/bets/bet.php?id=36
8. Connolly S, Brannigan A, Heffeman E, *et al.* (2002) Sigmoid volvulus: a 10-year-audit; *Ir J Med Sci.* Oct–Dec; **171**(4):216–17.
9. Williams AJ. (1998) Assessing and interpreting arterial blood gases and acid-base balance. *BMJ*; **317**: 1213–16.
10. American Gastroenterological Association Medical Position Statement: guidelines on intestinal ischemia. (2000) *Gastroenterology*; **118**:951.
11. Callum K, Bradbury A. (2000) ABC of arterial and venous disease: Acute limb ischaemia. *BMJ*; **320**:764–7.
12. Alvarado A. (1986) A practical score for the early diagnosis of acute appendicitis. *Ann Emerg Med*; **15**: 557–64.

TOXICOLOGY AND POISONING

Shumontha Dev

Introduction

Core topics

Management of the following overdoses and poisonings, including knowledge of the antidotes to common poisons:[1]

- paracetamol
- salicylate
- tricyclic antidepressants
- selective serotonin reuptake inhibitors (SSRIs)
- iron
- lithium
- the alcohols (ethanol, methanol and ethylene glycol)
- opiate
- ecstasy (MDMA)
- digoxin.

Recognition of the major toxidromes (groupings of signs and symptoms which suggest poisoning by a certain **class** of drug):[1]

- cholinergic
- anticholinergic
- sympathomimetic (adrenergic)
- serotonin
- opiate
- sedative.

The use of generic treatments in the poisoned patient:

- gut decontamination, e.g., with activated charcoal[3]
- haemodialysis.

SAQs based around poisoned patients may draw from a wide range of clinical data. Be familiar with important drug levels, such as those of paracetamol, salicylate and lithium. The ECG provides many clues in the poisoned patient. Look for tachycardias, bradycardias and commit to memory the series of ECG changes in tricyclic antidepressant overdose – an exam favourite. Commonly seen also are acid-base calculations (salicylates, tricyclics) and the determination of the osmolar gap and the anion gap (alcohol, methanol and ethylene glycol).

The most comprehensive and up to date resource for the diagnosis and management of poisons is the National Poisons Information Service (NPIS) currently accessible online as Toxbase at www.toxbase.org.[4] You do need a login and password to access this resource but all Emergency Departments (EDs) will have one.

And do not forget the psychiatric management of patients presenting with self-harm of any sort (*see* Chapter 11) as this may form part of any question on self-poisoning. In children with accidental poisoning, there may be social issues to attend to as well.

Case 1

A 35-year-old obese woman with a history of depression and previous self-harm comes to the ED after an unwitnessed overdose. She claims to have taken 30 tablets of paracetamol four hours previously, along with a bottle of wine. She has a history of chronic alcohol use and takes no regular medications.

a What is considered to be a potentially hepatotoxic dose of paracetamol for a typical adult? [1]

b Give three groups of patients for whom the high-risk treatment line on the paracetamol level normogram should be used when deciding whether treatment for paracetamol overdose is needed. [3]

c This patient's paracetamol level was above the normal treatment line when sampled at four hours post ingestion. Write the standard three part prescription for the full 20 hours of treatment with n-acetylcysteine (NAC) assuming the patient weighs 60 kg. Include in your answer the total amount of NAC, or the amount of NAC per kilogram weight, the quantity and type of fluid it is diluted in and the time course over which it is to be given. [6]

d What alternative drug may be used if the patient refuses intravenous treatment for paracetamol overdose? [2]

[12]

Case 2

You are asked to see a 17-year-old male who, after an argument with his girlfriend, has taken an overdose of aspirin. He was witnessed to grab and consume a whole bottle (32 × 300 mg aspirin) of his father's tablets roughly four hours ago.

His initial observations are: heart rate 120 bpm, blood pressure 110/65 mmHg, respiratory rate 20/min, oxygen saturations on air 98% and temperature 37.1 °C.

a Give three symptoms of **mild** salicylate toxicity that you might ask about. [3]

b You take blood for a plasma salicylate concentration immediately and your consultant advises a further blood test in two hours. Briefly explain the rationale for a repeat plasma salicylate concentration after two hours. [2]

c This patient's plasma salicylate concentration is 343 mg/L. Is this consistent with mild, moderate or severe toxicity? [1]

d Arterial blood gas analysis forms part of the assessment of salicylate overdose. What acid-base disturbances might you expect to see in a patient with salicylate poisoning? [4]

e Give two treatments for severe salicylate poisoning. [2]

[12]

Case 3

A 30-year-old woman is brought by ambulance having taken an overdose of her prescription antidepressant after finding out that she was to be made redundant. She has been taking the antidepressant, imipramine for over two years. Her partner found her in the house semi-conscious and called 999. On arrival in the ED, she is drowsy but maintaining her airway.

a List four anticholinergic effects of this type of antidepressant. [4]
b Give three abnormalities of the ECG consistent with the overdose taken. [3]
c Give four indications for treatment with sodium bicarbonate for this type of overdose. [3]
d Name two further antidepressants of the same class or type as imipramine. [2]
[12]

Case 4

An 80-year-old man arrives in the ED with acute abdominal pain and profuse vomiting of black vomitus and blood. He confesses to taking an overdose of one of his prescription medications, which he receives as part of symptomatic medical treatment of his recently diagnosed colon carcinoma. He states to you that he does not want to live anymore.

a What is the most likely tablet that the patient has taken in overdose? [1]
b Name two gut decontamination methods that can be used in this type of poisoning. [2]
c Other than those already described in this patient, give two early and one late (>one week later) feature of **severe** poisoning with this medication. [3]
d Briefly describe the investigations you would perform to assess the likely severity of this patient's overdose. [4]
e What is the name of the specific antidote for this poison and by what route is it given? [2]
[12]

Case 5

A five-year-old boy is brought to the ED with drowsiness and acute diarrhoea and vomiting. His grandmother says that she had left her bottle of digoxin out after taking her morning pills and that the boy has swallowed a number of the tablets from the bottle, thinking they were sweets.

a How long after ingestion do digoxin levels peak in the circulation? [1]
b What cardiovascular effects are seen in acute digoxin poisoning? [3]
c What electrolyte imbalance is associated with digoxin poisoning and how would you treat it? Give drugs you would use and drugs you would avoid. [3]

d Give three indications for administering Fab antibody fragments to patients
with digoxin poisoning. [3]
[10]

Case 6

A man calls an ambulance after finding his 33-year-old neighbour confused and
irritable in his car at midnight. He first assumed he was drunk but then noticed
an empty bottle of antifreeze in his hand, and became concerned his neighbour
may have drunk the contents. On arrival to the ED, the patient is drowsy but
maintaining his airway and has the following observations: heart rate 115 bpm,
blood pressure 145/75 mmHg, respiratory rate 22/min and oxygen saturations on
air 95%. Initial blood tests indicate the following:

Na^+	131 mmol/L
K^+	4.8 mmol/L
Urea	7.9 mmol/L
Creatinine	98 μmol/L.
Glucose	5.7 mmol/L
Serum osmolality	324 mosm/kg

a Calculate the osmolar gap using the above blood test results. Interpret your
result indicating the likely cause of any abnormality. [4]
b What are the clinical features of severe toxicity from methanol? [2]
c What happens to the anion gap in poisoning with antifreeze? [1]
d Give **two** specific treatments for antifreeze poisoning? [2]
e What further treatment may be required in severe poisoning with antifreeze? [1]
[10]

TOXICOLOGY AND POISONING – ANSWERS

Case 1

a Adult patients reporting overdoses of paracetamol greater than 150 mg/kg or 24 tablets (12 g) should be considered in danger of hepatotoxicity. For patients who are considered at **high-risk** of liver damage following paracetamol overdose (see below), it is advised to consider reports of 75 mg/kg or more as potentially toxic. In situations where measured paracetamol levels are of less value – staggered overdoses and delayed presentations – these benchmarks of potential liver toxicity are used to guide the need for initiating treatment.

b For most patients who present early after overdose, paracetamol levels can be taken from four hours post-ingestion and the result read from the universally used Rumack-Matthew normogram to decide the need for treatment. Certain patients, however, are at higher risk of liver damage from excess paracetamol due either to enzyme induction of cytochrome p450 CYPE1, the enzyme which metabolizes paracetamol to the hepatotoxic metabolite NAPQI, or due to reduced clearance of this harmful metabolite by glucorinidation. Thus, there is a lower threshold for treating such patients and the high-risk treatment line on the normogram is used when the following apply:

- chronic alcohol use
- anticonvulsant therapy with carbamazipine, phenytoin and barbiturates
- patients on rifampicin or isoniazid
- taking over the counter St. John's Wort
- anorexia or malnourishment.

c Write up the standard regime for treatment of paracetamol overdose with n-acetylcysteine (NAC) as follows:[3]

- 150 mg/kg (9.0 g in a 60 kg patient) in 200 mL 5% Dextrose IVI over 15 minutes, then
- 50 mg/kg (3.0 g in a 60 kg patient) in 500 mL 5% Dextrose IVI over four hours, then
- 100 mg/kg (6.0 g in a 60 kg patient) in 1000 mL 5% Dextrose IVI over 16 hours.

d In patients that either refuse intravenous access or have a previous allergy to NAC, the alternative is methionine. This preparation is given as 2.5 g orally every four hours up to a total of 10 g. Caution is required as methionine is less effective in vomiting patients or where there is a delay to treatment of more than eight hours. It is also less effective if the patent has been administered activated charcoal.

Case 2

a Salicylates are available both by prescription and as an over the counter medications in doses of 75, 150 and 300 mg aspirin and are frequently taken in overdose. Symptoms of salicylate toxicity depend on the degree of poisoning:

Table 19.1

Mild poisoning (typically >125 mg/kg ingested aspirin)	Moderate poisoning (typically >250 mg/kg ingested aspirin)	Severe poisoning (typically >500 mg/kg ingested aspirin)
Nausea	Dehydration	Hyperpyrexia
Vomiting	Restlessness/agitation	Confusion
Dizziness	Sweating	Coma
Lethargy	Vasodilatation	Convulsions
Tinnitus		Renal failure

b Large amounts of salicylates form concretions within the stomach that delay absorption making it difficult to predict from a single level when the peak plasma concentration of salicylate might occur. It is important, therefore, to recheck the plasma salicylate concentration two hours after the first level. If the salicylate concentration rises on repeat sampling, then the maximal toxicity has yet to come and the patient requires further plasma levels at two to four hour intervals until they begin to fall. Conversely, once the plasma salycylate level decreases between repeat bloods, the worst symptoms are likely to have passed.

c In overdose, serum salicylate concentrations roughly correlate with toxicity as follows:

Table 19.2

Plasma salicylate concentration (mg/L)	Likely toxicity
<350	Mild
>350–700	Moderate
>700	Severe and potentially fatal

d Early in salicylate poisoning, respiratory stimulation causes hyperventilation and blowing off of CO_2 with a consequent **respiratory alkalosis** detectable on arterial blood gas analysis.

Later, and in more serious poisoning, salicylates uncouple oxidative phosphorylation within cellular mitochondria leading to predominant anaerobic metabolism, and a **metabolic acidosis** becomes evident on blood gas analysis.

e Urinary alkalinization aids elimination of salicylates through the kidney and is indicated in moderate and severe toxicity (salicylate concentrations >450 mg/L in adults). The National Poisons Information Service (Toxbase)[4] recommends for adults either 225 mL of 8.4% sodium bicarbonate intravenously over

60 mins or 1.5 litre 1.26% sodium bicarbonate over two hours. Aim for urinary pH 7.5–8.5, checking hourly, and repeat dosage sodium bicarbonate may be required to maintain this.

Haemodialysis should also be used in highly symptomatic patients (coma, renal failure, severe acidosis) and those with potentially fatal plasma salicylate concentrations (>700 mg/L).

Case 3

a Imipramine is a tricyclic antidepressant (TCA). TCAs are less commonly used these days due to their narrow therapeutic window and poor side effect profile both at treatment doses and especially when taken in excess. The classic anticholinergic effects of TCAs (anticholinergic toxidrome) include:

- dry mouth
- warm and dry skin
- tachycardia
- blurred vision
- urinary retention
- large dilated pupils
- respiratory depression
- confusion
- coma.

increasing
—— tricyclic
toxicity

In addition, TCAs may give hypotension from alpha-adrenergic receptor blockade and cardiotoxicity from inhibition of fast sodium channels in myocardial cell membranes.

b Typical ECG changes of tricyclic overdose are most often a sinus tachycardia but more ominously a prolonged PR interval and a widened QRS complex. Remember that in the context of a TCA overdose, a QRS (>120 ms indicates likely toxicity and >160 ms indicates severe toxicity and high risk of arrhythmia. Widened QT interval and all forms of arrhythmia (VT, SVT and bradycardia) may also occur.

c The drug of choice for patients poisoned with TCAs is sodium bicarbonate. Indications for its use are:

- acidosis on the blood gas (pH <7.35)
- QRS >120 ms
- arrhythmia
- hypotension resistant to fluid resuscitation.

Serum alkalinization with sodium bicarbonate promotes protein binding of TCA molecules, thereby reducing their cardiotoxic effects. Give 50 mmol (50 mL of 8.4% bicarbonate) as an initial bolus. General wisdom suggests avoiding anti-arrhythmics; correct hypoxia and acidosis instead.

d Common tricyclic antidepressants include: amitriptyline, dothiepin, dosulepin imipramine, lofepramine and trimipramine. Although we have said the prescription of TCAs for depression is now less common, it should be remembered that certain TCAs are also increasingly used as analgesia in neuropathic and chronic pain and in the treatment of migraines, insomnia and irritable bowel syndrome such that a large population of patients are still using these medications.

Case 4

a The most likely poison in this patient is iron. In a patient diagnosed with cancer of the large bowel, anaemia is often present and requires iron supplementation. Furthermore, clinically iron overdose presents with:

- nausea
- vomiting (usually of grey or black vomitus)
- diarrhoea
- abdominal pain
- black stool
- haematemesis may also occur.

b Activated charcoal does not bind iron and is, therefore, of little use. Two alternative methods of gut decontamination to consider are:

- gastric lavage is indicated within one hour of significant iron ingestion (>20 mg/kg elemental iron).
- whole bowel irrigation with polyethylene glycol is also effective where undissolved iron tablets are still visible in the gut on plain abdominal X-ray.

c Iron can be extremely toxic in overdose with features of severe poisoning occuring at different times post-overdose. Typically:

Table 19.3

<12 hours	24–48 hours	>2 weeks
Haematemesis	Gastric erosion and GI bleeds	Gastric strictures and
Confusion	Metabolic acidosis	pyloric stenosis
Coma	Hepatocellular necrosis and acute liver	
Seizures	failure with jaundice, Encephalopathy and	
Haemodynamic shock	clotting disorders	
Metabolic acidosis		

d Measured serum iron concentrations at close to four hours post-ingestion correlates well with degree of poisoning as follows:

Table 19.4

Serum iron concentration (micromol/L)	Degree of poisoning
<55	Mild
55–90	Moderate
>90	Severe

Repeat iron levels should be taken after two hours to ensure peak concentration has passed (i.e., all ingested iron has been absorbed). Further useful investigations are blood glucose level and white cell count, both of which are raised with iron toxicity. An arterial blood gas is essential in all symptomatic patients.

e   Desferrioxamine is the antidote for severe iron poisoning and is given by IV infusion at a dose of 15 mg/kg body weight/hour (max dose 80 mg/kg in 24 hours). It acts as a chelating agent that binds with the iron and enhances its elimination within the urine. Classically, this causes the urine to change colour and become a pinkish red. Be sure to discuss all cases of severe poisoning with the National Poison Information Service.

Case 5

a   Digoxin is another drug with narrow therapeutic index and poor side-effect profile such that toxicity is seen in a variety of scenarios, including patients on regular digoxin therapy, those with accidental ingestion – as with the boy in this question – and also those taking digoxin in deliberate overdose.

Early on (one to two hours post-ingestion) digoxin toxicity causes nausea, vomiting and diarrhoea as well as headache, confusion and, rarely, disturbance of colour vision. Absorption of digoxin is slow, however, with peak effects delayed six hours or more and, after which time, cardiovascular symptoms become apparent. More than 2–3 mg in an adult (>50 mg/kg in a child) are associated with toxicity.

b   Cardiovascular effects of digitalis poisoning occur in all ages and are what you would expect:

- PR prolongation
- bradycardia
- A-V block of all types
- sinus arrest
- hypotension.

c   Digitalis inhibits the sodium-potassium ATPase pump in all cell membranes leading to potassium accumulation in the extracellular space. Thus, digoxin excess may lead to severe hyperkalaemia (>7 mmol/l), particularly in the presence of underlying renal impairment.

Hyperkalaemia of digoxin poisoning is treated with an insulin-dextrose infusion (50 mL 50% dextrose with 12 units of actrapid intravenously). In contrast to the normal treatment of hyperkalaemia, however, calcium gluconate or calcium chloride should be avoided because in the presence of digoxin excess, calcium **promotes** ventricular dysrhythmia rather than preventing it.

d   The purified Fab fragments of digoxin-specific antibodies can be given as the antidote for severe digoxin poisoning in the following circumstances:

- severe hyperkalaemia resistant to treatment with insulin-dextrose infusion
- bradycardia or heart block associated with hypotension resistant to treatment with atropine
- tachyarrhythmias associated with hypotension.

Case 6

a Commercial antifreeze may contain ethylene glycol or methanol or both , as well as in most cases a coloured dye to discourage desperate drinkers! Further sources of methanol and ethylene glycol include copy fluids, brake fluids and paint removers. Interestingly, both methanol and ethylene glycol are non-toxic until broken down into their harmful metabolites by alcohol dehydrogenase. Around 100 mL of ethylene glycol can be fatal in adults.

Both components of antifreeze are organic solutes and are readily absorbed into the bloodstream from the gut causing a rise in plasma osmolality during the first hours after ingestion. Thus we can calculate the osmolar gap as a sign of significant organic solute ingestion (Box 19.1):

Box 19.1 Calculating the osmolar gap

Osmolar gap = serum osmolality (measured) – calculated osmolality

Where calculated osmolality = $(2 \times Na^+)$ + glucose + urea
Thus, using the blood test results given in the question,
Osmolar gap = 324 − $((2 \times 131) + 5.7 + 7.9)$ = 48.4 mOsm/kg

The normal osmolar gap is <15 mOsm/kg, and values greater than 25 mOsm/kg indicate significant organic solute ingestion (alcohol, methanol, ethylene glycol, acetone and others)

---

b Mild toxicity with methanol produces symptoms similar to alcohol intoxication. Severe toxicity, however, causes profound metabolic acidosis with drowsiness, coma convulsions and acute renal failure. Ocular toxicity is often described in textbooks, with patients complaining of blurred vision with 'mistiness' or 'whiteness' within the visual field. Without treatment, this may lead to permanent visual impairment or blindness.

c Ingested ethylene glycol and methanol are converted into toxic organic acids, over several hours, by alcohol dehydrogenase enzyme present in liver hepatocytes. In contrast to their parent chemical, these organic acids have no effect on the osmolar gap but as circulating anions do influence the anion gap and acid/base status of the patient giving rise to a high anion gap acidosis (*see* Chapter 18, Question 8 for calculation and interpretation of anion gaps).

d It often comes as a surprise to many new doctors in the ED that most departments will keep a bottle of vodka or whiskey in the drug cupboard to be used as an antidote to methanol and ethylene glycol poisoning. Ethanol acts by saturating the alcohol dehydrogenase, thus slowing the breakdown of these poisons to their potent metabolites. Ethanol is usually given as an intravenous loading dose of 7.5 mL/kg of 10% ethanol in water or 5% dextrose over 30 minutes but an oral dose of 2.5 ml/kg of 40% ethanol (i.e., most spirits) diluted with water over 30 minutes works equally as well – in either case, the aim is a blood alcohol level of around 100 mg/dL. Caution is required in patients with CNS depression but the only absolute contraindication to ethanol therapy is current or recent use of disulfiram.

Fomepizole (4-methylpyrazole) is an alternative that also acts by inhibiting alcohol dehydrogenase. It is expensive (very!) but has the advantage of predictable pharmacokinetics and none of the CNS depression of ethanol.

e Haemodialysis removes both the organic solute and the harmful organic acid in ethylene glycol and methanol poisoning, and so is used in refractory or particularly severe cases (e.g., severe acidosis and/or renal failure). It is also worth remembering that haemodialysis can also be used to treat life-threatening overdose with ethanol itself.

Further Reading

1. Longmore M, Wilkinson I, Davidson E, *et al.* (2010) *Oxford Handbook of Clinical Medicine*, 8th edn. Oxford University Press. pp 850–6.
2. Jones AL and Dargan P. (2001) *Churchill's Pocketbook of Toxicology*. Churchill and Livingstone.
3. Emergency treatment of poisoning. (2010) British National Formulary. 60.
4. National Poisons Information Service database. Toxbase. Current versions found at www.toxbase.org.

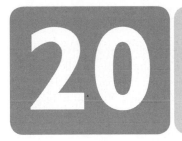

TRAUMA AND ORTHOPAEDICS

Elaine Harding and Mathew Hall

Introduction

Core Topics

- haemorrhage and hypovolaemic shock
- ATLS and major trauma (cervical spine injury, traumatic brain injury, penetrating and blunt chest and abdominal injury, pelvic fracture, spinal cord injury, compound fractures)
- trauma in special circumstances (paediatric, pregnancy, the elderly)
- significant fractures in adults and children (cervical spine, lumbar spine, clavicle humerus, supracondylar, distal radius, scaphoid, neck of femur, femoral, ankle, calcaneus etc.)
- clinical decision rules (Canadian C-spine rule, Ottowa ankle and Ottowa knee rules)
- shoulder dislocation
- compartment syndrome
- septic arthritis
- osteomyelitis
- back pain
- hand and finger infections
- wounds over key anatomical sites
- bite wounds
- complex wounds.

A large part of this topic is based on ATLS[1] and APLS[2] principles and so it pays to be familiar with the ATLS and APLS manuals or attend a course in the run up to the exam. Another useful resource for major trauma is the UK website www.trauma. org, while for practical orthopaedics a common reference is the *Pocket Book of Orthopaedics and Fractures* by R. McRae.[3]

Case 1

A 40-year-old female pedestrian has been hit by a car travelling at approximately 30 mph. On arrival in the Emergency Department (ED), she is able to talk to you, has a semi-rigid collar in place and is fully immobilized on a spinal board. Her observations are as follows: heart rate 120 bpm, blood pressure 90/50 mmHg, respiratory rate 30/min and oxygen saturations 99% on oxygen via reservoir mask. Primary survey reveals a prolonged CRT and tenderness and bruising over the lower abdomen and pelvis.

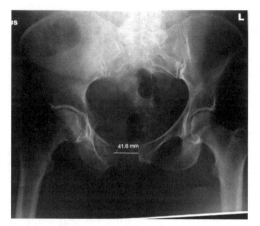

Figure 20.1

a Estimate the volume of blood loss suffered. [1]
b Outline your approach to fluid resuscitation in the ED. [3]
c As part of your primary survey you request a pelvic X-ray (Figure 20.1.). Describe the abnormality in the pelvic X-ray of this patient and comment on the likely stability of the pelvis. [2]
d Give three complications associated with the injury indicated in the X-ray (Figure 20.1). [3]
e What is the immediate management of this injury in the ED? [1]
[10]

Case 2

A 67-year-old woman with severe osteoarthritis has tripped and fallen forwards striking her face against a door frame and in the process hyper extending her neck. She felt immediate neck pain and could not get up from the floor due to weakness of her arms. She was alert when the paramedics arrived and promptly placed into a hard collar then immobilized for transfer on a spinal board. All her observations are stable on arrival in the ED and initial examination reveals a marked weakness of both arms.

a List three high risk factors of the Canadian C-spine rules that indicate radiographic imaging of the C-spine is required. [3]
b What is the sensitivity and specificity of the Canadian C-spine rules in correctly identifying potential cervical spine injuries requiring radiography? [2]
c Cervical spine X-rays followed by CT of the cervical spine reveals extensive degenerative changes but no acute bony injury. What diagnosis therefore might account for her clinical presentation? [1]
d Give the main clinical features of the diagnosis you give in answer to **c.** above. [3]
e What further investigation is required to confirm this suspected diagnosis? [1]
[10]

Case 3

A 16-year-old boy attends the ED with worsening left upper quadrant pain. The previous day, he had fallen from his pushbike and describes coming down on top of the handlebar which 'stuck' him in the upper abdomen. His airway and breathing are satisfactory but his heart rate is 135 bpm and blood pressure 85/40 mmHg.

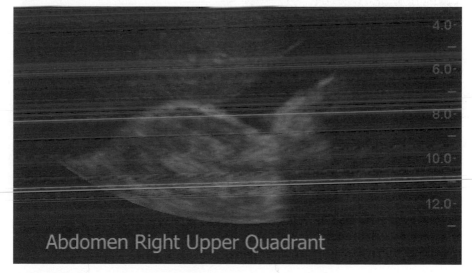

Figure 20.2
Ultrasound image courtesy of Sonosite

a What injury is suspected? [2]
b As part of your circulatory assessment you decide to perform a FAST scan at the bedside. Name the four views which make up the FAST scan. [4]
c Describe the findings in the image from the FAST scan shown in Figure 20.2 above. [2]
d What are the indications for a laparotomy following abdominal trauma? [2]
[10]

Case 4

A 25-year-old man attends the ED with a painful wrist after a fall whilst intoxicated the night before. The following X-ray (Figure 20.3) was taken by the emergency nurse practitioner who has come to you for advice.

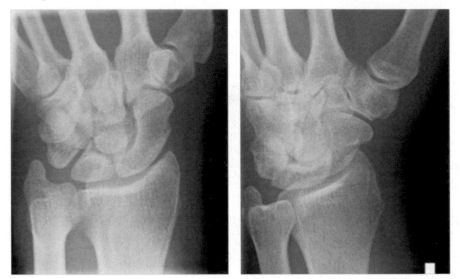

Figure 20.3

a Describe the abnormality on the X-ray above (Figure 20.3).   [2]
b Give two complications from this type of injury.   [2]
c How would you manage this injury?   [2]
d How should the hand and wrist be positioned for the specific plastercast
   that is appropriate for this injury?   [2]
                                                          [8]

Case 5

A four-year-old girl attends the ED with her mother. She has fallen while playing on a trampoline two hours earlier and, after the initial crying had died down, her mother noticed she was not using her left arm and would not let anyone touch it. She has no other apparent injuries. Her elbow X-ray is shown below (Figure 20.4).

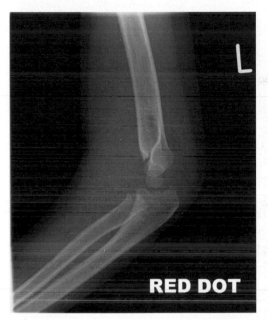

Figure 20.4

a Describe the abnormalities in the X-ray (Figure 20.4). [2]
b How should this child be managed by the ED (give three key steps)? [3]
c List two early and two late complications specifically associated with this injury. [4]
d Describe the order and age at which the ossification centres at the elbow appear in children. [3]

  [12]

Case 6

A 50-year-old woman has fallen down the stairs at home. She is crying out in pain and has an obvious swelling to her right thigh. After primary and secondary survey, her injuries appear localized to the left leg. Her observations are stable. An X-ray of the right femur is obtained (Figure 20.5)

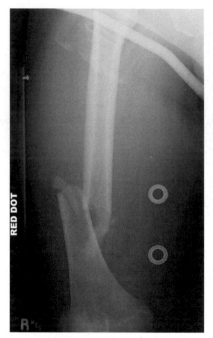

RED DOT

R

Figure 20.5

a Describe the abnormality in the X-ray (Figure 20.5).   [2]
b Outline your immediate management of this injury.   [3]
c Describe how you would perform a femoral nerve block.   [4]
d Give three advantages to placing the leg in traction.   [3]
                                                                    [12]

Case 7

A 21-year-old male was being pursued by the police and jumped out of a second floor window landing on his feet. He has been brought to the ED by the police as he is unable to weight bear on his right foot. A lateral X-ray of his right foot has been taken and available for review (Figure 20.6).

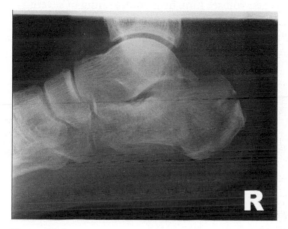

Figure 20.6

a Describe the abnormality in the X-ray (Figure 20.6). [1]
b From the X-ray, what is the approximate angle of compression (Bohler's angle). Explain the significance of your answer. [2]
c Give four other injuries you would actively examine for in this patient with this injury. [4]
d What further X-ray views would you request and what other investigation are the orthopaedic surgeons likely to ask for? [2]
e How is this injury managed? [3]
[12]

Case 8

A 23-year-old man arrives in the ED from Switzerland via medical repatriation. He had sustained a 'broken leg' while skiing two days earlier and attended the local hospital where a long leg plaster backslab was applied. Admission under the local orthopaedic team had been recommended but the patient had insisted on flying home on the next available flight. When you see him, he is complaining of severe pain in his right calf and once the plastercast is removed you note the calf is very tense and tender. Pedal pulses are present. He has brought a copy of his X-ray taken in Switzerland (Figure 20.7).

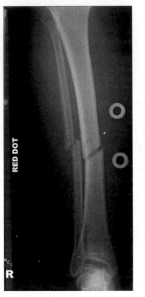

Figure 20.7

a What surgical emergency needs immediate consideration? [1]
b Other than swelling and tenderness give four further clinical signs that may be present with this emergency. [4]
c How is this diagnosis confirmed? [2]
d What definitive treatment does this patient now need? [1]
e Give two other complications associated with this diagnosis. [2]
[10]

Case 9

A semi-professional footballer was tackled from the side and crumpled to the ground, with immediate pain in the left knee. He reports his knee swelled up straight after the injury and that he can no longer bend it. On examination, he has a very swollen and tense right knee and is unable to actively flex or extend.

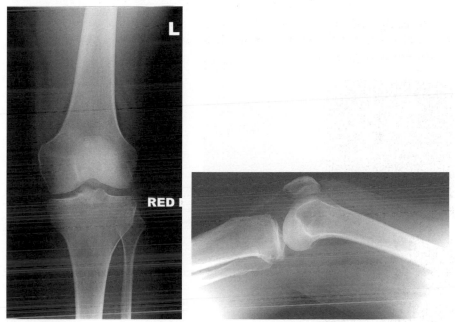

Figure 20.8

a List three of the clinical features from the Ottawa knee rules which are used in deciding whether plain films of the knee should be requested. [3]
b Describe the abnormalities in this patients knee X-ray (Figure 20.8). [2]
c Name three soft-tissue injuries that could be associated with this injury. [3]
d Outline how you would perform a knee aspiration. [4]

[12]

Case 10

A 21-year-old rugby player is bought into the ED after the rugby scrum collapsed on top of him. There is no sign of a head injury and his cervical spine has been cleared. He is complaining vociferously of pain to his right shoulder. An X-ray of the right shoulder has been obtained and is shown below (Figure 20.9).

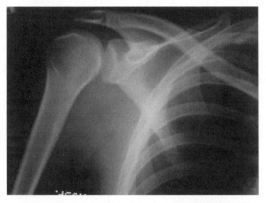

Figure 20.9

a List four non-bony structures that stabilise the gleno-humeral joint.   [2]
b On clinical examination, you note an empty glenoid fossa and suspect
   shoulder dislocation. What else can be examined for to help distinguish
   between anterior and posterior dislocation?   [4]
c Describe the abnormality in this patient's shoulder X-ray (Figure 20.9).
   What is the radiological diagnosis?   [2]
d Briefly describe two methods for reducing a dislocated shoulder.   [4]
                                                                                 [12]

Case 11

A 53-year-old woman involved in a head-on RTA is brought to the ED as a priority trauma call. She was not wearing a seatbelt, at the time of impact, and was thrown forwards striking the steering wheel with her chest. On arrival, primary survey reveals a clear airway but compromised breathing with a respiratory rate of 38 breaths/min. She is alert and groaning with pain.

a List four life-threatening thoracic injuries that may be present in this woman. [2]
b Give three signs of traumatic aortic disruption on the chest X-ray.   [3]
c The trauma series chest film shows a haemopneumothorax. Describe the
   anatomic (surface) landmarks for insertion of a chest drain.   [3]
d Outline in detail the main indication for performing an emergency
   thoracotomy in the ED.   [2]
                                                                                 [10]

Case 12

A 45-year-old publican attends the ED with acute severe low back pain which began after lifting heavy beer barrels in the pub cellar. He has had previous episodes of musculoskeletal back pain but this is far worse and he cannot walk at all.

a List five features of the history or examination – 'red flags' – which may alert
   you to a serious underlying pathology causing this patient's low back pain. [5]
b What are the clinical features of sciatic nerve root **irritation**? [2]
c What neurological signs may be present with nerve root **compression** from
   an acute prolapsed intervertebral disc at L4/L5 level? [2]
d This man has no red flags and normal neurological examination. Outline
   your management (give three important points). [3]

[12]

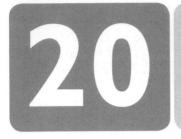

TRAUMA AND ORTHOPAEDICS – ANSWERS

Case 1

a From the mechanism of injury alone, serious injuries are suspected. Using ATLS[1] principles a primary survey is carried out. Remember: Airway with c-spine control, Breathing, Circulation, Disability, Exposure. However, the question specifically asks for the assessment and management of this patient's likely blood loss. Remember, hypovolaemic shock can be classified using clinical parameters as follows:

Table 20.1

	CLASS I	CLASS II	CLASS III	CLASS IV
Blood loss (mL)	<750	750–1500	1500–2000	>2000
Blood loss (%)	<15%	15–30%	30–40%	>40%
Pulse rate	<100	>100	>120	>140
Blood pressure (mmHg)	Normal	Normal	Decreased	Decreased
Pulse pressure (mmHg)	Normal or increased	Decreased	Decreased	Decreased
Respiratory rate	14–20	20–30	30–40	>35
Urine output (mL/hour)	>30	20–30	5–15	Negligible
CNS/Mental status	Slightly anxious	Mildly anxious	Anxious, confused	Confused, lethargic
Fluid replacement	Crystalloid	Crystalloid	Crystalloid and blood	Crystalloid and blood

This patient is tachycardic, hypotensive and has a respiratory rate of 30 and so is presumed to have lost 1.5–2.0 litres of blood (class III shock).

b Class III shock requires immediate fluid resuscitation. Cross-match for six to ten units of blood, give crystalloid immediately, and blood as soon as it is available.

The new ATLS guidelines[1] suggest that if the blood pressure is rapidly corrected before haemorrhage has been definitely controlled, there is an increased risk of bleeding. Balancing the goal of organ perfusion with the risks of re-bleeding accepts a lower than normal blood pressure, this is known as controlled resuscitation or hypotensive resuscitation.

c The pubic diastasis is widened indicating an A-P compression fracture of the pelvic ring (Figure 20.1). Traumatic A-P compression forces both hemi-pelvices into external rotation and disrupts the pubic diastasis, the sacroileac (SI) joints and the posterior ligaments of the SI joints. Young or Young and Burgess classified pelvic fractures[4] depending on mechanism of injury and radiological appearance allowing a prediction of likely pelvic stability to be made (Box 20.1):

Box 20.1 Young and Burgess' classification of pelvic fractures.[4]		
Category	Distinguishing characteristics	Pelvic stability
A-P compression type I	Pubic diastasis <2.5 cm, SI joint intact	Stable
A-P compression type II	Pubic diastasis >2.5 cm, anterior SI joint disruption	Rotationally unstable
A-P compression type III	Type II plus posterior SI joint disruption	Vertically unstable
A-P = anterior-posterior, SI= Sacroiliac		

Thus, the pelvic X-ray in this question (Figure 20.1) shows a pubic diastesis of >2.5 cm but without evidence of complete SI joint disruption making it a type II A-P compression fracture. It is therefore an unstable pelvic injury.

d Complications of unstable pelvic fracture include:

- haemorrhage – originates from the sacral venous plexus or internal iliac artery rupture
- urological injury – urethral laceration, bladder rupture
- gynaecological injury – vaginal laceration, uterine injury and, if the patient is pregnant, there is a high-risk of foetal loss
- rectal injuries – diagnosed on rectal examination by blood in the rectum
- ruptured diaphragm – which is thought to be under-diagnosed
- nerve injury – the lumbosacral plexus is vulnerable to sacral fractures.

e Apply circumferential pressure to the pelvis using a pelvic brace or bedsheet tied tightly around the pelvis. This reduces pelvic volume and helps tamponade bleeding vessels.

Case 2

a The Canadian C-spine rule is a clinical decision rule designed to avoid unnecessary cervical spine X-rays in selected trauma patients who are alert and stable and where cervical spine injury is a concern. (*See* Box 20.2)

Box 20.2 The Canadian C-spine rule

First ask, is there a **high risk** factor?

- age >65 years
- dangerous mechanism of injury (fall from >3 ft/5 stairs, axial load to head, high speed RTA, or RTA involving rollover or ejection of the patient from vehicle)
- paraesthesias in the extremities

If **YES** – radiographic imaging of the C-spine is required

If **NO** – then ask, is there a **low-risk** factor permitting safe assessment of range of movement at the neck?

- simple rear end RTA
- ambulatory since the event
- sitting position in the ED
- delayed onset of pain
- absence of any midline cervical tenderness

If there are **NO low-risk** factors then radiographic imaging of the C-spine is required.

If **there is ONE or more** low risk factors, then test the range of movement by asking the patient to actively rotate their neck 45° to the left and right. If the patient is unable to do this, then imaging of the cervical spine is required. If the patient can rotate the neck through 45° left and right, then no imaging is required and the neck is 'clear'.

b A large study of over 8000 trauma patients attending North American EDs reported that the Canadian C-spine rules had a sensitivity of 99% and a specificity of 45% for correctly identifying potential C-spine injuries requiring radiography.[5]

c Clinically, this patient has a spinal cord injury (SCI). Furthermore, as the plain X-rays and CT did not demonstrate a bony abnormality, we might say she has a spinal cord injury without radiological abnormality (SCIWORA). To get the marks here, though, we need to consider the clinical information in more detail and indicate the most likely diagnosis to be central cord syndrome.

d The central cord syndrome describes a pattern of spinal cord injury characterized by weakness, predominantly of the upper limbs compared to the lower limbs. The motor deficit is worst distally (i.e., hands > shoulders) and a variable sensory loss is present below the level of the injury. Dysasthaesia in the form of a burning feeling in the hands is often felt. The central cord syndrome most often arises from forced hyperextension of the neck in older patients with pre-existing cervical spondylosis and/or canal stenosis, although it can occur in the young, associated with cervical spine fracture of vertebral subluxation.

For completion, other spinal cord syndromes to be aware of include:

Table 20.2

Syndrome	Clinical features
Anterior cord syndrome	Paraplegia and dissociated sensory loss, whereby pain and temperature is lost but the posterior column function of position, vibration and deep pressure sense is preserved. It is usually due to infarction of the anterior spinal artery and carries the worst prognosis
Brown-sequard syndrome	Arises from hemi-section of the cord. There is ipsilateral hemiplegia and below the lesion accompanied by contralateral loss of pain and temperature sensation. Penetrating trauma and tumours are often to blame
Posterior cord syndrome	Loss of sensation but preserved power below the lesion

e The next step is MRI imaging of the cervical spine to show the location and extent of cord injury.

Case 3

a A delayed presentation of abdominal pain following blunt trauma to the left upper quadrant must make us suspicious of splenic rupture.
b The focused assessment by sonography in trauma (FAST) scan is increasingly used in EDs as an extension of the primary survey to look for intraperitoneal free fluid from abdominal organ injury (haemoperitoneum), as well as for pericardial tamponade from cardiac trauma. The following areas are examined:

- hepatorenal space (between the liver and right kidney)
- splenorenal space (between the spleen and left kidney)
- suprapubic or pelvic view (rectovesical space in males; Pouch of Douglas in females)
- substernal or pericardial view (look for fluid between the pericardium and heart).

c The ultrasound image (Figure 20.2) shows free fluid as a dark hypoechoic stripe between the liver and right kidney in the hepatorenal space. As little as 200 mL blood is detectable by a competent operator and FAST has nearly 100% sensitivity in detecting intraperitoneal blood loss in the **hypotensive** blunt trauma victim.
d Indications for emergency laparotomy in adult trauma patients include:

- signs of peritonitis
- shock or hypotension despite fluid resuscitation
- evisceration of bowel
- evidence intra-abdominal bleeding on FAST ultrasound, CT scan of the abdomen and pelvis or diagnostic peritoneal lavage (DPL)
- free air or retroperitoneal rupture of the hemi-diaphragm in blunt trauma
- contrast CT evidence of the gastro-intestinal tract, intra-peritoneal bladder injury, renal pedicle injury or severe visceral parenchymal injury after blunt or penetrating trauma.

Case 4

a The X-ray (Figure 20.3) demonstrates a fracture through the waist of the scaphoid bone. Scaphoid fractures occur in three places: the waist (66%), the proximal third (16–28%), pole or distal third (10%).

b Clinical signs indicative of a scaphoid fracture include:

- tenderness in the anatomical snuff box
- tenderness over the palmer aspect of the scaphoid tubercle
- scaphoid pain on compressing the thumb longitudinally
- scaphoid pain on gentle flexion and ulnar deviation of the wrist
- tenderness over the scaphoid tubercle.

c Complications of scaphoid fracture are non-union, avascular necrosis and osteoarthritis, all of which may compromise carpal function.

d Manage radiologically-evident scaphoid fractures by immobilization in a scaphoid plaster cast and fracture clinic follow-up.

    Where there is no visible fracture (10% of fractures are not visible on initial X-ray) the wrist should be placed in a wrist splint with a thumb extension and reviewed within 10–14 days. If there is no clinical evidence of a fracture, the patient should be discharged. If the pain continues repeat the X-rays, if a fracture is present treat in a plaster of Paris. If repeat X-rays are normal, continue in the splint and arrange a bone scan or MRI to confirm the diagnosis.

e A scaphoid plaster of Paris should be applied from the mid forearm to metacarpal heads and hold the wrist fully pronated and radially deviated. The thumb is held semi-abducted with the cast extending just proximal to the interphalangeal joint.

Case 5

a The X-ray (Figure 20.4) shows a displaced supracondylar fracture of the humerus; the distal fragment being displaced posteriorly. There is also a joint effusion evidenced by the large posterior fat pad. Supracondylor fractures occur commonly in children from a fall onto an outstretched hand.

b Supracondylar fractures in children are managed according to the level of displacement. Remember that on the lateral elbow radiograph a line drawn along the anterior humerus should transect the middle of the capitellum; if the capitellum lies posterior to this line, then the fracture is displaced. Gartland classified paediatric supracondylor fractures as follows:

- type I: undisplaced
- type II: displaced but with cortical contact posteriorly
- type III: displaced with no cortical contact.

Type I fractures can be managed with above elbow plastercast and follow-up, types II and III should be referred to the orthopaedic team for reduction and internal fixation.

The fracture in this child is a type II supracondylor fracture. Thus, following thorough neurovascular assessment of the distal limb, an above elbow backslab should be applied in the ED and referral made to the orthopaedic team. Ensure good pain relief (e.g., intranasal diamorphine with paracetamol and ibuprofen). Elevate at all times to reduce swelling.

c Supracondylor fractures abound with complications, the more so the more displaced the fracture.

Early complications:

- **brachial artery damage.** The brachial artery runs antero-medially to the elbow joint and may be compressed or lacerated by the sharp edge of the displaced proximal humeral fragment
- **nerve injury.** At most risk is the median nerve which crosses the elbow joint with the brachial artery
- **compartment syndrome** from rapid swelling around the injury; distal vascular compromise may result.

Late complications:

- Volkmann's ischaemic contracture due to unrecognized distal forearm vascular compromise
- malunion/non-union
- osteoarthritis
- cubitus varus deformity with restricted range of movement.

d Essential knowledge for exams (CRITOL is the mnemonic):
Capitellum – 2 years
Radial head – 4–5 years
Internal (medial) epicondyle – 4–6years
Trochlea – 8–10 years
Olecranon – 8–10 years
Lateral epicondyle – 10–12 years

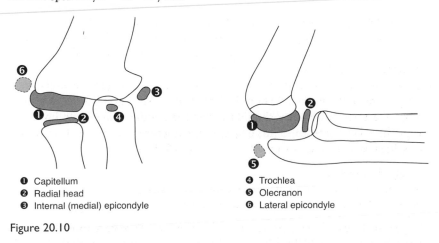

❶ Capitellum
❷ Radial head
❸ Internal (medial) epicondyle
❹ Trochlea
❺ Olecranon
❻ Lateral epicondyle

Figure 20.10

Case 6

a There is an oblique fracture through the distal third of the femoral shaft (Figure 20.5). Due to the powerful pull of the hip adductors and gastrocnemius, the distal fragment becomes displaced laterally and posteriorly.

b Immediate management of a patient with a fractured femur is with analgesia (morphine sulphate 2.5–10 mg titrated to pain) and full examination to identify any additional injuries sustained. The femur is highly vascularized and up to 1.5 litres of blood can be lost from a fracture. Thus, initiate fluid replacement with 1 litre normal saline.

c A femoral nerve block provides excellent analgesia for a femoral fracture as well as being quick and easy. The nerve lies always lateral to the femoral artery beneath the iliacus fascia. It is best approached anteriorly at the groin. Thus:

- sterilize the groin area
- uses a mixture of 5 mL of 1% lignocaine and 10–15 mL of 0.25% bupivicaine (practice varies)
- with a 21G needle, feel for the femoral artery just below the midpoint of the inguinal ligament. Insert the needle perpendicular to the skin 1 cm lateral to the artery to a depth of approximately 3 cm
- alternative methods use ultrasound to locate the nerve sheath or electrical stimulation to identify when the infiltration needle is close to the nerve
- aspirate for blood
- inject local anaesthetic moving the needle up and down and fan laterally
- full anaesthetic effect takes about 20 minutes to develop and lasts eight to ten hours

d Applying traction to a closed femoral fracture has significant benefits and should be performed in the ED ideally with a specialized traction splint (e.g., Thomas' splint). Separating and immobilizing the bone ends with tractions aims to:

- reduce pain
- minimize blood loss (bringing the bone ends back into the correct soft-tissue compartment tamponades bleeding vessels)
- prevents further damage to surrounding soft tissue from bony fragments
- reduces risk of further neurovascular damage.

Remember that traction splints are contraindicated in open femoral fractures where they may exacerbate neurovascular injury and, in these cases, the leg should be immobilized or splinted without traction.

Case 7

a The X-ray (Figure 20.6) shows a compression fracture of the calcaneum.

b Bohler's angle (tuber angle or angle of compression) describes the angle of 20–40 degrees which exists between the upper border of the calcaneal tuberosity and a line connecting the anterior and posterior articulating surfaces. With calcaneal fractures, particularly compression type fractures, this angle becomes more acute (less than 20 degrees), straighter, and can even reverse to a negative value. Bohler's angle is useful diagnostically to detect compression fractures of the calcaneum but also prognostically as the straighter the angle the poorer long-term result in terms of weight bearing.

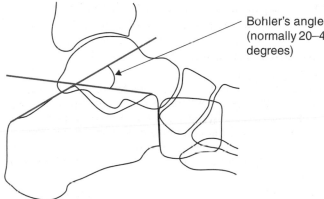

Bohler's angle
(normally 20–40
degrees)

Figure 20.11

In the X-ray used in the question, Bohler's angle is nearer five degrees indicating severe compression of the calcaneus.

c Calcaneal fractures most often occur in young males jumping from a height. It takes significant force to fracture the calcaneum and this force is also transmitted up the skeleton as it impacts the ground. Associated with calcaneal fracture therefore are:

- fractures of the other opposite calcaneum
- knee fracture femoral condyles, tibial plateau)
- hip fracture
- pelvic fracture
- lumbar spine fracture (compression of vertebral bodies)
- cervical spine fracture.

d You would ask for specific calcaneal views and the orthopaedic surgeons will likely need a CT of the calcaneum to aid in their reconstruction.

e Manage calcaneal fractures with analgesia (they are painful and may require morphine) and a below knee plaster of Paris backslab. Fractured calcanei swell considerably and elevation of the foot is an essential part of management. Refer to the orthopaedic team who will decide upon open reduction and internal fixation. Severe compression may require bone grafting.

Case 8

a A very painful, tense and tender calf following lower leg fracture (Figure 20.7) is a compartment syndrome, until proven otherwise. You may have thought of DVT, a haematoma or even a constrictive plastercast as answers here but compartment syndrome is the surgical emergency to be considered first and foremost.

b Further signs of a compartment syndrome include (the '6 P's'):

- severe **p**ain – out of proportion to the injury despite immobilization. Often exacerbated by passive stretch of the toes
- **p**araesthesias and sensory loss (vibration sense is lost first)
- **p**aresis (weakness of toe flexion or extension)
- **p**allor of the foot
- **p**oikilothermia (loss of thermoregulation)
- **p**ulselessness (this is a late sign that is rarely present).

The lower leg contains four muscles and soft-tissue compartments each constrained within a tight fascia. Bleeding and swelling from a fracture increases the pressure within these compartments, and tissue perfusion can become compromised either by loss of tone or collapse of thin-walled vessels. When the muscles become ischaemic, histamine is released promoting capillary dilation and fluid leakage into the tissue space and further increasing compartmental pressures. Normal compartment tissue pressures are 10 mmHg or less. Capillary blood flow is compromised at compartment pressures above 20 mmHg and muscles and nerves are at risk of ischaemia above 30–40 mmHg. Arteries and arterioles are at higher pressures and loss of arterial pulses does not happen until very late and after considerable tissue necrosis has already occurred.

c To diagnose compartment syndrome, the intra-compartmental pressure can be measured directly with a pressure gauge and needle probe inserted into the compartment. Generally:

- <15 mmHg is safe
- 20–30 mmHg may cause damage if left for several hours, the limb should be closely monitored
- 30–40 mmHg requires intervention.

d Compartment syndrome is treated with emergency fasciotomy performed by the orthopaedic surgeon in theatre. Two longitudinal incisions are made, one anterolateral and one posteromedial, to decompress the four major compartments of the lower leg. Necrotic muscle and tissue are excised and the fasciotomy left open until the pressure subsides. Skin grafting is often required to cover the resultant wound.

e Complications (with or without treatment) include:

- reperfusion injuries – hyperkalaemia
- hypocalcaemia
- acute renal failure – myoglobin released from muscle and urate crystals obstruct renal tubules
- Volkmann's ischaemia – necrosis with permanent post-traumatic muscle contracture.

Case 9

a The Ottawa knee rule is a clinical decision rule assisting clinicians decide whether an X-ray of an injured knee is required or not. X-ray if any of the following are present:

- age 55 or over
- there is isolated tenderness of the patella
- bony tenderness over the fibula head
- inability to flex the knee beyond 90°
- the patient cannot take at least four steps immediately after the injury and at the time of the examination.

b The X-ray (Figures 20.8a and b) shows a tibial plateau fracture and associated lipohaemarthrosis.

c Tibial plateau fractures can be associated with injury to any of the soft-tissue structures of the knee, though more often the following:

- anterior cruciate ligament
- medial collateral ligament
- lateral meniscus
- if the tibial plateau is depressed, then the posterior cruciate and lateral collateral ligaments may also be injured.

d Knee aspiration of a tense haemarthrosis provides both diagnostic information (blood indicates a more serious injury to the joint) and therapeutic advantage (reduces pain and improves range of movement where desirable). To perform:

- use strict aspetic conditions
- the approach can be either medial or lateral with the leg in full extension
- identify the midpoint of the patella and insert a green needle attached to a 20 mL syringe 1 cm below its lower border. Direct the needle underneath the patella and aspirate effusion fluid as you advance
- a large effusion may yield 40–60 mL of blood or effusion fluid
- send aspirate for MC&S and/or crystal microscopy, if required.

For completeness, management of undisplaced tibial plateau fractures is conservative with non-weight bearing splint immobilization. Depressed tibial plateau fractures with fragments of more than 5 mm require elevation and possibly bone grafting using either internal fixation with a combination of screws or plates. Complications associated with this injury, include the development of a deep venous thrombosis and the later onset of osteoarthritis.

Case 10

a The non-bony structures which stabilize the glenohumural joint are the rotator cuff muscles – supraspinatus, infraspinatus, teres minor, subscapularis. In addition, the inferior glenohumeral ligament is key in preventing inferior dislocation.

b Patients with anterior shoulder dislocation often hold the arm slightly abducted away from their body and externally rotated and they resist any attempt to internally rotate the arm. In contrast, patients with posterior dislocation are more comfortable with the arm fully adducted and internally rotated while they cannot externally rotate the arm at all.

c The X-ray (Figure 20.9) shows three abnormalities at the shoulder. First the humeral head appears round and symmetrical ('light bulb' sign) due to interior rotation of the humerus; second, the humeral head is separated from the articular surface of the glenoid and instead is resting on the posterior rim ('rim' sign); and third loss of parallelism of the humerus and the articular surface of the glenoid. These abnormalities are seen with posterior dislocation of the glenohumeral joint (the radiological diagnosis).

d There are a number of methods to relocate a dislocated shoulder. A brief description of a few of the most common is given below.

- Kocher's method – this is the commonest method used, the patient should be lying flat, flex the elbow to 90° and slowly externally rotate the shoulder. Adduct the upper arm across the chest still in external rotation, finally internally rotate
- external rotation – the patient should be reclined to 45°, slowly and gently externally rotate the shoulder to 90°, if this is not sufficient forward flex the shoulder
- modified Milch technique – in a supine patient, abduct and externally rotate the arm overhead. With the elbow fully extended, apply traction and manually replace the humeral head over the glenoid lip
- Stimson's method – with the patient prone the dislocated extremity should be hung over the edge of the bed and a 10 lb weight attached to the wrist. Complete relaxation occurs after 20–30 mins
- Hippocratic method – with the patient lying on the floor, the wrist of the affected arm is put under traction, while a shoeless foot is placed in the axilla acting as a fulcrum to relocate the head of the humerus.

e Complications of shoulder dislocations include:

- recurrence – more common in younger patients
- Bankart lesion (avulsion of the glenoid labrium at the insertion of the inferior glenohumeral ligament) which destabilizes the joint leading to recurrent dislocation
- axillary nerve injury – which is usually temporary due to traction during dislocation (test sensation over deltoid C5/C6)
- axillary artery injury (rare)
- concomitant damage to the humeral head, e.g. greater tuberosity fracture or a Hill–Sachs lesion (compression fracture causing flattening of the posterior aspect of the humeral head)
- rotator cuff injury.

Case 11

a Striking the steering wheel in a head-on vehicle collision is a high impact injury associated with sudden deceleration. Life-threatening chest injury is likely.[6]

- aortic disruption (shock + severe chest pain radiating to the back)
- cardiac contusion and/or tamponade (shock + ECG abnormalities and arrhythmia)
- tension pneumothorax (shock + respiratory distress with tracheal deviation away from and hyperresonance over the affected lung)
- massive haemothorax (shock + tracheal deviation away from and dull percussion over the affected lung)
- flail chest (paradoxical chest wall movement)
- tracheobronchal injury (airway compromise and surgical emphysema)
- ruptured diaphragm (bowel sounds in chest and abnormal chest expansion).

b Radiological signs suggestive of a major vascular injury in the chest include:

- widened mediastinum (most often seen)
- fracture of the first/second ribs or scapula
- tracheal deviation to the right
- oesophageal deviation to the right
- loss of the aortic knob
- obliteration of the space between the pulmonary artery and the aorta
- elevation right main bronchus/depression left main stem bronchus
- widening of the para-tracheal stripe
- presence of a pleural or apical cap (increased opacity at lung apex)
- left haemothorax.

c Traumatic pneumothorax, haemothorax and haemopneumothorax are indications for insertion of a chest drain (thoracostomy tube). ATLS gives the correct position as the fourth or fifth intercostal space in the midclavicular line.[6] The British Thoracic Society describes a 'safe triangle' – the triangle bordered by the anterior border of the latissimus dorsi, the lateral border of the pectoralis major muscle, a line superior to the horizontal level of the nipple, and an apex below the axilla – inside which chest drains should be placed to minimize complications.[7]

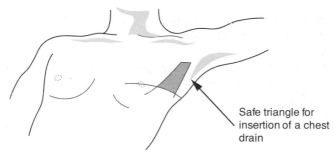

Safe triangle for insertion of a chest drain

Figure 20.12

d Emergency thoracotomy in the ED may be indicated for patients in **cardiac arrest** following **penetrating** trauma to the chest who have **organized electrical activity** on the ECG trace (PEA arrest). On the grounds of futility, ATLS advises against emergency thoracotomy in blunt trauma and in penetrating trauma in the absence of myocardial electrical activity. Other thoracic injuries such as aortic disruption, massive haemothorax, tracheobronchial injury and oesophageal rupture will also require opening the chest as an emergency but, in the live patient, this is done by cardiothoracic surgeons in theatre.

Case 12

a Most back pain presenting to the ED is simple or mechanical back pain. However, our assessment should always include asking about and looking for the 'red flags' which alert us to the potential for a more serious cause and that further action is required. There is no one definitive list but most agree on the following as 'red flags' in back pain:

- age <20 or >55 years
- precipitated by trauma
- non-mechanical pain (constant pain independent of movement)
- progressive pain
- night pain
- thoracic pain
- systemically unwell, e.g. fever
- weight loss or history of malignancy
- immunocompromise (long term steroids, HIV)
- intravenous drug abuse
- evidence cauda equina syndrome (difficulty with micturition, faecal incontinence, saddle anaesthesia, poor anal tone, weakness of the legs)
- evidence spinal cord lesion (limb weakness, gait disturbance, sensory level)
- features suggestive of ankylosing spondylitis (morning stiffness, rigidity of spine, progressive symptoms in the young adult).

b Sciatic neuralgia (sciatica) results from irritation of the nerve by intervertebral disc herniation (most often at L5/S1). Clinical features are of low back pain with pain radiating into the leg, from the buttock sometimes as far as the foot and toes. Pain on stretching the nerve root (e.g., straight leg raise) is characteristic. There is no motor or sensory loss.

c Prolapsed intervertebral discs impinge upon the nerve root below. Thus L4/L5 disc prolapse may compress the L5 nerve root to give the following neurology: weakness of knee flexion (hamstrings) and ankle dorsiflexion (tibialis anterior) as well as sensory loss down the lateral side of the calf. L5 has no associated deep tendon reflex.

d Simple or mechanical back pain without red flags can be managed conservatively and usually without further investigation. Advise the following:

- keep bed rest to a minimum (24–48 hours at most for those incapacitated by pain). Explain that prolonged immobility prolongs the problem
- prescribe analgesia (non-steroidal anti-inflammatories and paracetamol)
- early return to normal activities, particularly work
- discuss behaviour modification such as weight reduction, safe lifting techniques and posture improvement
- consider referral to a physiotherapist for advice on back exercises
- arrange for the GP to review progress in a week or so.

Further Reading

1. American College of Surgeons Committee on Trauma. (2008). *Advanced Trauma Life Support for Doctors*. 8th edn. American College of Surgeons.
2. Advanced Life Support Group. (January 2006). *Advanced Paediatric Life Support: The Practical Approach*. 4th edn. BMJ books and Blackwell Publishing.
3. McRae R. (1999) *Pocketbook of Orthopaedics and Fractures*. Churchill Livingstone.
4. Burgess AR, Eastridge BJ, Young JW. (1990) Pelvic ring disruptions: effective classification system and treatment protocols. *J Trauma*; **30**(7):848–56.
5. Stiell IG, Wells GA, Vandemheen K, *et al.* (2003) The Canadian C-Spine Rule versus the NEXUS Low-Risk Criteria in Patients with Trauma. *NEJM*; **349**: 2510.
6. American College of Surgeons Committee on Trauma. (2008). *Advanced Trauma Life Support For Doctors*. 8th edn. American College of Surgeons. pp 85–110.
7. BTS guidelines for the insertion of a chest drain. (2003) *Thorax*; **58**:ii53–ii59 or see www.brit thoracic.org.uk.

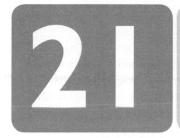

ENVIRONMENTAL EMERGENCIES

Shumontha Dev

Introduction

Core topics

- thermal burns
- chemical burns
- drowning and near drowning
- high voltage electrical burns/electric shock/lightning
- heat illness
- hypothermia/frostbite
- carbon monoxide poisoning
- radiation exposure
- altitude emergencies/diving
- major incident management.

Case 1

An 85-year-old man was found collapsed at home by his regular carer. The carer suspects he has been lying on the floor overnight. There was no heating in the house and the paramedics reported the patient felt very cold. On arrival in the Emergency Department (ED), the man was disoriented with a core temperature of 30 °C, pulse 60 bpm and blood pressure 80/50 mmHg. The patient was taken straight to the resuscitation room and during the initial workup a 12-lead ECG was performed as shown below (Figure 21.1)

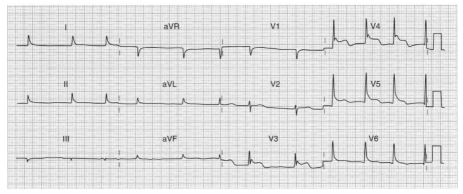

Figure 21.1

a Define hypothermia. Below what temperature do we consider a patient to have severe hypothermia? [2]

b Describe the abnormality on the ECG (Figure 21.1) which relates to this patient's clinical condition. [1]

c Describe three methods of re-warming a hypothermic patient, giving for each method a specific intervention to achieve re-warming. [6]

d When re-warming hypothermic patients in cardiac arrest at what temperature should you initiate the standard ALS algorithm with defibrillation and drug administration? [1]

e Give two specific blood tests you would request in this patient along with the reason for each of your two tests. [2]

[12]

Case 2

A three-year- old boy has been found face down in a shallow pond in a public park. He was rescued from the water by passers-by and he initially responded to rudimentary resuscitation measures at the side of the lake. He was brought to the ED as a priority call. The handover from the ambulance crew was that it was a 'near drowning' and the boy appears to be OK now.

a Define drowning and, by comparison, what is 'near drowning'? [2]

b What physiological differences exist between fresh-water and salt-water drowning? [2]

c Give two good prognostic and two poor prognostic factors in drowning or near drowning. [4]

d List four specific investigations you would ask for in this boy, a survivor of near drowning. [4]

[12]

Case 3

A 21-year-old man is brought to your ED feeling unwell after returning from a scuba diving expedition two hours previously.

a Briefly describe the pathophysiology of decompression illness. [3]

b What two main factors influence the risk of decompression sickness during a dive? [2]

c Give four symptoms of decompression illness. [4]

d What treatment would you urgently arrange for this man with decompression illness? [2]

e What other acute condition can be treated in the same way as decompression illness? [1]

[12]

Case 4

A 26-year-old woman collapses after 15 miles of running in hot weather during the London Marathon. She was attended on scene by medical volunteers who recorded her temperature as 40.7 °C. The ambulance crew transferred her as a priority to the nearest receiving hospital where she arrived in a confused state with initial observations of pulse 120 bpm and blood pressure 85/50 mmHg.

a From the information you are given about this patient, does she have heat exhaustion or heatstroke? Briefly explain your answer. [4]

b Describe the two types of heatstroke, indicating which persons are most at risk of each type. [2]

c How would you rapidly cool this patient down in the ED? [3]

d Give two complications of severe heat illness of this kind. [2]

e What brain structure is responsible for thermoregulation? [1]

[12]

Case 5

A 54-year-old construction worker has accidentally drilled into a high voltage underground power cable with a pneumatic drill and received a prolonged electrical shock from direct contact with the cable. He arrives by blue light ambulance and is alert, in pain throughout his upper limbs and chest and has scorched skin over his neck and face. His pulse is 139 bpm and blood pressure 156/98 mmHg.

a Define a 'high voltage' electrical injury. [1]
b Name three different mechanisms through which electricity causes injury. [3]
c What is your treatment priority in this man once he arrives in the resuscitation room? [2]
d Give four further complications of high voltage electrical injury that you would consider in this man. [4]
e What disposal is appropriate for this patient? [2]
[12]

Case 6

A priority call has come in from the ambulance service saying that a bomb has exploded at a major underground station near your hospital. As a result, a major incident has been declared at your hospital. You are the registrar in charge of the ED when the call comes through.

a Give a definition of 'major incident'. [2]
b Give three different ways in which major incidents are usefully categorized? [3]
c What is the communication structure that the emergency services use in a major incident? [3]
d Give four steps in **your** initial preparation for a major incident at your hospital? [4]
[12]

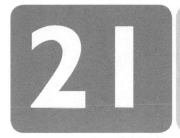

ENVIRONMENTAL EMERGENCIES – ANSWERS

Case 1

a Hypothermia exists when the core (rectal) temperature is <35 °C. Hypothermia can be further classified as:

Mild hypothermia	32–35ºC
Moderate hypothermia	30–32ºC
Severe hypothermia	<30ºC

b Close examination of the ECG (Figure 21.1) reveals extra waves immediately following the QRS complexes, best seen in the lateral leads. These are known as J-waves and are a specific to hypothermia. Otherwise, the ECG shows atrial fibrillation of rate around 60 bpm.

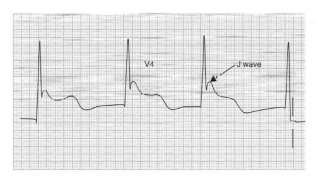

Figure 21.2

c The choice of re-warming method depends upon the severity and duration of the condition, available facilities and the individual patient. The three main methods are:

- **passive warming:** easy, non-invasive and suitable for mild cases (>32 °C). Wrap in warm blankets ± polythene sheets. Endogenous metabolism and shivering generates enough heat to allow spontaneous rewarming. Aim for a rate of 0.5 to 2°C/hour. The elderly with prolonged hypothermia should not be rewarmed too rapidly as hypotension or cerebral or pulmonary oedema may develop

- **active rewarming:** A water bath at 37–41°C is rapid and useful for acute immersion hypothermia. A hot air blanket (Bair Hugger) is more convenient and often helpful
- **core rewarming:** airway warming (humidified heated oxygen at 40–45°C; peritoneal lavage (simple to use and the method of choice in severe hypothermia or cardiac arrest); extracorporeal rewarming (cardiopulmonary bypass maintains brain and vital organ perfusion and can result in rapid rewarming).

d In cardiac arrest, the heart may be unresponsive to defibrillation, pacing and drug therapy below 30°C while drug metabolism is decreased and unpredictable. The Resuscitation Council UK recommends initiating standard management of cardiac arrest with defibrillation and drug administration after the patient has been rewarmed to above 30°C.[1]

e Specific blood tests in this patient might include:

- blood glucose
- urea and electrolytes (to exclude dehydration)
- CK (for rhabdomyolosis as patient has been on the floor for a number of hours); amylase (pancreatitis secondary to hypothermia)
- coagulation screen (hypothermia cause or aggravate coagulation disturbance).

Case 2

a Drowning is death by suffocation/asphyxiation from submersion in any liquid. Near drowning is survival of such, at least temporarily.

b Drowning or serious near-drowning often involves ingestion of water and also, following asphyxia induced laryngeal relaxation, aspiration of water. Sudden ingestion and aspiration of large volumes of fresh-water cause osmotic imbalances resulting in haemolysis, electrolyte disturbances and intravascular overload. Large volumes of salt water have the opposite effect, drawing water from the vasculature and causing hypovolaemia and haemoconcentration of blood constituents. However, despite these differences, the management of both types of drowning are similar.

c Table 21.1

Good prognostic factors in drowning	Poor prognostic factors in drowning
Alert on admission	Extremes of age
Hypothermia (protective effect)	Severe acidosis
Older children/adults	Immersion for more than five minutes
Brief submersion time	Coma on admission
Receiving prompt basic life support	Cardiac arrest
Good response to initial resuscitation	

d Even in well-looking survivors of near drowning, there may be significant lung injury and the potential for deterioration and the following should be performed as part of the assessment:

- blood glucose
- electrolytes (see above)
- chest X-ray (looking for aspiration)
- arterial blood gases (or a capillary gas in a young child) as marked hypoxia and/or acidosis may be present with few clinical signs.

Case 3

a Decompression illness results from too rapid depressurization of the body. This may occur from quickly exiting a high pressure environment (e.g., sudden depressurization of an aircraft cabin at high altitude, or a diver ascending from depth) or through rapid ascent into lower atmospheric pressures of altitude. As the pressure on the body reduces, inert gases (nitrogen, helium), dissolved in tissue fluid and blood, come out of solution and form bubbles in the tissues and vasculature – this is termed decompression sickness. A second form of decompression illness, arterial gas embolism, is caused by larger air bubbles forming in the arterial circulation from direct barotrauma to the lung exposed to sharp external pressure change.

b The two main risk factors for decompression sickness after a dive are:

- longer depth and duration of dive (increases dissolved gases)
- increased rate of ascent from dive (allows less time for gases to come out of solution and disperse without forming bubbles).

c Symptoms in decompression illness depend on where in the body the gas bubbles form.

Table 21.2

Location	Symptoms	Signs
Joints	Joint and back pains	Painful passive movement of the joint
Skin	Pruritis, commonly of the face and upper body	Mottled appearance. pitting oedema
Lungs	Cough, pleuritic chest pain and shortness of breath	Respiratory distress, dyspnoea, and cyanosis Pulmonary barotrauma may give frothy haemoptysis
Ear	Vertigo, balance dysfunction	Peripheral labyrinthitis
CNS	Mild – headache and amnesia Severe – behavioural change, confusion, seizure and coma. Arterial gas emboli may give stroke (cerebral artery involvement) or ascending paralysis (spinal artery involvement)	Disorientation, impaired consciousness, coma Focal neurological deficit

d The treatment of decompression illness is recompression in a hyperbaric chamber with 100% oxygen (hyperbaric oxygen therapy), then gradual staged decompression back to ambient pressures over hours. In addition, aspirin or dextran solutions help decrease the capillary sludging that accompanies severe decompression sickness.

e Hyperbaric oxygen therapy is also used to treat severe carbon monoxide poisoning.

Case 4

a Heat exhaustion and heatstroke are serious manifestations of the failure of the body's cooling mechanisms (vasodilation, sweating and behavioural changes) to cope with heat stress. Heat exhaustion occurs when these cooling mechanisms are not sufficient to adequately control rising body temperature. Further, the body may not be able to compensate for the water and salt depletion caused by heat stress. Heat exhaustion may progress rapidly to heatstroke where the body's cooling mechanisms fail completely and body temperature rises unchecked, to potentially fatal levels.

Clinically, both forms of heat illness (heat exhaustion and heatstroke) may give excess sweating, pyrexia, dehydration, nausea and vomiting, fainting, headache, lethargy and muscle cramps. However, heatstroke is more serious and is recognized with additional features of:

- hyperpyrexia (temperatures >40.5 °C)
- neurological dysfunction
- hypotension
- dry hot skin from absent sweating (failure of heat dissipation mechanisms).

Thus, the woman runner in this question has the signs and symptoms of heatstroke.

b Heatstroke can be categorised as classic or exertional.

Classic heatstroke occurs most often in elderly or debilitated persons passively exposed to significant heat stress. Their ability to respond to heat stress is compromised and the normal thermoregulatory mechanisms easily overwhelmed to the point of failure. Other groups at risk include the very young (age <4 years), those with cardiovascular diseases, neurologic diseases, endocrine disorders and previous heatstroke.

Exertional heatstroke occurs in young physically fit persons with normal thermoregulatory systems who perform strenuous exercise in hot weather. Exogenous heat stress together with exertional heat production, can also overwhelm the body's heat loss mechanism. In most cases, the ability to sweat remains intact allowing some degree of recovery once exercise ceases. More at risk of exertional heatstroke are those unaccustomed to exercise in hot weather and overweight individuals.

c Patients with heatstroke are at risk of multi-organ failure the longer they remain with dangerously elevated core temperatures, and they must be cooled as rapidly as possible (i.e. within 30–40 minutes) to below 39 °C. The two most common methods of rapid cooling are immersion therapy or evaporation.

- in the ED, evaporation is the most practical and effective method. Warm water mist is continuously applied to the patient's exposed skin with a handheld spray bottle with cool airflow from a strong fan directed across the patient's skin to promote evaporation

- complete immersion is difficult to achieve in the ED but ice packs (bags of iced water) applied to groins and axillae work well, although take care to avoid cold damage to the exposed skin
- internal or invasive cooling methods, such as gastric lavage, bladder irrigation, or peritoneal lavage should only be used after there has been no response to external treatments.

d At temperatures above 41°C, cellular proteins begin to denature leading predictably to multi-organ failure. The longer the temperature remains elevated to this extreme, the greater the damage. Thus, in addition to death, complications of severe heatstroke include rhabdomyolysis, renal failure, liver failure, heart failure and coma.

e The anterior hypothalamus is the body's thermostat for heat regulation.

Case 5

a The electrical injuries can be classified as high-voltage (>1000 volts) and low-voltage (<1000 volts). An obvious generalization, high-voltage injuries are more serious than low-voltage injuries but, bear in mind, other factors affect the nature and severity of injury such as type of current (DC or AC), resistance of tissues, current, current pathway and duration of contact.

b The different mechanisms of electrical injury include direct contact, arc, flash, thermal and traumatic.

- the victim becomes part of the electrical circuit in **direct contact** injuries. The injury reflects the passage of current through the body causing electrothermal damage to both skin and deep tissues and is demarcated by entrance and exit wounds
- **arc burns** from current sparks causes high temperature thermal burns at point of contact
- **electrical flashes** cause superficial, partial-thickness burns due to the current striking the skin but without entering the body
- **secondary thermal injuries** may occur from fire started by high temperature electricity
- **traumatic injuries** arise from the violent tetanic muscle contraction associated with AC sources or after being thrown from a high voltage DC source.

c The treatment priority with this patient is the assessment and securing of the airway. Although he may have no initial airway compromise, where there is evidence of high voltage electrical injury above the shoulders, electrical injury to deep tissues can be assumed and resultant airway swelling is a life-threatening hazard. Call for an urgent anaesthetic review.

d Further complications of high-voltage injury to consider include:

- cardiac injury and arrhythmia (perform an ECG and check the troponin)
- full thickness electrothermal burns to the skin, most commonly at current entry and exit points

- partial thickness flash burns to the skin
- most of the current in high voltage electrical burns travels in lower resistance tissues below the skin, and the extensive deep tissue damage it causes is not immediately apparent. Muscle necrosis is common leading to rhabdomyolysis and subsequent renal failure. Check the CK
- compartment syndrome requiring fasciotomy also arises from muscle necrosis within fascial compartments
- neurological sequelae can include amnesia and impaired concentration (similar to concussion type syndrome).

e Disposal is to a specialist burns unit with HDU/ITU facilities. Due to the danger of airway swelling and compromise, transfer certainly requires pre-transfer anaesthetic assessment and, not infrequently, prophylactic intubation for transfer is recommended.

Case 6

a The definition of 'major incident' is 'an incident where location, number, severity or type of live casualties requires extraordinary resources'.

b Major incidents may be variously classified as follows:

- natural (floods or earthquakes) or man-made (bomb explosions, chemical spillage)
- simple (where infrastructure is intact) or compound (where infrastructure such as roads or electricity supply is damaged)
- compensated (resources are sufficient to cope with the demands of the major incident, e.g., coach crash) or uncompensated (where resources are insufficient, e.g., nuclear blast).

c The communication structure that is used in a major incident is **METHANE**:

- **m**ajor incident standby or declared
- **e**xact location
- **t**ype of incident (i.e., road crash, chemical incident, etc.)
- **h**azards (i.e., chemicals, fire, etc.)
- **a**ccess (how can the scene be reached)
- **n**umber of casualties (total number of victims of the incident)
- **e**mergency services (what services are present at the incident and what services are required).

d All hospital major incident plans follow a common pattern with the first steps in preparing for a major incident outlined as follows:[2]

Call switchboard and initiate the major incident call out procedure (switchboard will contact all relevant people including the ED consultant)

⇩

Go to, open and set up the major incident control room (usually in or near to the ED). Do not leave this room until relieved of your role in leading the incident response.

⤋

Open the major incident folder and follow the instructions!

⤋

Allocate roles to personnel arriving at the control room using the pre-prepared instruction cards contained in the major incident pack.

Remember, all necessary actions such as triage, clearing the department to accept mass casualties, press management etc., are set out for the relevant persons in these cards and are not the primary responsibility of the incident leader.

Further Reading

1. The Advanced Life support Group (2010). *Advanced Life Support.* 6th edn. Resuscitation Council (UK).
2. Major incident folder of your hospital is an excellent resource!